PRAISE FOR

*What It Takes to Pull Me Through*

"Fascinating. More than simply a cautionary tale, this extremely well written book provides useful insight and a welcome dose of hope."

— Augusten Burroughs, author of *Running with Scissors*

"These kids breathe fire and hope, break your heart and heal it, and then show how teenagers can wander through the darkest woods toward sunlight. In all, a profoundly moving journey."

— Ron Suskind, author of *A Hope in the Unseen*

"One of the most revealing insights in this wonderful book is how familiar these troubled kids are to us. It shows just how thin the line is between the world of the normal adolescent and those who are fighting for their emotional health."

— Daniel J. Kindlon, coauthor of *Raising Cain*

"Startling, heartbreaking, and finally redemptive."

— Alison Smith, author of *Name All the Animals*

"*What It Takes to Pull Me Through* will surely inspire soul-searching discussions among teens, teachers, and parents."

— Madeleine Blais, author of *In These Girls, Hope Is a Muscle*

"Compelling, empathetic, and hopeful . . . for parents and teens alike. It will be of special use to families experiencing emotional trauma or fracture, offering both solace and a road map of survival that goes far beyond self-help."

— Alissa Quart, author of *Branded: The Buying and Selling of Teenagers*

"Revealing and engrossing."   — *Booklist*

"The reporting is detailed and gripping, the analysis thoughtful."

— *Library Journal*, starred review

"Lots of honest observations on being a teen today. The stories from kids and anguished parents are both harrowing and hopeful."

— *Parade,* "Parade Picks"

"Marcus is a cool-eyed reporter whose perceptions we trust . . . gripping."

— *New York Sun*

"A staggering number of today's teens are depressed, doped up, online, and off the hook. David L. Marcus takes the psychic temperature of the youth culture in the chilling *What It Takes to Pull Me Through*."

— *Vanity Fair*

"A fascinating read."

— Lester Holt, coanchor, *Weekend Today,* NBC

"A tightly woven and extremely engaging book."

— *Brain Child*

"*What It Takes to Pull Me Through* shines with compassion."

— *Pages*

"Marcus deftly intersperses his sharp observations with heart-wrenching statistics about the often crushing pressures of modern teenage life."

— *Publishers Weekly*

# What It Takes to Pull Me Through

### WHY TEENAGERS GET IN TROUBLE
### — AND HOW FOUR OF THEM GOT OUT

## DAVID L. MARCUS

HOUGHTON MIFFLIN COMPANY

BOSTON   NEW YORK

FIRST HOUGHTON MIFFLIN PAPERBACK EDITION 2006

*Library of Congress Cataloging-in-Publication Data*

Marcus, David L.
What it takes to pull me through : why teenagers get in trouble — and
how four of them got out / David L. Marcus.
p. cm.
ISBN 0-618-14545-1
1. Problem youth — Counseling of. 2. Problem youth — Education.
3. Academy at Swift River (Mass.) — Students — Biography.
4. Teenagers — Massachusetts — Biography. 5. Adventure therapy.
6. Therapeutic schools — Massachusetts. 7. Marcus, David L.
I. Title.

RJ506.P63M37 2005
362.7'083 — dc22      2004054076

ISBN-13: 978-0-618-77202-5 (pbk.)
ISBN-10: 0-618-77202-2 (pbk.)

Book design by Anne Chalmers; typefaces: Minion, Scala Sans

Printed in the United States of America
MP 10 9 8 7 6 5 4 3 2 1

*For the kids in Peer Group 23,*
*who taught me so much about parenting,*
*and for Benjie and Tatiana,*
*who help me practice what I learned*
*and who inspire me to learn more*

When my mama ask me will I change
I tell her yeah, but it's clear I'll always be tha same
Until the end of time.
— Tupac Shakur, "Until the End of Time"

# CONTENTS

# Summer Vacation

The midnight curfew came and went. No car pulled up, no doors creaked open. Burns Chambliss called his daughter Mary Alice's cell phone. Still no answer. He left his wife, Lillian, asleep in the master bedroom of their vacation condominium in the mountains and paced the halls. For the second time in three days, he drank coffee, peering out the window for headlights.

Burns worked long hours at his Dallas business but made time for his four children. Lillian had quit her job as a dermatologist in order to spend more time at home. They'd given the kids the best of everything: private schools, riding lessons, family trips to Hawaii. Mary Alice was a natural athlete and Burns loved coaching her basketball team, taking her water-skiing, cheering her at gymnastics meets.

As she finished middle school, though, Mary Alice became a foreigner in her own home. She treated her parents like an ATM; she'd tear in for a cash withdrawal, then vanish. When she didn't get her way, she'd pout and scream. Strange new friends called the house at strange hours, leaving strange messages.

Just after two in the morning, Burns walked downstairs, past a row of framed photos: Mary Alice snowboarding, Mary Alice soaring over a mogul, Mary Alice beaming from a pool like a little blond angel. Precious Angel — that was her nickname when she was younger. Burns surveyed the chaos in her room. Mascara and lip gloss covered a bureau. Bathing suits, shorts, and tank tops spilled out of drawers. Burns sat amid the heaps of sheets and pillows on the unmade bed. He figured he'd close his eyes until Mary Alice arrived and he could inform her of the latest development: She was grounded for the rest of the summer.

On the night table, he noticed a spiral notebook with a grinning

Garfield on the cover. He picked it up. The rings were bent, the pages worn at the edges. The word "Confidential" was scribbled in marker on the cover. At sixteen, Mary Alice indiscriminately mixed capital and lowercase as she had since elementary school. She had kept diaries back then, too. Burns and Lillian occasionally sneaked a look, chuckling at the giddy tone she used in charting her crushes.

Burns flipped open the diary and read the first paragraph: "SANTA FE, NEW MEXICO. The ride here was 19 hours. I bought an ounce of weed and was high beyond my mind the whole time." Mary Alice had written this during a church trip early in the summer. She'd told her parents that the trip — a busload of teenagers touring the West and studying the Bible — had changed her life.

Burns kept reading. In La Jolla, California, Mary Alice wrote about sneaking away from the church group to get her tongue pierced. A day later she took out the stud because "I smoked and drank and it swelled a shitload." Over the next pages, Mary Alice mentioned using acid, cocaine, nitrous oxide, Ecstasy, painkillers, mushrooms, and more marijuana. Burns did the math: In just over a month, she had used seven kinds of drugs. She referred to trying something else, but she didn't even put down a word for it, just a jagged mark. It looked like a lightning bolt. Burns puzzled over that, trying to think what the mark signified: bolt . . . broken . . . crack. She had come up with a symbol for crack. Burns's hands trembled. *Mary Alice did crack*. "But I will never do it again," she had resolved. "It isn't that great."

At Yosemite, she wrote about pretending to be sick so she could skip the youth group activities. She met a twenty-three-year-old mountain climber. "One thing led to another," she wrote, "and all my clothes were off."

Something began to churn inside Burns. It was a raw mixture of rage and fear and guilt — he didn't know what to call it, but it was so intense that his heart pounded wildly. He felt dizzy. As he read, he lost count of how many sexual partners Mary Alice had during the month she'd kept the diary. Mary Alice herself couldn't keep track. Before taking the Western tour, she had spent a few days with her family at a beach resort. She remembered having sex with four guys during that time: "The gorgeous asshole/drug addict." "The cute jock." "The sweetie." "The innocent hottie." Then she realized she had overlooked another. "Ugghh! Regret that one. Fag! Rapist! Slut!"

Burns kept thinking one thing: They had failed. He stepped over the clothes and makeup on Mary Alice's floor and tiptoed to the bedrooms where the three younger children were sleeping. He looked in at each one. Then he went upstairs to wake his wife.

# What It Takes
## to Pull Me Through

# INTRODUCTION

THE GIRL on the phone, a reporter for a high school newspaper, had just read an article about teenagers I'd written for a national newsmagazine. One of her best friends was crushing Adderall pills and snorting them. Another friend had such severe bulimia that she purged every day. "You don't know what it's like to be a teenager now," she said. If I didn't know, I was getting an idea. A doctor from Florida called to say that his sixteen-year-old daughter had just been expelled from school for selling Ecstasy. A mother in California wrote that her fourteen-year-old boy had run away after using the family's credit card to download pornography.

Adolescence has always been turbulent, but it is more complicated today than it was just a couple of generations ago. An extensive study published in the journal *Pediatrics* found that nearly one in five children and adolescents suffers from some sort of behavioral or emotional illness — nearly triple the level of twenty years before. Another study found that the onset of bipolar disorder, once called manic depression, has fallen from the early thirties to the late teens. At the same time, the number of young people in America who committed suicide tripled over thirty years before leveling off in the 1990s.

While researching the magazine story, I dropped into meetings of parents in the suburbs of Washington, D.C., where I lived. Befuddled mothers and fathers agonized about their kids' Internet addictions, eating disorders, and attention deficit–hyperactivity disorder. They worried about studies showing that hyperactive, impulsive kids have higher-than-normal rates of school failure, drug use, and delinquency. Some of the parents turned to books such as *Now I Know Why Tigers Eat Their Young: Surviving a New Generation of Teenagers*. Other parents sought solace in online chat rooms that seemed to start every month: DifficultChild.com, Defiant-

1

Teen.com, HelpYourTeens.com. One of the most popular, Struggling Teens.com, attracted mothers and fathers from across the country. The message lines hinted at heartbreaking stories: "Help needed for 12-year-old," "16-year-old son needs rehab," "13-year-old with anorexia," "What's next for my 14-year-old truant?" "Out of control 15-year-old daughter," "Ripping my hair out," "Teen giving up on school — help!" "How can I help this child? How can I help me?" "What do I do?"

In many ways, of course, middle- and upper-class concerns differed from those of the poor. Less than twenty miles from my neighborhood, in Washington's blighted Southeast side, parents worried about basics such as decrepit classrooms and abysmal graduation rates. In both affluent and poor areas, though, parents agreed that teenagers have less support than they used to. Families are overstressed, many schools resemble factories, and few communities have adults around in the afternoon. Traveling the country as a reporter covering education, I kept meeting teenagers from all income and ethnic backgrounds who were falling through the cracks.

To deal with these kids, more than two dozen special schools have opened across the country since the 1970s. Called emotional-growth or therapeutic schools, they are spartan versions of traditional boarding schools. They remove students from a toxic environment — a home where they clash with their parents, a high school where they are bullied, a neighborhood where they hang out with drug dealers — and offer adult role models and a new set of peers. The schools cram their schedules with academic classes, exercise, and six or more hours a week for group therapy. Counselors lead seminars on time management, responsible sexual behavior, and addictions.

The special schools form one sector of a burgeoning industry. Not long ago, parents could send disruptive boys to a military academy or to Aunt Mabel's farm to work off energy. Now educational consultants charge thousands of dollars to help overwhelmed families decide what's best for their kids. Nonprofit agencies and for-profit corporations have opened wilderness academies in the mountains of Utah, boot camps on the Texas plains, equine therapy ranches in Wisconsin, cocaine detox programs in the Arizona desert, and fundamentalist Christian reform schools in Missouri. Jamaica and the Czech Republic have behavioral modification programs for American kids. Transporters, also called "escorts," employ muscular men and women to take hostile kids away from home.

All this captivated me as a parent as well as a journalist. After bouncing around the world for nearly a decade as a foreign correspondent, I returned in the 1990s to an America I barely recognized — a country that had been strip-malled and Wal-Marted. Soulless, look-alike exurbs were sprouting everywhere as downtowns died; companies were downsizing faithful employees right out the door. While on a fellowship at Harvard in 1995, I invited a history professor named Robert Putnam to dinner. He had just written a provocative essay, "Bowling Alone," which analyzed declining participation in PTAs, bridge clubs, and other groups. Putnam put into words something I'd noticed: In the era of the five-hundred-channel TV and the ubiquitous franchise, Americans were disengaged and disenfranchised.

Putnam's theory continued to haunt me as I struggled to balance a family and a demanding job. I settled in the suburbs for the quality of the schools but found myself disillusioned with the quality of life. When I managed to get home from work early, I spent afternoons crawling through traffic with my kids — the Monday-swim-lessons, Tuesday-library, Thursday-gymnastics circuit — cell phone in hand for calls from the office. My relatives and in-laws were scattered far away; my son and daughter didn't have the frequent contact with extended family that I'd taken for granted growing up. I kept wondering what I could do to instill resilience in my children — to inoculate them from the harried, consumption-crazed society around them.

⟋⟍

I decided to write in depth about teenagers who'd gotten in a crunch and who, along with their parents, were getting help. I wanted to look mostly at the sons and daughters of the middle class, but I hoped for a broad sample, from urban working-class kids to teens from bustling suburbs where families appear to have it all. Following a group of students through a therapeutic boarding school seemed the best way to get inside a world that most adults never see. Again and again psychologists and educational consultants recommended the Academy at Swift River, a school I had visited for my magazine article. Tucked in the hills of western Massachusetts, Swift River started with a wilderness program and concluded fourteen months later with a service-learning project in Costa Rica.

Swift River charged $5,000 a month for tuition, room, and board (at the time, Harvard cost $3,800 a month). Nonetheless, the school was so deluged with applications that it rejected two-thirds of prospective students. Like many other therapeutic programs, Swift River was a for-profit business. Its corporate parent was a privately held California company that had started in the hospital and healthcare business but had turned into the nation's fastest-growing provider of adolescent treatment programs.

When Swift River admitted a student, in many ways it was also admitting the mother and father. Parents had to write frequent letters and talk regularly on the phone with their child and with counselors. Something had gone wrong in the family, and the parents had to own up to their responsibility. Every three months they had to come to campus for seminars and group therapy; then they joined their sons and daughters for the final days in Costa Rica. By the end of the fourteen months, the parents in a group knew the details of each other's lives — from alcoholism to affairs, from dad's fiery temper to mom's anxiety disorder.

Several parents declared that Swift River had rescued their children. Mike Nakkula, a professor at Harvard's Graduate School of Education and an expert on intervention programs, called the therapeutic schools "parenting by proxy." He explained: "Some people who feel they have failed as parents face the fact that they can't adequately help their children. They turn to those who can provide a tougher form of love." Other experts I contacted took a more cynical view, saying that parents were simply outsourcing nettlesome children the way they turned to a lawn service to get rid of crabgrass. Anyway, the critics said, a year or so in a residential program could do only so much to treat depression, alcoholism, or other illnesses with complex biological and environmental origins. These conflicting messages of hope and caution made me more curious.

In June 2001, I began observing as the Swift River admissions department selected a peer group — a dozen students who would go through the program together. Swift River allowed me complete access to group therapy, classes, and supervisors' meetings. The parents let me sit in on their seminars and informal discussions. The most important access came from the kids, who allowed me to immerse myself in their lives while they played guitars, threw snowballs, and hashed things out during family therapy. On breaks, I accompanied them to their neighborhoods, their old high schools, and hangouts. During the last phase of the program, the five-week trip to Costa Rica, I joined them in kayaks, on mountain bikes, and on horseback.

By the end of the fourteen months, I'd heard about the traumas they'd endured, the friends they'd made and lost, the dreams they clung to. I learned the secrets that they had kept for years from their parents, teachers, and guidance counselors — the very people who might have helped them.

When I began my research, America was finishing a decade-long boom. By quite a few measures, teenagers were doing extraordinarily well. Teen pregnancy rates were declining, as were deaths from drunk-driving accidents; college enrollment was soaring. Teenagers I knew were far more sophisticated than my friends and I had been in the 1970s. They knew sushi from sashimi. They debugged Windows, memorized the lines from entire episodes of *Buffy the Vampire Slayer,* and volunteered at the soup kitchen after soccer practice.

For some reason, though, the students at Swift River had taken more risks than their brothers and sisters or their childhood friends. They did hard drugs; they got drunk and sneaked out in mom's car for a ninety-mile-per-hour spin; they went through a dozen sexual partners in a few weeks. Or they simply gave up on everything and withdrew to a world of electronic games. But they weren't freaks. I found kids like them at massive public schools and at elite private academies. Every teenager in America sits in classrooms with them and ends up at parties with them. Seeing snapshots of them dressed as camels in kindergarten skits, or watching videos of them pitching in Dad's Club baseball tournaments, I'm struck by how much they remind me of boys and girls I grew up with in another generation, one that was defined by the Kennedys, Watergate, and Vietnam rather than Columbine, 9/11, and war in Iraq. We can all learn from them.

From the start of this project, three questions seemed the most important:

Why had the kids gotten into so much trouble at home and at school even as their friends and siblings thrived?
How could their families have helped earlier?
What lessons can the rest of us — parents, teachers, religious leaders, lawmakers — draw from a fourteen-month program that most people can't afford?

I hope the stories that follow — the true stories of what happened to these complicated, misunderstood, extraordinarily talented boys and girls — offer some answers.

# Part I

# Truths and
# Half-Truths

# 1

## "I Hate You, Dad"

BIANCA BITTMAN'S FATHER knocked gently and opened her bedroom door. "Bianca, you need to get up."

Bianca awoke with a start, trying to remember what day it was. Sunday, the second day of summer vacation. "I don't want to go to church today," she mumbled. She squinted at the light coming from the hall. Her father was framed in the doorway. Behind him stood two husky strangers, a man and a woman. She glanced at the digital clock: four in the morning. It was still dark outside.

"Who the hell are these people?" she said.

"Listen, Bianca," her father said. "You have to go to . . ." His voice drifted off.

The woman spoke. "It's okay. We're gonna help you."

Bianca lived with her dad and twin brother in a stucco ranch house in West Palm Beach, Florida. She was sixteen and had just finished tenth grade. She rolled out of bed, ran across the hall, and grabbed a phone. She punched in her boyfriend's number. "There are two people in my house. I don't know where —"

The man jabbed a finger at the phone, disconnecting the call. "Okay, that's enough." The woman hovered by Bianca's room, ordering her to get dressed. Bianca's father retreated to the kitchen table.

Bianca asked for a minute to change. She knew she needed half that time to slide out of the window, squeeze through a gap in the hedge outside, and disappear. She'd done it many times while her father slept.

"Don't close the door all the way," the woman said.

"I want privacy!" Bianca yelled, trying to slam the door. The woman wedged her foot in.

Shelves filled the wall over Bianca's bed. The top one was packed with the dolls she had slept with as a child. The next-highest brimmed with soccer and debate trophies. On the bottom shelf, amid shiny metallic balloons from her boyfriend, was a boom box. She'd come home the previous night from her summer job as a waitress and fallen asleep to Tupac's "Until the End of Time." Tupac — the late, great Tupac Shakur — managed to say it all in a few words: "Somewhere inside my childhood witnessed my heart die."

The woman called out that Bianca needed a hairbrush, a toothbrush, and a portable CD player. Nothing more.

"Where am I going?"

"You'll find out when you get there."

Bianca's sliding closet door was missing because not long ago she'd kicked it so hard in a fury that she'd smashed it. At the top of the closet, Bianca had hidden a suitcase packed with clothes and a passport, ready for the day when she and her boyfriend had enough money to run away. Grabbing a few things, she stomped out of her room, past her father. When he tried to speak, she interrupted. "I hate you, Dad! Don't ever talk to me again!" He bowed his head, his eyes red and teary. She walked by the upright piano her mother used to play before she got cancer. Next to it was Bianca's favorite picture, the one of her mom in a white blouse, smiling on vacation in Portugal. Usually, as a way of holding on to her mother, Bianca would stop and say a few words to the photo, but now she kept going.

A Chevy Suburban idled in the driveway. Bianca slumped in the back seat and tried to open the door from the inside. It wouldn't budge. "Where the fuck are we going?"

"Just cooperate," the woman said. "You'll come back soon."

They must be taking her to a boot camp like the one she'd seen on MTV. "This is bullshit!"

"We're not going to take that kind of language from you," the man said sharply. "Stop cursing."

"Fine, I'll stop right away." Bianca sneered. "Who the hell are you, you fuckin' fat assholes? Fuck this shit!" The man drove them out of her neighborhood. They passed by the park where she used to play hopscotch with her mother. They passed her boyfriend's house, her high school, the eighteen-screen movieplex where she got arrested on a misdemeanor charge one night. Bianca listened to Tupac on her headphones.

At the West Palm Beach airport, the three joined a line at the Delta counter. Bianca pretended to study a departure schedule on a screen, then leaned forward to tell a cleaning lady that she was being kidnapped. Bianca whispered in the Spanish she remembered from classes and TV shows: *"Secuestro! Ayudame!"*

The cleaning lady looked at Bianca, then at the couple. *"Dios mio!"* As the cleaning lady bustled toward sheriff's deputies at the front entrance, the man intercepted her. He flashed a few notarized documents: "It's all right. We've got custody."

The line moved forward as the couple, flanking Bianca, waited to pass through the metal detectors. Departure was in twenty minutes.

Damien John Pandowski, wearing dark sunglasses, squirmed on a chair in the admissions office of a boarding school in Connecticut. He sat between his parents. The three had driven up from New Jersey. D.J. was fifteen, short, and skinny, wearing baggy pants with zippers around the knees. The pants were so long that he stepped on them when he walked. He wore five rings on his hands; his favorite bore an alien's head. His mother had made him take off the chain and padlock he usually draped around his neck.

D.J. had been sullen on the ride up, and he was sullen now. He'd always floundered at school and pushed the limits at home, but the past year had been his worst by far. He had barely squeaked through ninth grade, he had endangered the family by playing with fire, and he'd run away. The Pandowskis decided to take drastic action before he got into more trouble. A boarding school that set hour-by-hour schedules and offered group therapy seemed the best option; they were going to tour two campuses in two days.

The admissions officer, a woman with a no-nonsense attitude, fixed her gaze on D.J. "What do you think is good about yourself?"

"I don't know."

"What would you want to accomplish here?"

"I don't know."

"How are your relations with your parents?"

D.J. looked at his mom as he tried to assemble his thoughts.

"I'm not interested in what your mother has to say," the admissions officer said. "Speak for yourself."

Back in the car, D.J. offered his reaction to the Connecticut school: "It sucks."

The next morning, D.J. and his parents drove through the foothills of the Berkshires. They came to a small wooden sign marking the Academy at Swift River and turned into a driveway to face low-slung white buildings with green shutters gleaming in the sun. Plum trees with lavender blossoms and black-eyed susans flanked the double doors at the front entrance. The corridors were lined with photos of students tossing Frisbees, paddling sea kayaks, and riding horseback in a Central American rain forest.

D.J. was still wearing his sunglasses, still sullen. The admissions director asked how he was doing. He stared at the floor, mumbling.

"Speak up, D.J.," his father said.

Silence.

"D.J., please look at her," his mother coaxed.

D.J. glanced up and said he was fine. His fingers jiggled by the side of the chair. He looked at the floor again.

The admissions director had read the application file. She asked if D.J. was prepared to discuss his adoption and what it meant to him.

"Adoption isn't the issue here," his father said.

"Yeah, it's no big deal," D.J. said.

"We've talked it over numerous times," his father said.

"When I was six, I found a book in my room called *The Adopted Child.* That's how I knew I was adopted."

"D.J., that's how you remember it," his mother said. "We talked with you about it long before that."

The admissions director picked up on the tension. And more: She picked up on D.J.'s confusion and loneliness.

It was eighty degrees out, and Tyrone Harriston was sweating. He had been hiking for a half hour with a forty-pound pack. He was heading toward a wilderness camp where he would fetch drinking water from a river, run every day, and do writing assignments about his life back home. That is how everyone started at Swift River — with a few weeks of reflection and exercise in the hundreds of acres of woods behind the main campus.

Like all enrolling students, he first had to go through a strip search in a wooden shed. Counselors turned Tyrone's clothes inside out looking for hidden pockets or suspicious lumps in the inseams containing knives or telltale packets. The search was cursory because the admissions file said Tyrone didn't carry weapons or do drugs. They had him change into blue cargo pants, a white T-shirt, and hiking boots. Tyrone went along without complaint, which was his nature.

Everyone else Tyrone had seen was white — the counselors, the admissions officers, the nurse and secretary. Tyrone was black. He was sixteen and six feet tall, with close-cut curly hair and a handsome face that seemed permanently set in a serious look. Most of his life he had been raised by his mother, who had driven him up from their home in Queens, New York, in her dented old Toyota.

Another student, a pale, lanky boy with tortoiseshell glasses, walked alongside him, and a counselor stayed a few steps behind. The boy was from a New England town. He was close to finishing his fourteen months at Swift River, and he had volunteered to tell Tyrone what awaited him.

"Why are you here?" he asked.

"My mom made me."

"I know. I mean, what are you here for?"

"Academics."

"That's all?"

Tyrone hesitated. "Depression," he said, finally, because that's what his mother said: *If you sleep all day long, you must have depression.* He didn't like uttering it — the word itself sounded depressing — but it was better than a long explanation about his parents' marriage falling apart.

"Did you do drugs?"

Tyrone shook his head.

"Drink?"

He shook his head again. He was tired. He'd stayed up all night, in the thick of a final game of Street Fighter on his PlayStation. It was noon, a time when he was usually sound asleep.

The lanky kid told Tyrone that when he was eleven, friends of his older sister had let him try pot. Soon he was smoking regularly. By the time he was thirteen, he was using acid and mushrooms, and a year later he got hooked on Ecstasy and crystal meth. Then he got into Special K.

Tyrone looked at him quizzically.

"You know, Ketamine. It's like a tranquilizer that vets use. You cook it." His story continued: At sixteen he'd overdosed on heroin in his bedroom.

His parents made him go to rehab. When that failed, they sent him to Swift River.

They crossed a narrow wooden bridge over a stream. The kid asked whether Tyrone knew the three major agreements of Swift River. Tyrone shook his head. The kid rattled off the highlights. The first was no sex. That meant no kissing, no flirting, no petting, no groping. The second was no drugs. Not just hard drugs, but also inhalants, cigarettes, and beer. The third was no violence, including teasing, bullying, and threatening others, cutting, or other self-mutilation. Did Tyrone have any questions? He didn't.

The counselor, listening behind them, had had enough of Tyrone's silence. "You're not happy to be here, are you?" Tyrone shook his head. Or maybe he nodded; it was hard to tell.

She tried to rile him. "Aren't you angry?" He didn't bite. "Look," she groaned, "we're not going another step until you start talking about yourself. Tell me *something*. Give me a sentence to describe what you feel about being sent here."

Tyrone thought for a few moments. "It's a new experience."

"That's lame," she sighed. "You're going to have to learn to be more open."

She said Tyrone would go through the wilderness program at his own pace. The average stay was thirty-two days, but some students had taken three times as long. They arrived at a clearing with the remnants of a campfire. The counselor showed how to set up an A-frame, a blue tarp suspended by ropes over a sleeping bag. Then she took Tyrone to a trench up the hill from camp that would serve as the boys' bathroom, and showed him the five-gallon jugs where he'd fill his water bottle.

For the first two days, every kid was a "shadow." A shadow couldn't talk to other kids. A shadow didn't do the morning exercises or join in the meals the others prepared. Mainly, a shadow watched everything and silently took it in.

Tyrone didn't have a problem with that. He'd been doing it his whole life.

After her father found the diary with the Garfield cover, Mary Alice Chambliss vowed to change. She put her promises in writing: She'd act responsibly; she'd stop doing drugs; she'd go back to Bible study. She knew her parents would give her a second chance; she just needed to perk up and be a precious angel, as they used to call her. And if she messed up again, they'd let her have a third chance. With her parents, there was always one more chance.

This time, though, they held firm. They couldn't trust her, and they couldn't watch her twenty-four hours a day. Instead, she was going to a special boarding school, a strict school where every minute was scheduled; where smoking, drinking, and sex were prohibited; and where she would go to therapy to see why she kept endangering herself.

On her last night in Dallas, Mary Alice begged her parents to let her have a little send-off. Just a few friends dropping by. Her father hesitated — there wasn't much point in celebrating a kid's being sent away — but her mom said it was better to have friends at the house than to let Mary Alice go out. Her father agreed to a party as long as there was no rowdiness, no pot. And Mary Alice had *better* be up and ready to go at dawn, when they had to fly to Massachusetts.

A few hours before the party, Mary Alice drove to Toys 'R' Us and bought three PlayStation sets for $380 with her parents' MasterCard. Then she took them, still unopened, to a pawnshop, using a fake ID that put her age at twenty-one instead of sixteen. She used the money — a hundred dollars in cash — to buy cocaine.

As night fell, Cherokees, Range Rovers, and Beemers filled the driveway and spilled onto the street. A dozen of Mary Alice's old friends showed up. The guys were built, the girls thin and long-legged. It was like a convention of jocks and preps from Dallas's best private schools. By eleven o'clock, when Mary Alice's parents went upstairs to bed, the kids were lounging out back by the pool, chugging beer. In the basement rec room, a couple fondled each other under the black lights of the playroom. Someone passed around a joint.

Wearing a one-piece bathing suit, Mary Alice scrambled back and forth, sipping Diet Coke, puffing cigarettes, and taking in the gossip about who was hooking up with whom. Her blond hair was bleached platinum, her muscular five-foot-ten frame was down to 112. She didn't hide her Parliament Lights or spray aerosol to disguise the smell of pot. Thoughts ricocheted through her mind: *I am the family fuck-up . . . an embarrassment to my parents . . . they want to get rid of me . . .* She did a line of coke in the basement bathroom but didn't bother locking the door. What could her mom and dad do to her at this point?

Several kids got out their cell phones, and word spread about the going-away party. A new group came — slackers and stoners from a couple of schools. They stumbled past the pictures of the Chambliss family on an African safari, the Chambliss family skiing, the Chambliss family dressed up for dinner at the club. One of the new guys was a cute twenty-one-year-old who sold weed. He paid a lot of attention to Mary Alice as the rest of the kids drifted away. Still barefoot and in her bathing suit, she found herself alone with the guy. Just before sunrise the two of them slipped out of the house and drove off.

These four teenagers — Bianca Bittman, D.J. Pandowski, Tyrone Harriston, and Mary Alice Chambliss — ended up in Peer Group 23, the twenty-third group to go through the Academy at Swift River. Although all four had been falling and failing, they had little else in common. Bianca lived in a ranch house in the outer suburbs of West Palm Beach. She had turned from an A student and enthusiastic soccer player to an angry, foul-mouthed, truant who cut school, sneaked out with strange boys, and lied constantly. What made her downward spiral especially puzzling was that her older sister and her twin brother had avoided trouble. D.J. came from a picturesque town in the middle of New Jersey horse country. His parents, both teachers, wanted to do something for an impulsive kid before he harmed himself. They had to ask their relatives to pitch in with Swift River's $70,000 tuition, room, and board. Mary Alice grew up in an enclave in Dallas where houses had pools, nanny's suites, and three-car garages. She drove her own SUV with leather seats. Her parents wanted their beautiful, athletic daughter to understand why she considered herself fat and ugly, and why she sought solace in drugs and boys who used her.

Tyrone came from another world. He lived with his mother and stepfather, and occasionally his unmarried sister and her baby, in a cramped row house facing a wall of housing projects in Queens. Tyrone's mother wanted her son, an African-American boy growing up in a tough neighborhood, to emerge from a funk that had ground him down so much that he'd barely emerged from his bedroom for two years. He was on the verge of being a school dropout with an eighth-grade education. Even as he hiked out to the woods, his mother was still figuring out how to pay for Swift River, which cost twice her annual take-home pay from the phone company.

The mothers and fathers put their trust in a last-chance school surrounded by farms and forests. The kids would begin by looking at what had caused things to go awry. The parents wanted to give their sons and daughters something to grab on to, so that at last they could start pulling themselves back up. At the same time, the parents would have a chance to reconsider how they were raising their sons and daughters. The parents had come to realize that they, too, needed help.

# 2

# PSYCHOLOGICAL
# SCAVENGER HUNT

ON A BREEZY Thursday morning in July 2001, a mother and her sixteen-year-old daughter drove through Northampton, a quaint little city filled with bookshops and coffee bars lined with fliers for massage therapists. It was here, in 1730, that Jonathan Edwards wrote, "Licentiousness for some years greatly prevailed among the youth of the town." He clucked disapprovingly at the loosening of family bonds, which led to young residents "very much addicted to night walking, and frequenting the tavern, and lewd practices."

The mother and daughter continued on a winding state road past stables, a llama farm, and a dairy with an enormous faded milk jug on its roof. After twenty-five minutes, they reached Cummington, a western Massachusetts town with the kind of roiling rapids, undulating cornfields, and county fairs that prompt city tourists to fantasize about leaving the rat race and opening a bed-and-breakfast. With its sagging farmhouses and two-pump gas station, Cummington had the comfortable feeling of a well-worn flannel shirt. It had a particular New England live-and-let-live mentality (one longtime resident liked to read Chaucer, then step outside to go skeet shooting with his 12-gauge shotgun). The general store was owned by a lesbian couple who sold chewing tobacco and seventy-five-dollar bottles of balsamic vinegar.

The mother and daughter pulled into a driveway that was marked by a simple wooden sign with raised letters: THE ACADEMY AT SWIFT RIVER. To the girl's surprise, there were no fences or gates. The main structure, a long white and green clapboard building topped by a towering octagonal cupola, appeared to have the dignified air of an institution that had been around for generations and would last for generations more.

Soon the pair settled into wing chairs in the admissions office, in a cozy, carpeted nook by a fireplace. The girl wore a snakeskin-patterned tank top that hugged her bony frame. Two earrings drooped from her right earlobe, eight bracelets jangled on her left wrist. A dozen crimson marks, each half an inch long, cross-hatched the wrist. The admissions officer explained that kids who were sent to Swift River had consistently taken higher-than-normal risks. Most were diagnosed with ODD, he said, using the acronym for oppositional defiant disorder — a clinical term for hostile behavior, including repeated arguments, temper tantrums, and rule breaking.

"You look up ODD in the dictionary and my picture's there," the girl quipped.

The admissions officer said that Swift River stood out from similar places — therapeutic or emotional-growth schools, as they were known. Swift River was the only one that opened with a monthlong wilderness program and concluded with a five-week community service project in Costa Rica. The staff wanted kids to start and finish by spending time in simple surroundings, where they could reflect on what had gone wrong and what kind of people they wanted to be.

About a dozen students entered and went through the program together, and this "peer group," as it was called, became like a family. They took part in group therapy as well as all-day workshops on anger, forgiveness, and other subjects. They also attended classes; the level depended on how often they'd skipped school at home. The mother didn't say much at first, but she smiled as she looked around during a tour. At lunch in the dining hall, she and her daughter sat with student volunteers who talked openly about drinking, drug use, and fights with siblings and parents.

After three hours, the mother was a believer. She and her husband would find a way to pay Swift River's cost — $70,000 for fourteen months' room, board, and tuition.

All applicants needed the approval of the admissions director, the headmaster, and the special education coordinator. The admissions officer said the staff would review the girl's application, school transcripts, and medical records. He didn't say that although he had found the girl smart and articulate, he was worried about her history. She had cut herself on several occasions, and she had tried to commit suicide at least once.

As the mother and daughter walked to their car, another family arrived for an interview.

In an office looking onto a courtyard splashed with red and yellow begonias, headmaster Rudy Bentz locked his door and slid a CD of medieval chants into his computer tower. A floor-to-ceiling bookshelf was filled with books such as *Anxiety Disorders in Children and Adolescents* and *Suicide*. At eye level was a reference book published by the American Psychiatric Association, the *Diagnostic and Statistical Manual for Mental Disorders,* fourth edition, known as the *DSM-IV.*

It was a Friday afternoon in July. As he did at the end of most weeks, Rudy was reviewing a stack of applications. He needed to approve applicants for the last spots in Group 23. The summer had been turbulent. The staff had caught several students trying to smuggle in drugs while others plotted an escape. More than ever, Rudy needed to find students who were workable.

He took a couple of minutes to consider D.J. Pandowski, the adopted kid from New Jersey. D.J. had been diagnosed with ADHD when he was in kindergarten. He'd run away from home a few months ago. Swift River could handle that. But there was something else: He had played with matches ever since he was little, and recently he had set something on fire in his room. Did that make him a pyromaniac? Pyromaniacs and arsonists weren't allowed on a campus with hundred-year-old wooden buildings. Rudy thought back to his own adolescence, when he got so wrapped up making experimental rockets that he burned down the garage. There was a difference, Rudy knew, between playing with fire and being a pyromaniac.

D.J. was falling behind in school; smoking cigarettes; arguing with his parents; spending his nights on the Internet looking for friends, love, something. If he kept going, he could end up in real trouble. But Rudy had no doubt that D.J. was workable. The counselors could help him understand himself, develop confidence, and find a passion.

Rudy turned to the file of the girl who had joked that her picture was in the dictionary under ODD. Swift River was for kids with emotional problems; it wasn't set up to deal with severe psychiatric disorders. Quite a few girls had lightly cut themselves once or twice before coming to the school, but on a wide-open campus where students weren't locked up, a compulsive cutter could die.

Rudy agreed with the admissions staff: this girl was too risky. Her family would receive a polite call saying Swift River wasn't the appropriate place at the present time.

&#x261E;

In the summer of 2001, the Academy at Swift River was hot. Investment bankers and a fashion designer had turned to the school in the foothills of the Berkshires when they couldn't handle their kids. Dozens of parents recommended it on electronic chat rooms. Educational consultants, who helped families place troubled children, praised Swift River (one consultant called it "the Princeton of therapeutic schools").

Because it was designed for kids in crisis, Swift River didn't run on a standard academic calendar. The campus never closed; classes and group therapy continued throughout the year, and it had rolling admissions. The admissions office had a predictable daily rhythm. Interested parents started to call around 8:00 A.M., when their kids left for school. Another wave began in the late morning — parents phoning furtively during coffee breaks at work, asking vague questions in case colleagues were eavesdropping. Day after day, the receptionists gave the same responses:

"If your daughter is smoking that much marijuana, there could be a deeper issue you want to look at."

"You and your ex-husband will have to come here every three months . . . Yes, at the *same* time."

"We're familiar with that; a lot of boys have both ADHD and depression."

"I understand the urgency, but there's nothing available immediately. Right now we're taking applications for after Labor Day."

Swift River looked especially good because the therapeutic-program industry had been tainted by scandal. The most maligned were the outdoor programs, dubbed "hoods in the woods." Arizona investigators were trying to find the cause of death of a fourteen-year-old boy who collapsed in 111-degree heat at a boot camp where he was "observed eating dirt." In Florida, a 320-pound counselor had crushed a twelve-year-old boy to death while restraining him. In Virginia, a fourteen-year-old Boy Scout who loved reading history hanged himself in a wilderness program. He had been sent

away for a few months, his despondent father said in a letter posted on one
site, StrugglingTeens.com, "because he had a learning disability and needed
a positive experience to bolster his self-confidence." In Samoa, two dozen
American families accused staff members of groping and assaulting teenagers in a program that promised a "kind and loving environment." Newspaper accounts said the Samoa program's chief marketing consultant had
run nonprofit programs that had been shut down in Hawaii, Puerto Rico,
the Virgin Islands, and Costa Rica. The papers said he had also run a camp
in Utah where a sixteen-year-old girl died of heat exhaustion on a forced
hike.

Less than an hour from Swift River, a jury had acquitted two employees of a therapeutic school for administering the wrong dosage of lithium
to a girl. And Elan, a therapeutic school in Maine, appeared in the news because police were reopening the murder investigation of a girl in Greenwich, Connecticut, who had attended the school. One of the suspects was a
nephew of Robert F. Kennedy who had been sent to Elan in the 1970s. Tales
surfaced of students at Elan jeering at each other and settling disputes with
boxing matches.

Amid the controversies, a site called TeenLiberty.org demanded that
states shut down all the therapeutic "gulags."

Although therapeutic boarding schools had become a multimillion-dollar
business in a dozen states by the twenty-first century, they had humble origins. In 1965, a furniture store owner named Mel Wasserman in Palm
Springs, California, spotted a strung-out young man with wild hair sitting
on the steps of a building across the street. Wasserman decided to bridge
the generation gap. He and his wife invited the young man to dinner. Before long, others were joining the charismatic Wassermans to discuss Vietnam, racism, and other issues of the day. All were welcome except those using or carrying drugs. After a few months a dozen twentysomething men
and women had moved in with the family. Everyone helped with chores,
and the house buzzed with conversation late into the night.

In 1969, Wasserman bought a ranch in the hills east of Los Angeles and
relocated his family, along with their flock of houseguests. It didn't take
long before a woman showed up with her teenage son and asked if she
could pay to have him stay at the ranch. The Wassermans agreed. Soon

other parents were sending their troubled teens. Several of the twenty-year-old boarders became counselors.

Wasserman called his program CEDU (pronounced *see-do*), shorthand for a phrase the staff used: "See yourself as you are and do something about it." He drew from the humanistic psychology movement that was popular at the time; kids discussed their fears and traumas in frequent group sessions, or raps. The raps often lasted for hours and ended with participants in tears. As word of CEDU spread, social service agencies started paying the Wassermans to take in teenagers who had gotten in scrapes with the police.

A six-foot-three, 250-pound bear of a man, Wasserman often sat in a large chair, sometimes on a riser left over from drama productions. He towered over the counselors assembled around him during meetings. He flew the staff to retreats at his lakefront house in Idaho, which he named Dunrovin' (because he was "done roving" from place to place). As a boss, he alternately praised and ridiculed the staff; when enrollment slipped and money was tight, he bellowed, "We need asses in beds!" Rudy Bentz, who started working at CEDU in the late 1970s, found Wasserman brilliant, exasperating, inspiring, and arrogant.

CEDU staff members scattered around the country to found other programs. Many of the new programs had corporate structures, with executive directors, headmasters, and academic deans, in order to avoid becoming cults revolving around one charismatic leader. They hired trained therapists, licensed social workers, and consulting psychiatrists. They used traditional talk therapy to help kids identify and cope with sources of stress, and they borrowed addiction-fighting techniques from twelve-step programs. They included high school–level classes in the curriculum. Although CEDU had encouraged counselors to wrestle with their own resentments and anxieties in groups, the newer programs required the staff to focus on the kids. Whereas CEDU had banned psychiatric medicines, the next generation of programs welcomed kids on antidepressants and antipsychotic meds.

As in the rest of the healthcare business, for-profit companies moved in. One was College Health Enterprises, which owned several adolescent programs in the West. In 1997, the company paid $2.5 million for 640 acres and several wooden buildings in rural Massachusetts. Straddling the border between Cummington and another sparsely populated town, it had sweeping views of a wooded valley. The main buildings had been con-structed nearly a century before as a dairy and stables. After the dairy went bust, a summer camp opened on the site. Then, in the 1980s, it was turned into a cross-country ski resort, which quickly went bankrupt. The next owner, an entrepreneur from Northampton, had made a fortune inventing the Teenage Mutant Ninja Turtles, the "heroes in a half-shell." The resort closed after several unseasonably warm winters.

College Health Enterprises (later renamed Aspen Education Group) opened a therapeutic boarding school on the property, promising to create a flagship campus drawing from the best techniques of other programs. The first seven students arrived after driving across the country in vans from a school that the company owned in Oregon. The seven had applied for the privilege of transferring to the new campus, the Academy at Swift River.

As the resort was transformed to a school of last resort, the ski trails in the forest became wilderness trails, the bar became a library, and a com-mercial kitchen became a chemistry lab. The property still had a pool, ten-nis courts, athletic fields, ponds, and marshes brimming with cattails. Swift River itself was more like a fast-running stream, usually four or five feet wide, coursing through a rocky bed surrounded by fir and ash trees that blocked out sunlight for most of the day. Fishing for brook trout from a wooden footbridge, counselors and students had glimpsed beavers, moose, and brown bears wandering along the riverbank. The water was a source of irritation and pleasure. Great swarms of black flies rose from its surface each spring, but it also spoke its own language, a timeless gurgle and babble that lulled frightened, forlorn boys and girls to sleep when they'd been sent far from home.

Swift River had a large campus where anyone bent on getting into trouble could find it. Kids weren't locked up, and the school ran on trust. Much of the job of the admissions office was screening out applicants who would be likely to violate the trust, such as rapists or burglars. Anyone who had been cruel to animals was turned down because that often indicated conduct disorder — a condition for those who have trouble feeling and express-ing empathy and who persistently threaten others or cause property dam-age. The school didn't take students with severe mental illnesses, such as schizophrenia, that required regular monitoring. Those with major physical handicaps or frequent seizures weren't allowed because of the arduous hikes in base camp and in Costa Rica. The academics were demanding, so kids with IQs under 95, slightly below average, weren't admitted.

Swift River had a few rules about parents, too. They had to bring their kids to the intake shed to start base camp; they couldn't use escorts or transporters. That was a symbol that they weren't simply shoving bothersome children out of their lives. (However, Swift River couldn't prevent families from using escorts to take their children to other programs, as happened when Bianca's father first sent her to a wilderness camp in North Carolina.) During the fourteen months, parents had to participate in meetings and family therapy on campus as well as try marriage counseling, Alcoholics Anonymous, or something else at home to work on their own problems.

The admissions officers' job was made more complicated because parents often couldn't own up to the extent of their kids' troubles. If the parents thought their son was smoking pot, he probably was using acid. If the parents reported that their daughter had tried acid, she probably was snorting coke. Staff members were constantly amazed by what parents didn't know about their kids — and what they didn't want to know.

By the time parents applied to Swift River, they felt their lives careening out of control. One morning in July a couple with dark pouches under their eyes arrived at the admissions office. Their eight-year-old son trailed behind; their fifteen-year-old daughter had refused to come. While the parents talked with the admissions officer, they left their son in an office to draw pictures and play computer games.

The father summed up their story with the efficiency of a trial lawyer (which he was): their once sweet daughter had soured in ninth grade. She stole money so often that they had to put a lock on their bedroom door. She taunted her little brother, who was dyslexic, calling him a "retard." She sneaked out of school with a friend, took the family Volvo for a drive on a highway, and crashed into another car. Now she needed a safe place to go so her parents could return to work after Labor Day.

The girl sounded like many students at Swift River, the admissions officer said. He was confident she'd be admitted. The problem was timing. The admissions process for Group 23 was closing; the first kids had started in the woods and more were on their way to campus. Unless a family got cold feet, Swift River wouldn't have room for anyone else until the next group formed, in late September, two months away. The mother and father looked crestfallen.

After the trio had departed, the admissions officer glanced at a calendar that hung four and a half feet above the floor — eye level for an eight-year-old boy. There, in red marker, were seven block letters:

FU
CK
YOU

*⚬*

When putting together a peer group, Swift River didn't try to achieve a balance of genders or backgrounds, drug users versus abstainers, anorexics versus obese kids. The school did not try for ethnic or economic diversity, either. Like most for-profit therapeutic programs, it didn't offer scholarships. Many families took out educational loans or second mortgages. Others dipped into funds they'd been socking away for a child's college education. For about 10 percent of the students, public school districts picked up the tuition. Under the 1990 Individuals with Disabilities Education Act (IDEA), schools were required to provide free, appropriate education for all disabled children. If a school district didn't have the right facilities, it had to pay for a student to attend a program elsewhere. The legislation was intended to help blind, deaf, and severely handicapped children, but the wording wasn't precise. Over the years courts had broadened the definition to include those with learning disabilities and emotional disorders. A surprising number of school districts picked up the tab for programs like Swift River — sometimes simply to avoid costly legal battles with parents.

Despite the tens of millions of dollars parents and school boards had paid Swift River over the years, nobody could say with assurance how well the program worked. Everyone on the staff had a favorite anecdote about a drug addict who stayed clean after graduation or a high school dropout who went on to excel at college. The anecdotes were true, but that wasn't the whole truth. For every one hundred students who entered, twelve left before graduation. Some were expelled for breaking rules; others couldn't keep up with the academic work; still others needed the intensive support of a residential treatment center.

Determining the success rates of graduates was difficult. The staff didn't volunteer statistics; the school's brochures, with their gauzy pictures of beaming kids strumming guitars and studying on the lawn, didn't make any claims. When asked, admissions director Anne Favre said the success rate was 10-80-10: 10 percent of the kids soared; 80 percent stumbled back into trouble but ultimately managed to get on with their lives. The remaining 10 percent ended up the way they'd started out — drifting, isolated, or strung out on drugs. An admissions officer who sat in the adjoining office put the rate at a less promising 20-60-20. Down the hall, Swift River's executive director was the most optimistic. He said the success rate approached "the low 90 percent."

These figures were nothing more than estimates. Although nearly four hundred students had passed through the school in its four years, Swift River had never done a follow-up study. Administrators couldn't even agree on what questions to ask. Did success mean that a former Ecstasy user now limited his indulgence to pot? Did it mean that a boy who used to crash the family car and lie about it was now crashing it and telling his parents? Did success mean that a girl who used to have unprotected sex with a stranger every couple of weeks had decided to abstain? Or that she was restricting herself to boyfriends who used condoms and stayed around for a few months?

In any case, few parents demanded data. Even attorneys and executives who made a living asking tough questions lost their edge when they sank into the admissions office's wing chairs. After a couple of hours on campus, most parents were sold. The students shook hands, spoke politely, tucked in their shirts, combed their hair, and made their beds. They seemed so, well, *normal* (a poster by a math class confirmed that: Swift River's median SAT scores matched the nationwide average). Desperate parents didn't want cautionary tales or statistical caveats. They wanted hope.

The unspoken fact was that fourteen months of therapy and workshops often weren't enough. Quite a few kids could fake their way through and seem fine, only to fall apart after graduation. Some counselors didn't know how to reach certain kinds of kids. And even the best programs and the most savvy counselors had spectacular failures. If a child returned to the same toxic environment that caused problems — an abusive sibling, parents in emotional distress, a ready supply of alcohol and drugs — the outlook was dire. The admissions staff didn't mention the boy from the South who had arrived on campus after using drugs and dropping out of school. As a child, he said, he had often been locked in the basement for hours as punishment by his mother. His estranged father was a drinker. The boy had plenty of potential: He was a self-taught computer programmer who voluntarily set up Swift River's computer network. He said he hated English class, but at the urging of a teacher he wrote and starred in a play based on Gabriel García Marquez's novel *One Hundred Years of Solitude.* A few days before graduation, he was ordered to leave because he kept breaking into the computer room. As he left, he said he was scared of his mother.

A few months later, his mother ordered him to take revenge on a man who had abused his sister. Instead, the boy grabbed a gun, drove to a deserted field, and killed himself.

Rudy Bentz, forty-seven, had started his career twenty-two years before as a drama teacher at CEDU in California, known as the original emotional-growth school. There he met his wife, Jill, who taught art. They moved on to direct a start-up therapeutic school in Georgia, then joined Swift River in 1998, less than a year after it opened. Rudy oversaw a staff of about twenty counselors and four supervisors, one for each phase of the program. Jill trained the counselors.

To Rudy, each package of paperwork — the eighteen-page application, the report cards, the guidance counselor's letters, personality tests, and medical records — constituted a series of clues in a psychological scavenger hunt. With all students, the challenge was to figure out why things had gone amiss. Then, and only then, counselors could help them learn how to live without taking excessive risks.

Rudy described the typical admitted kid as a bright, underachieving fourteen- to seventeen-year-old with very low self-esteem and few close friends. About 60 percent of the students regularly took drugs or drank; at least a third of those kids were addicts or "addiction-prone." About 20 percent had police records for offenses ranging from vandalism to drug possession.

Just over 60 percent were boys, not because boys were more troubled but because they were more likely to act out and attract attention. Girls tended to cut or starve themselves. Those distinctions were blurring, however. Rudy had noticed an increasing number of boys coming in with eating disorders.

Seventy percent had psychiatric issues such as depression, ADD-ADHD, ODD, OCD (obsessive-compulsive disorder), PTSD (post-traumatic stress disorder), bipolar disorder, or anxiety disorder — and often a combination of one or more because the conditions frequently overlapped. Every year, more students came with diagnoses from doctors and psychologists; Rudy didn't know whether experts were getting better at identifying adolescent issues or whether health insurance companies and school districts were more eager to label kids. At least half of the students had some kind of disability, from dyslexia to nonverbal learning disorders. Quite a few had a nonverbal learning disability — difficulty perceiving concepts or reading facial expressions. A small but growing number of students had a class of conditions known as PDD, pervasive developmental disorder. PDD is characterized by problems in communication, repetitive behaviors, poor social skills, and a limited range of interests (at its most extreme, PDD includes autism and Asperger's syndrome).

Sometimes the cause of a kid's downfall appeared obvious. A history of depression in the family, and a mother who retreated to her room every day, overwhelmed by life. A distant, workaholic father. A learning disability that made a student in a competitive high school feel dim-witted. Sixty percent were children of divorce. Thirty percent of the kids were adopted; adoptees' feelings of abandonment and confusion often were exacerbated just as adolescence hit. But sometimes it was harder to explain why things had gone awry: no financial strains, no marital splits, no difficulties in the first years of school, no signs of instability. The students didn't lend themselves to psychiatrists' labels and diagnoses. These were the "mystery kids" — regular teenagers who had made one bad choice after another for no apparent reason.

Rudy flipped open the inch-thick folder of the sixteen-year-old from Dallas, Mary Alice Chambliss. Her parents had brought her in for an interview earlier in the summer. At the time, Rudy had taken one look at her — an emaciated waif with listless eyes, blond hair dyed even blonder, brand-name clothes reeking of cigarettes — and he'd almost blurted, "This girl looks ready to die."

Rudy had an assortment of sayings — Rudyisms — that he tossed around. Mary Alice was, as he put it, an "emotional terrorist." She had not only hijacked the safety of her family, she had also endangered herself by repeatedly bingeing and purging. He turned to the key questions near the beginning of the application.

> Are parents divorced/separated? *No*
> Is your son/daughter adopted? *No*
> Were there any complications during pregnancy, birth, or early years?
>   *N/A*
> Describe any major traumatic events or changes in your son/
>   daughter's life:
> Abuse? *No*
> Illness? *No*
> Death? *No*
> Rape? *No*

Nothing jumped out to explain the causes of her self-destructive ways. Unlike Bianca, she hadn't lost a mother. Unlike D.J., she didn't have to deal with an adoption. She didn't have an absentee father like Tyrone's. Mary Alice was a mystery kid. "From the outside, these kids look like the picture-perfect Barbie dolls," Rudy often said. "They're wonderful kids from tremendous families, with all the love in the world."

Behind his desk, Rudy had a white erasable board covered with a series of concentric circles. He called it "Layers Covering Core Identity." Each circle was labeled, starting from the center:

Adoption
Drug/alcohol abuse
Learning difference
Attention deficit–hyperactivity disorder
Death/loss
Bipolar/mood swings
Victim of violence
Divorce/legal issues
Financial crisis
Major trauma
Racial incidents
Parental dysfunction, including alcohol/drugs

Many developmental psychologists had studied the layers that make up identity. But Rudy's chart was more than an academic exercise. It was an attempt to figure out what kind of kid would respond to Swift River's mixture of talk therapy and writing exercises. The experts had all sorts of ways of assessing kids: the WISC III (Wechsler Intelligence Scale for Children, third edition); the Beck Depression Inventory; the Minnesota Multiphasic Personality Inventory, adolescent version; the Woodcock-Johnson Test of Cognitive Ability. Often, though, Rudy had to set aside the mountains of tests and psychologists' reports and rely on his gut.

His gut had told him to say no to an application that came nine months earlier. It was Tyrone's. In ninth grade, Tyrone had simply stopped going to his school in Queens. He was fifteen and writing at the level of an eleven-year-old. "His special learning needs are considerable," said an assessment by Swift River's special ed team. Tyrone's mother, Natalie, had insisted on bringing her son for an interview, but then Tyrone sat languidly while his mom talked. Afterward, Rudy had said it was as if someone had propped up a blow-up doll in Tyrone's chair. Rudy worried that Tyrone would lag behind not only in classes but also in the cognitive work — the all-day workshops that counselors ran every three months to help the kids understand their behavior. Besides, Rudy doubted that Tyrone's father would show up for the required parents' seminars.

The admissions office had vigorously backed Tyrone, arguing that tests of reading comprehension and other subjects showed that he was very bright. He probably had struggled at school because he lived in a fog of depression. "This is the kind of child who, if he gets an education, can really go somewhere," admissions director Anne Favre insisted.

The staff was impressed by Natalie. She was so damned persistent. She had called frequently to ask about Tyrone's application, she had arranged for every psychological and academic test that the school requested, she'd driven Tyrone to campus in her thirteen-year-old Toyota for a second interview. Natalie planned to make the New York City schools pick up the cost of Swift River because they'd failed to provide classrooms where Tyrone felt safe. If she couldn't get the Board of Education funds, she'd find a way to pay out of her nest egg and her $20-per-hour wages from the phone company. "I've been saving money since the day I started working," she explained. She was a short woman — four foot eight — and from her first minute on campus she talked to everyone in her strong New York accent as if she were an old friend. During visits to the admissions office she held court, sharing her theories on parenting and the differences between genders (she thought men were less responsible than women because boys were often allowed to urinate anywhere outside while girls had to learn to be discreet and find the right place). She could account for every penny she'd spent, and gladly dispensed shopping secrets. On one visit she interrupted a story of bargain hunting for Tyrone's clothes at J. C. Penney just long enough to remind a receptionist to buy bulk packages of generic food.

The headmaster constantly exhorted parents to "trust the process." After close to a year of debates about the kid from Queens, Rudy reluctantly decided to trust the process himself. Tyrone was admitted to Group 23. He would be the most unlikely member of the unlikely bunch of kids that was assembling in the woods in back of the former dairy barn in western Massachusetts. If they had attended the same high school back home, they probably would have passed in the hallways without so much as a nod. Now they were going to spend fourteen months learning every facet of one another's lives.

# 3
# BACK TO BASICS

THE FIRST THING Tyrone noticed at base camp was the smell — teenagers reeking of sweat, unwashed clothes, and acrid campfire smoke. On Sundays, the kids went to the rocky bed of the five-foot-wide Swift River to bathe, the boys upstream and the girls downstream, but the water was frigid and no one really got clean.

The second thing was the eerie quiet. Tyrone could detect the whine of a single mosquito four feet away. At night, he heard wolves, or something that sounded wolfish, anyway. Then there was what some kids called the "Dutch Weatherman," a voice with a mechanical accent that broadcast storm warnings on a radio channel. The other noise came from the counselors' walkie-talkies, which occasionally crackled with chatter from supervisors on the main campus. The kids at base camp tried to decipher the conversations to find out if anyone was attempting to run away, as happened a few times a year. Most of the talk, though, was about logistics such as restocking broccoli. Tyrone missed the background music of summer in the city — people shouting, basketballs slamming through hoops draped with chains, gypsy cabs whooshing up the streets, car alarms wailing.

The third thing he noticed was the deprivation. There were no radios or watches, no electricity or toilets. No pizza, no burgers, no chicken wings (the other kids griped about the absence of cell phones, pagers, laptops, e-mail, instant messaging, Web access and DVDs, but Tyrone couldn't miss something he'd never had). There weren't even chairs; the kids sat on the ground to eat and do writing assignments. When it rained, everyone crowded under tarps strung from branches. It took Tyrone about five seconds to count all his possessions. The most important was a bag of food meant to last two days: granola, dried fruit, an unpeeled carrot, and a can of tuna. He also had a notebook and a pencil, a water bottle and a toothbrush, and a sleeping bag. The counselors explained that base camp was meant to remove the distractions from life. That way, the kids could focus on their emotions.

Base camp had five phases: shadow, turtle, coyote, beaver, hawk. Each required readings and writings in a "growth book" as well as mastery of skills such as tying knots. Turtles, coyotes, and beavers had to ask a counselor's permission for things as basic as going to the pee hole. Hawks had the most freedom. They could help themselves to extra scoops of brown sugar on their morning oatmeal and walk by themselves whenever they wanted.

Shadows were the lowest of the low. They were on "bans" with the other kids, which meant they couldn't communicate in any way. They had to sit and watch while the others did PT, physical training. They had to be brought to the pee hole. They couldn't even glance at the growth book yet.

The only thing they could do was write a "letter of responsibility," explaining why they had been sent to Swift River and what they could contribute to the group. Tyrone started the letter as soon as he set up his A-frame. He wrote slowly, in big letters:

> Hi, my name is Tyrone. I am 16teen years old. I am from NY. The reason why I was here because I have a depretion that I don't know what it is. I blamed most of my problems on school. It took me awhile to rlizes that I had a depretion. I always said that I was tired that was that. My mom tried to talk to me, but I always shut her out. I stoped going to school in 9th grade. I lied to my mom and told her I went and they had a problem with the atandants sheet.
>
> What I can contribute to the group is. I am a person you can trust. I will always fallow the rules. I don't point or blame people if thay mess up. I will finish what I start.

That would be his guiding rule: he'd finish Swift River, no matter how aggravating it got.

For teenagers raised in a world of virtual reality, base camp was the forest primeval, far from fast food and other signs of civilization. Adding to the mystique, the counselors made kids crisscross paths in a pretzel pattern when they arrived. Newcomers were so disoriented anyway that they almost never noticed that any given campsite was rarely more than a half-mile walk from the main campus. The sites seemed isolated because the canopy of leaves was so thick that the August sunlight started to fade by 5:00 P.M. — two hours early. Gradually, though, the kids figured that they were in a patch of woods, not a real forest. On some nights, Tyrone heard music wafting from fairgrounds across a valley. By listening to the walkie-talkie exchanges, he and the others figured out how long it took for an all-terrain vehicle to come from campus (about six minutes).

The days at base camp had a monotonous pattern: Wake at dawn, drink a bottle of water, brush teeth, go to the pee hole. The kids gathered at the fire circle for a "feelings check" — describing their moods on a scale of 1 to 10. Then they'd eat an apple and hike to the physical training field for forty-five minutes of jogging or pushups, stomach crunches, leg lifts, and pull-ups. Twice a week, if everyone was punctual, the counselors replaced routine PT with boisterous games of Wiffleball or touch football. Then back to the fire circle for breakfast: oatmeal with powdered milk (anyone who had followed the rules could add a spoonful of brown sugar — and amid all the bland food, brown sugar acquired the exquisite taste of a gourmet treat). They talked about the day's "Gs & Cs," or goals and concerns. A boy would announce a goal of being honest in group therapy. A girl would share her concern that someone else was chattering too much and slowing down the group. Then, in midmorning, the chores started: chopping and hauling firewood, filtering river water with a hand pump. After lunch, everyone scattered to write in journals or read selections from Emerson's "Self-Reliance," Khalil Gibran's *The Prophet*, a Robert Frost poem about the woods. Then the kids split into crews to build a fire, cook dinner, and clean up.

Base camp was run by a short-haired, broad-shouldered guy who had served in an army infantry unit (another staff member called him "jar-head," though actually that was the term for a Marine). Teams of three counselors rotated in and out for three-day shifts. They talked with the kids during hikes and work projects. The staff had a zero-tolerance approach, which was a jolt to kids who had gotten away with quite a bit at home. If campers were caught filching a pear or throwing trash in the brush, they were punished with extra PT. If they didn't wash their bowls spotlessly after a meal, they lost privileges; they might be put on spice bans so they had to eat bland food with no salt, pepper, or garlic powder for a couple of days. If a boy and girl flirted, they were put on bans — no talking to each other, no notes, no clandestine hand signals. Repeat offenders got extra PT.

A few kids from the previous group, 22, were finishing in base camp and getting ready to go to main campus. They were friendly enough, Tyrone thought. But the only other member of his group, a girl who had arrived the previous day, barely gave him a glance. Tyrone heard the counselors talking about her escapades: at the entrance to base camp, she had cursed out her parents and threatened to kill herself. She had refused to put on the standard cargo pants, T-shirt, and boots, and then she sprinted toward the road, pursued by the staff.

A day in the woods hadn't made her any tamer. At wake-up time, she rolled over and went back to sleep. When she finally straggled to the fire circle, the counselors reminded her that she had to drink a full bottle of water to hydrate for the morning's activities. "Try to make me!" she taunted. She prattled on — something about a watchtower and pagans. At the PT field, she planted herself in the grass while the others did exercises. She dawdled during the walk back. Because of the girl's intransigence, the counselors made everyone stop and do thirty gorilla jumps — a combination of jumping jacks and toe-touches. The other kids were indignant.

A frizzy-haired, even-tempered counselor known as the "den mother," who had raised two teenagers of her own, spoke softly with the watchtower girl. No luck. Jarhead, the former soldier, came out and bellowed, "Get with the program or we'll make you a shadow again!"

"Your intimidation shit isn't going to work with me," the girl shot back. She refused to eat for a day, and the following day. She didn't care if she spent the rest of her life at a hoods-in-the-woods camp.

Admissions officers made it sound as if base camp had always been an integral part of Swift River's curriculum. In fact, though, base camp was an afterthought.

Swift River was in chaos as soon as it opened in the summer of 1997. The school had started in such a frenetic rush that there wasn't time for the usual staff recruiting. One evening the director was at a restaurant when he heard a waiter mention his love of poetry. The waiter was hired as Swift River's first teacher — a fortuitous move because students and parents alike praised him. The thirty-seven students scoffed at the dress code by wearing baggy, low-riding pants (the "ghetto style" originated in prisons, where belts aren't allowed). They sniffed paint thinner in a maintenance shed. While wandering through the underbrush on his first day of work, a teacher tripped over a heavy backpack. He opened it and found that it was stuffed with pot. Then came an unsolved crime a couple of miles away: Someone broke into a store to steal cigarettes and candy. The director of Swift River phoned the state police to say that he had a hunch about the burglars' identities but he'd need a few days. The counselors called in the students, one by one, and asked them to come clean about Swift River's underground. Several boys confessed to breaking into the store; other kids admitted to getting high on pot and mushrooms.

Between them, Rudy and Jill Bentz had nearly forty years of experience at therapeutic schools, starting with the original one in California. When they came the following spring to interview for jobs at Swift River, they stopped for breakfast in Northampton and picked up a copy of the *Valley Advocate*, the weekly alternative paper. They stared at it in disbelief. The cover story was an exposé of Swift River. Based on interviews with a man who had worked as a cook at the school, the article accused the staff of using sleep deprivation in all-night workshops, shouting obscenities at kids, and forcing them to do degrading work projects such as cleaning a staircase with a toothbrush for a day. The former employee "saw bored students who seemed to be growing increasingly unhappy and agitated," the article said, noting that he had complained to the state Office of Child Care Services.

The school was in such turmoil that administrators postponed the Bentzes' visit, leaving them to sit in a hotel. Arriving on campus a day later, the Bentzes were told that the former cook had exaggerated Swift River's problems. Still, students boasted to Rudy that they had done acid in the woods and developed a hazing technique that involved heating the mouths of soda bottles with a lighter and branding each other's arms. Asked what he would do to improve the school, Rudy replied, half-jokingly, "Burn it down and start over." He was hired.

With losses increasing, the administrators decided to revamp the whole program. They expelled a dozen students; anxious parents pulled out several others. Soon only twenty remained. Swift River declared a three-month freeze on admissions, then borrowed wilderness counselors from other programs owned by the Aspen company and dispatched them with the remaining students to the Appalachian Trail for three weeks to hike and camp. During a three-week blitz the Bentzes helped write a curriculum that combined exercises from other therapeutic schools and twelve-step programs like Alcoholics Anonymous to assist the kids in dealing with anger, fears, and forgiveness.

Then something unexpected happened: The twenty students returned from the Appalachian trek, looking invigorated. Rather than grumbling about being banished to the woods, they proudly swapped stories about kayaking through rapids and battling horse flies. The idea of a Swift River wilderness camp emerged. Rudy and Jill didn't have their own children, but after dealing with hundreds of teenagers in therapeutic schools they'd decided there was something cleansing about living simply in nature. "Instead of the headphones pounding the Tupac shit, kids need to listen to the elegance of the aeolian harp," Rudy said, using the ancient Greek image of a harp gently plucked by the winds. Swift River already owned an ideal site: the hundreds of hilly acres that had been used for cross-country skiing and, years before that, for grazing cattle.

The way Rudy saw it, a month or so outdoors had four benefits. First, it removed kids from the mindless materialism of their daily lives — the "mall crawl." In the serenity of the forest, kids could start to focus on what had gone wrong. Second, base camp gave a group a chance to bond without the pressures that came from trying to impress dozens of peers on the main campus. In the woods, they could open up in therapy; gradually they'd learn to rely on one another for the remainder of the program, all the way through Costa Rica. At best, the counselors and fellow students would become a supportive family.

Third, base camp allowed counselors to use behavior modification, rewarding positive actions in a controlled environment. In nature, every misstep had a stark consequence. A boy who didn't hang up his wet clothes at night would slosh around in sodden socks the next morning. A girl who was too lazy to zip up her sleeping bag and store it during the day might find toads cavorting inside at dusk. No whining, no histrionics could change what happened outdoors; mom and dad couldn't call the principal and ask for a second chance. Kids were given one spoon and one bowl. If they lost either, they had to carve a replacement from a log. As the logistics coordinator of base camp explained, "If we go crazy over a lost spoon, kids think, 'Whoa, imagine what they do over the big things.' That way, they're not out in the woods banging each other."

The admissions office didn't dwell on the fourth purpose of base camp. It was a trial period, a time for winnowing out unsuitable kids. Occasionally someone who wasn't right for Swift River made it through the application process. More than one set of parents, frantic to place a difficult child, had deceived the admissions staff by neglecting to mention schizophrenia, conduct disorder, or drug use so heavy that it had done neurological damage. And some bright, extremely defiant kids simply refused to change. There was a saying that 20 percent of the kids took 80 percent of the counselors' time. Every so often a truly hard case — a "vortex" kid, as one staff member put it — came along and sucked up all the counselors' energy, creating so many disruptions and distractions that they couldn't focus on anyone else.

The girl who nattered about watchtowers was a vortex kid. As she continued her self-imposed fast, the supervisors were so worried that they put her in the all-terrain vehicle and took her to the nurse's office on the main campus. She didn't return to base camp. The kids soon heard that she had been sent to another program — a "lockdown." Group 23 was off to an inauspicious start; the first kid to enter became the first to be kicked out. She hadn't lasted even a week.

Tyrone resigned himself to base camp. If he was supposed to do forty push-ups, he did sixty. If he had to chop two logs for firewood, he'd chop four. "At home, I barely moved," he shrugged. "At least I'm getting in shape." Anyway, once his mother made up her mind about something, she wouldn't change. She had decided that he would stay at Swift River till graduation. End of conversation.

Base camp was all about focusing on the past, not the future, so the counselors brushed off questions about life on the main campus. Still, the kids quietly exchanged information they'd gleaned during admissions tours. Everyone agreed that Swift River could've been a lot harsher; they rattled off the names of programs with isolation wards and a therapeutic school where kids were sent into a ring with boxing gloves to work out quarrels. The consensus was that Swift River's underground was pathetic: It was nearly impossible to get a joint or even a cigarette on campus; there was always some suck-up spilling everything on a "truth list" for the counselors.

Tyrone had been to a place where the underground was completely aboveground. At his high school in Queens, a massive, five-story brick building with more than three thousand students, drugs were sold in bathrooms, stairwells, and locker rooms. If Swift River cracked down on drugs, he was glad. But he kept it to himself.

Tyrone could take only so much of the nosy counselors. Every couple of days the kids sat in a circle on the ground for group therapy session as the counselors asked question after question: What was it like when your father went away on all those business trips? How did you feel when your grandmother died? Why did you have to impress the cool kids at school? Group lasted three hours. You couldn't lie down or even rest your back against a log; no one could leave. If you wanted to say something about the person next to you, you had to move at least two spaces away. That was so no one could get in anyone's space and be threatening. There was no sugarcoating — you had to tell the "harder truth" about yourself and others.

If you wanted to agree with someone else, you used a Native American expression, *Ho.* It stood for "I know what you mean."

After Tyrone mumbled responses to other kids' questions during a few groups, a counselor held up her hand. Hadn't he ever showed emotion? Yes, Tyrone said, sometimes he'd gotten so pissed off that he'd yelled at his mom. The woman faced Tyrone. "Okay, I'm your mother. Come on, Tyrone. Tell me why you're so pissed off!"

"I'm mad at you 'cause I can't see dad."

"Let it out!"

"I'm mad."

"Let's *hear* it!"

"I'm mad at you!"

The counselor folded her arms. "There's a lot of anger and resentment stuck in there, and it's paralyzing you. One day it's going to come gushing out."

The watchtower girl had announced that group therapy was bullshit. Tyrone gave that a silent *Ho!*

After a few days in the forest, it was time to write a life story. The kids had to describe their highlights and low points, starting with infancy. Life stories usually lasted for a dozen handwritten pages. After writing, they read the story out loud and talked about what had gone wrong.

In his life story, Tyrone stuck to the necessary facts: He was born in

Queens, and that's where he'd grown up. He had an older sister. His mom worked days, his dad worked nights. When he was nine, his mom kicked his dad out. Tyrone had gone to a noisy, crowded elementary school and middle school. Sometimes there were more than thirty kids in a class. Then he went to a huge high school. He couldn't describe it well because he'd basically skipped all his classes. He usually stayed up till 4:00 A.M. playing video games, then slept for a couple of hours, got dressed, and pretended to go to school, but in fact he just circled the block and waited for his mom to go to work at the phone company. It was a pretty simple life story when you got down to it.

After dropping off a child at base camp, the parents wrote what the counselors called an "impact letter." It was supposed to say how the child's behavior had impacted the rest of the family. Each kid had to read and discuss the letter with a counselor and "process" it. After a day or two of processing, the kid read the letter to the group.

Tyrone's mother wrote a sentimental letter saying how much she missed having him at home. Instead of passing it to Tyrone, the counselors told her to think back on why she'd sent Tyrone away, then write a stronger letter. She wrote six pages of looping script, describing how worried she was when Tyrone stayed home from school and passed entire days in front of the TV, barely uttering a sentence. As the sun set on a Saturday night, Tyrone held the pages. He knelt by the fire and read aloud:

> Tyrone, I've always worked very hard for my family. I worked at the phone company and at home. These two jobs took up all of my time and energy. My son needed help. Which of my two jobs could I take time from? How much will the family suffer as a result of whatever decision I choose?
>
> I was afraid that you were hurting so much that you didn't want to live. I prayed at work, I prayed in Church, I prayed on the train, I prayed waiting for the bus, I prayed at night, and I woke up praying to God for the strength to think clearly, for the words that would make a positive difference, for Him to watch over you day and night and for you to be able to hang in there until I was able to get help for you.

"Your mom sounds chill," one of the kids said when Tyrone finished. "She is chill."

Mary Alice Chambliss showed up at base camp a day later than expected. Her parents had spent a morning calling friends after she left her going-away party wearing nothing but a bathing suit. They'd tracked her down at the house of the twenty-one-year-old pot dealer.

One look told Tyrone the basics. Mary Alice was blond and thin, her hair falling like straw over her gaunt face. Her back was arched as if she was about to start a gymnastics routine. Her face was still smudged with makeup, but its weariness suggested that she'd seen and done a lot more than most sixteen-year-olds. From the way she walked — certain that all eyes were on her — it was obvious that she was rich and popular, the kind of girl who wouldn't have time for someone whose family didn't belong to the country club. She'd apparently made quite a first impression on the staff; Tyrone heard them saying that she'd thrown a fit at the intake shed when she found out she couldn't bring a mirror to base camp.

Mary Alice was supposed to spend her forty-eight hours as a shadow writing a letter of responsibility. But the counselors spotted her furtively working on the growth book, trying to get a jump on base camp. They took it away and said she'd have to wait an extra day as a consequence for breaking the rules. She passed the time staring at the others, as if she were confined to the edges of a party. One of the supervisors of the base camp counselors had grown up in Dallas and knew a lot about the social pressure in Mary Alice's elegant neighborhood north of downtown. "You've spent your whole life trying to be accepted by others," he told Mary Alice. "Swift River is about dealing with your own stuff, not about impressing everyone else for a Miss Congeniality contest."

To make sure she did some thinking, he put her on "look bans." She couldn't look over at the others, not even a glance. Soon, she motioned for another counselor to come over. She had a request. Her skin was dry. She needed her parents to send tanning lotion; she knew a brand that contained moisturizer that would be just right for the arid New England summer.

The counselor explained that base camp was about getting rid of extraneous things, about reducing life to the barest essentials. Moisturizer was not essential.

❧

Labor Day was a month away, so the pace was picking up in the base camp enrollment shed, a rickety structure lit by a bulb dangling from the ceiling.

At least three, sometimes four kids were arriving every week. It happened at this time every year. Students had been told they were not welcome at their old schools. With the end of summer in sight, their parents were panicking.

The day after Mary Alice arrived, Bianca Bittman came to the intake shed. After the man and woman had taken her from her home in West Palm Beach, she spent six weeks in a wilderness program in North Carolina. She learned to "bust" a fire using nothing more than a flint and a twig. She hiked stolidly for hours with a heavy pack. Participants also were supposed to talk about what went wrong at home. That's where Bianca drew the line. She'd walk but she wouldn't talk. She had managed to grab one memento before leaving her bedroom: a photo of her mother hugging her. She'd wrapped it in plastic and kept it in her backpack the whole time. Bianca had counted on going back to West Palm Beach, back to her waiting boyfriend, as soon as she finished the North Carolina program. Instead, her father picked her up and they flew to Massachusetts. Bianca sat rigidly, listening to a Walkman and occasionally grunting at her dad, who was so tense that he left his cell phone on the plane.

As he said good-bye at the shed, Bianca's father reminded her she still hadn't dealt with whatever demons were plaguing her. She needed to take Swift River's therapy seriously —

"Fuck this place," Bianca interjected. They could stick her in the woods again. They could march her around with a damned pack. But no one — not a new batch of granola-munching counselors, not another bunch of screwed-up druggies, and certainly not her father — could force her to talk. Anyway, her dad was clueless. He didn't know the half of it.

# 4

# THE COUNSELOR
# AND THE TEACHER

THE AD in the *Daily Hampshire Gazette* said a therapeutic boarding school in western Massachusetts was seeking a counselor. Tanya Beecher had never heard of a therapeutic boarding school, but she had grown up as a faculty brat at a traditional boarding school and she'd studied to be a therapist. She had worked with elementary school kids in an inner city, she'd counseled college students during a fellowship at Harvard, and she'd mentored adults in a group home for the mentally ill. Teenagers were the one group she hadn't worked with. In her application letter to the Academy at Swift River, she said her studies and on-the-job experience had trained her to deal with all kinds of issues, from abuse to depression.

When Tanya came for a daylong series of interviews with supervisors and students, she was struck by the school's stately appearance. The main building was laid out like a giant "E." The top prong held an infirmary and computer room, the middle prong housed the boys, and the bottom prong contained girls' dorms. The long backbone of the "E" was made up of a kitchen, the dining hall, and administrative offices. Above the dining hall, a soaring hayloft had been converted into a great room used for meetings and study halls.

Tanya stepped into a foyer decorated by a framed newspaper story from 1917 announcing the opening of a farm on the site (at the time, the land, the dairy, the barn, and the stables cost $50,000 — less than one year's tuition in 2001). The exposed beams and stone fireplaces still gave the feel of an understated ski lodge where hot chocolate brewed day and night. The dorm rooms were clean and there wasn't a speck of graffiti anywhere. It was as if the students had a stake in the place. Staff members explained that the kids started each weekday by vacuuming the carpets, mopping floors, and cleaning windows. In addition, anyone who had broken rules had to serve on a weekend work crew. Swift River didn't have a janitor; it didn't need one.

To Tanya, the campus felt safe — not just safe in that a student wouldn't assault others, but emotionally safe. The kids seemed to trust their peers and the staff enough to talk honestly about their past troubles. After a meeting in the great room, which had a Ping-Pong and foosball table and a dozen couches, students stood around hugging one another. In college, Tanya had been set on a career as a doctor, but she'd grown disillusioned with the grade grubbing and the frosty personalities of her premed classmates. She wanted a job that would allow her to help people. Idealism ran in her blood, she figured. One of her ancestors was Harriet Beecher Stowe, author of *Uncle Tom's Cabin,* and her grandfather had worked in a New Deal project building houses for migrant workers. Her sister served in the Peace Corps in New Guinea, and her brother was a social worker.

Tanya admired her father and her mother, who were art teachers; her father had been active in the free-speech movement in the 1960s. Her family volunteered at soup kitchens during the holidays long before that became almost a cliché. Her father rejected pretension. He hadn't eaten at a restaurant since the 1980s. Tanya had gone to Thailand at age eighteen to help build a village school. She had seen a world with no electricity, where men left at 4:00 A.M. to work in rice paddies and children walked ten miles to school. In Thailand, she'd come to understand that a lot of the things that obsessed her in high school — how she curled her hair, how she fit in with the popular crowd, what someone said about somebody else's boyfriend — were awfully petty.

As she looked around Swift River, Tanya noticed small measures that seemed like good ideas for any school. New kids were paired with those who were finishing the program to have the kind of positive role models that most lacked at home. The school encouraged every student to find an adult — a counselor, teacher, dining hall worker — who could be a mentor. The administration urged the counseling staff and the academic staff to work together. If a kid had just disclosed that she had been abused by a stepfather, the counselors were supposed to let the teachers know she was going through a hard time. For her master's thesis, Tanya had studied the relationship between social workers and teachers at a public school in a poor industrial city. She'd quickly seen that the teachers knew little about the students' lives outside of school, while social workers didn't understand what went on in the classroom. Rather than collaborating, the two groups undermined each other.

Swift River also gave kids chances to succeed. Anyone who behaved well in the woods could come to the comforts of the main campus. Anyone who behaved well on campus could take part in the adventure in Costa Rica. And anyone who did well in Costa Rica could graduate, with the whole school cheering. For kids who had dropped off of teams, quit after-school clubs, and floundered in classes, graduation was an important milestone. It showed they could stick with something difficult to the end.

Rudy Bentz interviewed four finalists for every opening for a counselor. The headmaster wanted to know how they would respond to hypothetical situations: What would you do if a kid threatens to run away? Knowing that a girl has a history of suicidal ideation, how will you react if she says she no longer wants to live? Most applicants sputtered after an hour or so. Some were reeling from their own rocky childhoods or divorces and seemed to be looking for a job that would, as Rudy put it, let them work out their own shit. Many had racked up stellar grades in psychology classes but had no idea what to do if things went wrong and failed to follow textbook cases. And things inevitably would go wrong on a campus filled with so many teenagers who had been, to use the Rudyism, emotional terrorists. "You'll have to make perfect decisions," he said, "based on imperfect information."

Rudy set candidates off balance by saying, "Why are you here? For a job? Go away." He paused. "For a career? Let's talk." Pause. "For a calling? That's more like it." He liked to tell the story of a job interview at the previous therapeutic school where he'd worked, in Georgia. He'd been ushering around a woman who had extraordinary credentials on paper. A boy stopped them.

"What are you doing here?" the boy demanded.

"I want to work as a therapist."

"I know that. What are you doing here?"

"I like working with adolescents."

"I know that, but what are you *doing here?*"

The woman looked helplessly at her interrogator. "Are you a fuck-up?" the boy continued. "Because I'm a fuck-up and I'm here."

After the woman stammered, Rudy cut the interview short and wished her well. From that time on, he looked for qualities that often didn't come through on a résumé and transcripts — poise, candor, wit. He wanted someone interesting, someone who inspired kids. Swift River's staff included a published poet, a photographer who had done a documentary about the homeless, and a rock climber who was so obsessed that he built a climbing wall in his attic. It wasn't a coincidence that several staff members had been Peace Corps volunteers; they were adventurous spirits.

Tanya Beecher stood out from the other finalists in the summer of 2001. Not only did she have top academic credentials — a master's in social work from Smith College and the Harvard fellowship — but she had a wide range of practical experience. While working with college students, she had dealt with three issues that cropped up frequently at Swift River: grief, eating disorders, and trauma. Rudy quickly found out something else: Tanya spent her free time dancing the Argentine tango.

Jill Bentz, who trained the counselors, liked the six-foot-tall applicant. At age twenty-nine, Tanya knew enough to admit that she needed to know more; she was willing to ask for guidance. "She's got great sensitivity," Jill said. "There's something about the way she was raised that gives her real balance."

Tanya accepted an offer to be the head counselor of Group 23. She didn't let on that she felt nervous because she wondered whether she could connect with adolescents. She still had bad memories of being shunned and taunted as a tall, awkward girl surrounded by rich kids at the prep school where her parents taught.

Tanya had been taught to listen to clients without talking about herself. Self-disclosure, her professors had warned, was treacherous. By sharing something personal, a therapist influenced what a client might say. It was especially tricky with adolescents. Some therapists wrongly used self-disclosure to gain acceptance with teenagers, to manipulate them into revealing more or to scare them into changing their behavior. At Swift River, she saw, she was going to have to go against her training. Rudy Bentz encouraged counselors to share anecdotes from their own lives. He liked to say that this wasn't a shrink's office where clients came for fifty minutes, got billed for an hour, and reappeared a week later. It was a living, interdependent community grounded in "relational-based, 24/7 therapy." Besides, Rudy said, teenagers respond to adults who are genuine, and being genuine means dealing honestly with personal issues. Of course, the self-disclosure had to be appropriate, and the counselors had to be clear about the purpose of opening up. One counselor occasionally mentioned his struggles as a recovering alcoholic. But he didn't say, "Man, I miss getting shit-faced."

Gennarose Pope had big brown eyes — artist's eyes that seemed to take everything in. She had gone to art school, then transferred to Columbia University to study English literature. In her free time, she painted portraits. She was lithe and moved as fluidly as a dancer, which she was. She also sang, wrote lyrics, and played rock, jazz, and R & B on the guitar and piano.

While volunteering in an adult literacy program, she discovered that teaching was like performing. Then she took a course with a professor who talked so passionately about literature that even the driest Puritan memoirs seemed scintillating. After graduating from Columbia, she moved to western Massachusetts to follow a boyfriend who was in grad school. She had no firm plans but figured she'd teach for a year before working on a master's and a doctorate. When she heard that the Academy at Swift River was looking for an English teacher, she sent a letter and résumé. They'd already found someone, but Gennarose asked to stop by and introduce herself anyway.

As soon as she arrived, she liked the small classes and the feisty students. They had gone through so much group therapy that they seemed hyperarticulate, unlike average kids who grunted their way through adolescence. She admired the school's mission statement, posted on the walls: *To educate them, guide them, direct them, get them through these dangerous ordeals until their development of intelligence can catch up to their awakening wants and drives.* The promise of a holistic education, working with the mind and the emotions at the same time, intrigued Gennarose. At her public high school in New Jersey, most teachers and students had known each other superficially from their fifty-five-minute blocks of daily face time. But one person stuck out: a teacher who helped Gennarose and her friends start an after-school coffeehouse where kids gathered to read aloud and perform music. Swift River seemed like a nonstop coffeehouse: Teachers ate with kids in the dining hall, they attended group therapy, and they worked late one night a week.

As soon as she got home from her Swift River visit, she dashed off a three-page follow-up letter to the academic dean. "The philosophy, pedagogy, work ethic and intense personal investments that drive your school make good sense. I'm convinced that I can help you develop what you're trying to do to make a real difference in the lives of your students. I'm also convinced that working at Swift River would make a profound difference in my own life." She meant it, though she didn't go into the details. When she was ten, her father left home after a stormy marriage. She and her mother fought constantly. She felt confident that her own struggles would make her more empathetic to the Swift River kids.

She kept calling and faxing. The dean said he'd never seen such a persistent applicant, and if Swift River teachers needed anything it was persistence. He retracted the offer to the other teacher and hired Gennarose.

Every teacher also served as the liaison between the academic faculty and the counselors for a particular peer group. Gennarose was assigned to Group 23. The dozen or so boys and girls in the group would get to know all sorts of adults at Swift River, including special education experts, wilderness counselors, and cooks in the dining hall. If their parents requested, they'd also see a consulting psychiatrist once a week. But only Tanya and Gennarose would be with them through the entire program, starting with visits to base camp and ending with the Costa Rica trip.

The cries echoed through the woods — low-pitched, like those of a wounded animal. It was late August and Tanya, finishing her first month at Swift River, was visiting Group 23 at base camp. The morning air had a snap — summer was already losing its potency. Tanya looked up to a bluff and traced the sound. It was coming from a blue A-frame tied between two trees. She walked over and looked inside. There, curled up, was the newest shadow, D.J. Pandowski, from New Jersey. He was a slight, skinny boy with wiry black hair and acne on his cheeks and forehead. He looked scared. The wilderness counselors said he'd been crying pretty much since he reached base camp the day before. It didn't help that one of the girls had said loudly, "Dudes, that kid is like *twelve*." D.J. was fifteen, actually.

Tanya had an urge to reassure him. Instead, she knelt and waited for him to speak. His eyes were puffy. "I don't understand why I'm here," D.J. sniffed. His eyebrows, which looked like bushy brown caterpillars on his pale skin, arched as if to emphasize his words.

After a month at Swift River, that was a new one. Usually kids could sum up their transgressions in a sentence fragment: "Selling pot on school property" . . . "Promiscuity and drinking" . . . "Crashing my dad's convertible."

"If you didn't do anything, why would you be here?"

"I don't know."

D.J. said he'd run away from home once, but that was all. While he talked, he kept poking through his backpack, looking for his glasses or his bag of shadow rations. He'd have things in order, then he'd pull out the granola and the can of tuna and start all over. His hands, and his brain, had to be in constant motion. Tanya picked up on something else: D.J. kept saying he missed his dog, Firecracker. He didn't mention his parents.

During her visit to base camp, Tanya had the kids build walls out of whatever they could find on the forest floor. They scurried about, gathering handfuls of mud and sticks, and then went to work. After an hour, Tanya had them talk about how their creations reflected the walls they put up around themselves to keep others from prying. D.J. worked zealously, making a low-slung, solidly packed hodgepodge of twigs, dirt, and leaves. Tyrone's was six inches thick, plain and simple. Made of densely packed mud, it was almost impenetrable.

Mary Alice, the Dallas girl, built a thin, flimsy wall, then adorned it with flowers. "That's me," Mary Alice declared, her intense green eyes looking for Tanya's approval. "I didn't take care of myself and everyone walked all over me."

As they talked, Tanya noticed that Mary Alice had a fake persona, a false self. She wore it like a mask. Even her smile was frozen in an everything-is-great expression. It would be easy to judge Mary Alice by what therapists called the "presenting problems" — her drinking, drugs, smoking, wanton sex, and eating disorder. Back in high school, Tanya probably would have dismissed someone like Mary Alice as an airheaded debutante. Yet while talking about her wall, she radiated something, a vulnerability. Mary Alice ached to be accepted and loved. Deep inside, she *wanted* to change before she ended up killing herself. Tanya could see that working with adolescents was going to be even more intriguing, and more complicated, than she'd imagined.

# 5

## MARY ALICE:

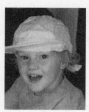 "EVERY PARENT'S
WORST NIGHTMARE"

IT WAS ALL a silly communication problem.

Really, Mary Alice assured the base camp counselors, things hadn't been that bad at home. She'd made a few mistakes, yes, but she'd learned her lessons. Her parents hadn't realized that her foolishness was over. If she could talk to them for a few minutes — just a quick call — they'd understand that she was ready to come back.

Her parents' impact letters told another story. Her mother wrote about a night when Mary Alice went out with her best friend but ditched the friend without explanation and disappeared. Her parents stayed up until dawn calling other families, trying to find Mary Alice. They learned that she was with an older boy. "To have a child, especially a daughter, that is so vulnerable and not know where she is in the middle of the night tears your heart out," her mother wrote. "We hoped the Lone Star Youth Ministry Western Tour would turn you around. Another DISASTER. According to your own words, it was sex, drugs, and alcohol. Your behaviors are every parent's worst nightmare."

The letter from Mary Alice's father stung even more. He had written it outside juvenile court, where he was waiting to fight a ticket that Mary Alice had received for smashing into the car of an off-duty cop. Her father said that he'd been hearing from friends who had spotted Mary Alice drinking and smoking pot. She was lucky she hadn't been arrested for drunk driving or drug possession, he wrote, "but I am positive it was just a matter of time."

The counselors noticed that Mary Alice was all over the place. She was

51

glad to have a chance to think . . . She was miserable . . . She loved nature and felt refreshed . . . She felt homesick . . . They said she needed to slow down. When she wrote her life story, she'd need to think carefully about what she believed. Rudy Bentz often talked about kids who had an "abundance of prosperity and a scarcity of internal life." That sounded a lot like Mary Alice.

Burns and Lillian Chambliss had one child after another — four in six years. The firstborn, Mary Alice, would burst into a room singing when she was a toddler. She didn't just walk somewhere, she'd amble along, greeting strangers and doing cartwheels. She was a Precious Angel.

Mary Alice's place in the family changed when the fourth child was born with a heart condition and spent weeks in intensive care followed by months recovering at home. Everyone focused on the crisis. When Mary Alice's mother went back to work, a housekeeper took over. She cooed at the baby and yelled at Mary Alice, who was constantly trying to get attention. Watching Mary Alice gobble food, the housekeeper boomed, "You eat any more of that and you're gonna be fat like me."

Mary Alice's suburban Dallas neighborhood put a premium on keeping up appearances. Houses had elegant gardens; everyone drove gleaming cars loaded with extras. Fathers worked and played golf, while mothers lunched at the club and went to water aerobics, Pilates, or whatever was in that year. Mary Alice explained it: "It's the kind of neighborhood where women put on lipstick before walking out to pick up the mail." Her mother was unusual. She had grown up in a working-class family and put herself through medical school. She worked as a dermatologist. A nanny, not Mary Alice's mom, came to shows and other events at Mary Alice's school. One day, Mary Alice blurted out that her nanny was more like her mom than her own mother. Soon after, Lillian quit her practice.

The Chambliss household had nine televisions, five computers, four phone lines, and six cell phones, along with two dogs, three cats, two ferrets, and a rabbit. The family also owned a lake house and a ski chalet in Utah. They were always taking carloads of friends waterskiing, tubing, and horseback riding. More than one friend said that Mary Alice had it all. It didn't seem that way to Mary Alice because she felt so much pressure to be perfect. Her father, who ran a business, expected everyone in the family to be upbeat. He got flustered when Mary Alice said she felt sad. Her mother was thin and fit and incessantly cheerful. She whisked Mary Alice from one activity to another: cheerleading, ballet, riding lessons. She chose Mary Alice's friends, too. She didn't like kids whose parents were divorced because they weren't well supervised. She kept arranging for Mary Alice to spend time with two sisters, the Sanderson twins, down the street. They were smart, upstanding girls from a good family. She didn't want to hear Mary Alice's opinion that they were prissy.

Things weren't all bad. On her parents' birthdays, it was Mary Alice who organized all the siblings to wake up and serenade mom or dad. And teachers noticed that Mary Alice had unusual talent in drawing and painting. In other school subjects, though, she had trouble keeping up with the work, so her parents switched her to another school, and then a third.

In ninth grade, Mary Alice threw a party when her parents were out of town. Her mother returned home to find a vase broken and beer cans in the trash. Mary Alice's father had made allowances for her behavior because he believed that his side of the family had a wild streak. He, too, had been a hard-partying kid. Then the housekeeper found a baggie of pot in Mary Alice's closet. She was grounded for the rest of the school year — at least in principle. If there was a party on a Friday, Mary Alice would make a deal with her mom; she'd go out on that Friday and be grounded Saturday. She knew that her mom, who had grown up as the only child of a divorced mother with very little money, didn't want Mary Alice to feel like an outcast.

The summer after ninth grade, Mary Alice went on an Outward Bound trip to Montana. At one point, she wrote a letter to herself. "On this trip, I have found *me* again — fun to be with, sensitive, loving, down to earth, good leader." That fall, she threw herself into photography and cheerleading. By then, she was at one of Dallas's best private schools — her father was on the board of directors — and she made the honor roll. Then, abruptly, three months into her sophomore year, Mary Alice lost interest in just about everything. She made the junior varsity soccer team instead of the varsity team, and she quit in a pique. She dropped cheerleading. One afternoon, a teacher caught Mary Alice passing a note to a friend. It was an invitation to go "rolling" on the weekend. School administrators thought that referred to pot and told her parents to arrange monthly drug tests. (The school's knowledge of drug slang was outdated. If they had realized that "rolling" meant taking Ecstasy, Mary Alice would have been suspended.)

The urine tests were supposed to be random, but Mary Alice's parents always scheduled the visit to the clinic a few days in advance, as if it were just one more after-school activity. She knew from friends that pot's mind-altering chemical, delta-9-tetrahydrocannobinol, or THC, is absorbed by fatty tissues in various organs. Most urine testing couldn't detect traces of a joint or two that had been smoked a few days earlier. Mary Alice drank a lot of water because friends who had done research on the Internet claimed that water diluted THC traces. Most important, Mary Alice's parents didn't have her tested for Ecstasy and other drugs. Month after month the tests always came out clean, so she celebrated in style — by getting stoned.

One day, Mary Alice used her father's credit card to charge a state-of-the-art bong, which she gave to a guy she had a crush on. Her father yelled at her when he noticed the $200 charge. She wrote him a letter, saying, "Shit needs to change in the way I'm living." She suggested a plan: "I need to take care of myself first such as working out, doing my homework, cleaning my room, eating healthy." Her father gave her another chance.

In May 2001, as sophomore year wound down, Mary Alice started a new diary. She titled it "My Fucked Up Life." She wrote the first sentence: "Well, what can I say, I'm 16 and living life on the edge."

She left the rest of the pages blank.

Swift River's application asked parents to summarize the goals for their child. Mary Alice's mother and father had put into words the thoughts of many beleaguered parents: "To improve self-esteem, get in touch with her issues, respect herself and others, property and life, find direction and a sense of purpose, gain healthy skills for dealing with anxiety and stress, to make better decisions."

At base camp, the supervisors decided to work on Mary Alice's self-esteem. One day, a counselor told her to bust a fire — strike a piece of coal with a bow drill just so to make a spark, then wedge in a piece of birch bark, let it ignite, and use that to light a bunch of sticks. The bark flared briefly, but then the flame faded. Mary Alice bent over and shielded the bark. The flame flickered briefly. She peeled a different piece of bark. The sparks flew into the ground and died.

"I can't do this!" she said.

The counselor reminded Mary Alice that, not long before, she had managed to light joints in the wind, or keep bongs going in moving cars with the windows open. Certainly she could do a task that primitive peoples had mastered.

"It's impossible," she insisted. "I can't do it!"

The counselors gave her a large tin can — they called it the "I can" — and painted *I CAN* in red across the side. Mary Alice had to lug it everywhere. One of the counselors recounted the children's story about the little engine that chugged up a mountain pulling toys while saying, "I think I can, I think I can . . ."

They made the message explicit: To get through the Academy at Swift River — to get through life — Mary Alice would have to change her attitude. She needed to rely on herself, on her own wiles, not on pawnshop scams with her parents' credit card.

Mary Alice held the can away from herself, as if it contained dirty diapers. But after a day, she started to rely on it like a personal organizer. Soon she tied a string on it and wore it over her shoulder — the base-camp version of a Kate Spade purse, smart and practical. During the next week, she kept her water bottle, spoon, pencil, and reading assignments in it. She went back to trying to bust the fire. After a dozen, then two dozen attempts, the spark at last lit the birch bark, the birch bark ignited the kindling, and the kindling lit the logs.

# 6

## BIANCA:

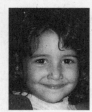

## "I CAN'T DO ANYTHING RIGHT"

SWIFT RIVER'S CURRICULUM defied easy explanations. It was a patchwork of the theories of the leading behavioral psychologists of the twentieth century, mixed with techniques from twelve-step programs, California feel-good movements, Big Sur group processing, and Esalen-style encounters. The curriculum drew from the pioneering Swiss philosopher and psychologist Jean Piaget, who believed that children must learn at their own pace. And Erik Erikson, who argued that a person's ability to resolve conflicts during critical transitions early in life is an indicator for later happiness. And, especially at base camp, Swift River borrowed from Abraham Maslow. He had charted a hierarchy of needs, starting with the physical — air, food, water — and ascending through self-esteem, belonging, love, and finally to truth and beauty.

The school wasn't trying to turn rampaging teenagers into cherubic clones. It was trying to help kids rediscover their talents, to give them the tools to deal with inevitable setbacks and pain. Swift River started by reducing newcomers to coping with primordial needs — potable water, shelter, a comfortable temperature. As they fulfilled Maslow's hierarchy, they started to think about who they really were.

Bianca, like everyone, changed her personality depending on who was around. With her aunts, she was the pleasant churchgoer. With her teachers, she was polite but distant. With her father, she was downright deceptive. "The most disturbing behavior is her proclivity to lie, tell half-truths," her father wrote in the application to Swift River. "Bianca is very good at saying what you want to hear for short periods and lulling you into a sense

56

of peace. Minutes, hours, or days later she will revert to unacceptable behavior." He admitted that he wasn't entirely sure what that behavior consisted of — though he had some unsettling hints.

The two-page impact letter from Bianca's father arrived on an August afternoon when the clouds had promised rain but failed to deliver. Bianca sat by the fire circle holding the letter, which opened with an explanation of why her father had sent her away to Massachusetts even after she'd completed the North Carolina wilderness program.

"If I had let you come back home," he wrote, "I think that within a minimal amount of time you would have been right back where you started: lying, sneaking out, skipping school, alienating yourself, defying authority, and verbally assaulting me or others."

I can't supervise you at home 24 hours a day. I have to be confident that during my absences you won't be just looking for ways around the rules. Right now, Bianca, I can't be confident in that.

The last few months it seems our communication consisted of loud arguments or you saying you didn't want to talk. You've refused to talk about a lot of things and that causes me to worry more, wondering about what really happened. It makes it impossible, too, for me to do my job as a Dad: to advise, comfort and protect you. We've never really talked about the gym incident or even Mom's death. We need to learn how to talk about both the big and little and we can't do that with you isolating yourself.

As Bianca read the letter to the other campers, her voice cracked. In the North Carolina wilderness program, she'd listened to kids grouse about fathers who left home without a word; fathers who drank and beat their kids; fathers who gambled away the family nest egg at casinos. Bianca was pissed at her dad, but she was starting to believe that what had happened wasn't his fault. She didn't know whom to blame anymore. She was certain of only one thing: If her mother had been around, none of this would have happened.

Almost as soon as she took her first breath, Bianca Bittman was a caretaker.

When she was born in November 1984, it was as if she came first to make sure things were safe for her twin brother, Bruno, born fourteen minutes later. As a toddler, Bruno had a toy vacuum cleaner that made an annoying whine. Their parents hid it every few days, but each time Bianca scoured the house and proudly carried it back to Bruno. In first grade, Bianca walked Bruno to his classroom before going to her own, and she did the same thing every first day of school after that, even in high school. Bianca wasn't close to her big sister, Claudia, but she felt lucky to have a twin. "You've known me for nine months longer than anyone else," she liked to tell Bruno.

Bianca liked poetry, acting, and singing, like her mother, Teresa, who had been invited to national singing competitions in high school. Bianca and her mom also shared the same gregarious personality, the same light-hearted laugh, the same Portuguese features, including burnished copper skin, and black, wavy hair. Teresa was a labor and delivery nurse at the hospital where Bianca and Bruno were born. Bianca liked to visit the hospital and hold the newborns when her mom was on duty. Because of her schedule, Teresa often had to leave the house at dawn. Bianca's father, Alan, made breakfast and dressed the kids for school. When Teresa was working a long shift, Alan took care of the kids in the afternoons and evenings as well.

Teresa was a devout Roman Catholic, and Alan, who was half-Jewish and half-Methodist, had converted to Catholicism. Bianca was more religious than her brother and sister, so the excursions to Mass on Sundays gave her time to have her mom to herself. After church, the two always baked biscuits.

When Bianca was eight, her mom sat the kids down to explain that doctors had found a lump in her breast. She had two months of chemotherapy at the hospital where she worked. Her hair fell out, but Bianca always saw her in a wig. And before long, Teresa was home, back to normal.

A year later, when Bianca was in fourth grade, her mom told them the doctors had found a lump in her other breast. This time, she needed to go to a hospital five hours away for a bone marrow transplant. The children weren't allowed in the hospital room. They had to watch their mother through a window because her immunity was low. Teresa came home after three and a half months. For four days, Bianca raced home from school every afternoon to hug her mom. On the fifth day, her grandma was waiting alone, looking pallid. Bianca's mother had become dehydrated and gone back to the local hospital. There Bianca saw her mother lying unconscious in the ICU. Her dad took the kids to a conference room and told them the bone marrow transplant had failed. Cancer had spread through Teresa's body, the doctors said. Teresa had a week to live. Bianca refused to believe it. Her mother always got better after being in the hospital. At the end of the third week, she died in her sleep.

In the months after the funeral, Bianca's father kept saying he was amazed by Bianca's strength. She didn't break down or get angry like her brother and sister. Instead, she continued to rack up A's. When she wrote a paper about Anne Frank, a teacher scrawled on it, "Wow!!! You are a star and I feel lucky to have encountered you as one of my students." Alan saved the papers.

Bianca didn't feel as good as she looked. She didn't tell anyone, not even the priest at confession, but she had decided that she had done something so horrible that God had taken away her mother. "I was a bad daughter," she told herself.

Shortly after his wife died, Alan married a teacher he'd met. Bianca's brother and sister ignored her. Their maternal grandmother, who lived a few blocks away, moved to a town three hours away to give Alan space to rebuild his family. But Bianca liked her new stepmother; they baked together and made scrapbooks and chatted about school. The marriage lasted less than two years. Alan told his children that he had jumped in too quickly. The other two were elated, but Bianca stopped speaking to her father.

Her mother was dead, her grandmother had left, and her stepmother was now her ex-stepmother. Why should she get close to anyone?

Just as students were getting comfortable in base camp, the counselors shook things up. That would happen throughout the program: As soon as the kids got used to the routine, they would be jolted by the parents' visit, known as the family resolution, or a "Social Skills Seminar" on sex and dating, or a theatrical performance in front of the whole school. Rudy Bentz described it as artificially igniting fear and anxiety. When the students were uncomfortable, they'd go "back to pattern" — hyper kids would start bounding out of their chairs; ornery ones would get stubborn about niggling things; druggies would try to get a buzz from anything on hand. Rudy reasoned that they would face all kinds of challenges in their lives, and they needed to deal with strange situations in a mature way, without reverting to their old games.

The wilderness counselors worried about Bianca because she was so clever at playing by the rules. Base camp was set up in part to get loud-mouthed or rambunctious kids to settle down. Bianca, though, didn't throw fits or refuse her food. She didn't pick fights. Quite the opposite. She was always mothering, always encouraging other kids to talk about their own frustrations. She spoke up in group so often that it was easy to forget that she rarely talked about herself.

During her first days in the woods, Bianca spent much of her time with Tyrone. Because she had raven hair and a perpetual tan from her mom's Portuguese ancestors, she identified with the blacks, Haitians, Puerto Ricans, and Dominicans back home in Florida. The races didn't mix at her school, and though she was technically white she felt rejected by the snotty white kids who lived in mini-mansions surrounded by golf courses. Whenever she was asked her ethnic identity she said "Hispanic," or "La-tina" — that's how she saw herself and how others saw her. Tyrone's skin was dark, like hers. He, too, minded his own business and didn't draw attention to himself. Back home, neither Bianca nor Tyrone had done drugs. They thought beer tasted bitter. Without exchanging a word — just a knowing glance once in a while — they concurred on the subject of Mary Alice: She was a selfish snob.

The supervisors had read the admissions office summary of Bianca. It said that in the six years since her mother's death, she had avoided dealing with her sadness. "If a kid is grieving about something as significant as the death of a parent, she's a mess, no matter what kind of front she puts on," one of the supervisors said. "If she won't talk about it, she's not even ready to grieve."

It was time, he said, to turn up the heat.

In group one morning, as a boy spoke of his pangs for cocaine, Bianca said, "Why can't you just try being sober?" The supervisor let the conversa-tion play out for a few minutes. Then he looked at Bianca. "What about you? I don't want you talking about everyone else because basically we kind of forget about you. What's going on?"

"I'm worried about my brother. He's starting school, and I've always been there to walk him to class on the first —"

"Tell us about you, not your brother."

"My father says —"

"Let's hear about *you*."

As if Bianca had been waiting for someone to ask, she sighed. "I miss my mom."

"Go ahead," the supervisor urged.

She looked off to the side and said she felt alone and unprotected without her mother. She was scared. The supervisor asked her to take a deep breath and think about her mother. What did she remember?

Bianca remembered Teresa playing the piano. She remembered her arranging yellow gladiolas in a vase and talking to patients in the maternity ward. But her most vivid memories featured her mother as a patient. "One day when I was at the hospital visiting my mom, my grandma asked if I wanted to help with the laundry. We went to the laundry room. I remember my grandma putting in a quilt my mom had on her bed. It had hair, blood and throw-up all over it. "I asked grandma why, and all she said was that my mom was very sick. I'll never forget what that blanket looked like."

At the start of tenth grade, Bianca began to go out with a seventeen-year-old named Darnell. From the start, her father didn't like the relationship because, he said, Darnell was older than Bianca, and he had dropped out of school. "He's not going anywhere, he's just going to bring you down."

Her dad never mentioned the most obvious thing: Darnell, who grew up in Jamaica, was black. Bianca had no doubt the fuss was about race, despite her father's denials. Nana Sarah, her grandmother on her father's side, was blunt. The day after Bianca's father met Darnell, Nana Sarah stopped by to see Bianca. They sat outside. "What are you doing?" Nana Sarah said. "You need to stay with your own kind."

"What kind am I?" Bianca snapped. "Dad was Jewish and he dated a Catholic. He didn't stay with his own kind. If he did, I wouldn't exist."

She didn't see any point in telling her father and grandmother about Darnell. He hadn't really dropped out of high school. He'd been expelled for carrying a knife. He said it was for protection, in case anyone messed with him, but the school had a one-strike policy on weapons. Darnell was always coming up with plans, though he didn't follow through on them. He was going to attend community college, but he put off registering. He was going to join the Job Corps or enlist in the army, but he didn't. "You're so smart, babe," he cooed. "I don't know why you want to be with me." She didn't say the main reason: Compared with other guys she'd known, he was a knight on a white horse.

Bianca played soccer and starred on the speech and debate team, where she specialized in memorizing scripts and impersonating others. Her signature act was the "La-La Awards," a Latin American tribute that had been shown on MTV. As the announcer, she rolled her *RRRR*s with proficiency; she switched to the sultry voice of Charo; she impersonated a suave Antonio Banderas. Her English teacher, who coached the team, pushed Bianca to practice for two or three hours a day, saying, "You're the best I have." Bianca competed in three states and won a national competition in New York.

While she kept up an easygoing, I'm-just-fine facade at school, she fell apart at home. She called Darnell so often that her father took her cell phone away. A few days later he ripped out the phone jack in her room. Undeterred, she'd wait till her dad went to bed, then she'd take the cordless phone from the kitchen. Sometimes she fell asleep listening to Darnell's lilting voice.

In the fall of tenth grade, Bianca stopped caring whether she won or lost in a debate. She fed the coach an excuse about being busy with schoolwork. And though she had been thrilled to make the girl's varsity soccer team, she quit in a huff after a senior made a crack about having underclass players on the team.

Bianca was too embarrassed to tell her English teacher or soccer coach what had happened a few days before. On a Friday night, Bianca and Darnell had been making out at theater number 18 of a nearby multiplex. A five-year-old glanced back at the last row and saw them doing something strange. After the child's father complained, the theater manager found Bianca and Darnell groping each other, half-clothed. They ran outside, but the police found them and charged them with disorderly conduct. After being arrested, Bianca confided in a girl whom she considered a friend. Within a day, the school was abuzz with stories about the arrest. Boys who had never acknowledged Bianca made pumping motions with their hands as they approached her, rolling their tongues over their lips. Others called out, "Hey, wanna do me at the nine o'clock show?" They'd walk away, snickering with their friends.

After the arrest, Bianca's father confiscated her keys for the old Honda Accord she shared with Bruno. "You don't fuckin' care about me!" Bianca said. She continued with something she knew would rile him: "Everything wouldn't be so fucked up if mom was alive." She punched a hole in her bedroom wall. She secretly made a duplicate car key.

Bianca and her dad barely spoke. At night she often slipped out her window, which was just a couple of feet above the ground, then wriggled through the hedge and walked a half-mile to the house Darnell shared with his father. When her dad caught on, he screwed her windows shut. She loosened the screws, and he drove them in tighter. No big deal. Bianca simply padded down the hallway to her sister's old bedroom, from which she could shimmy out the window, then walked carefully with her back against the side of the house to avoid the motion sensor that turned on the floodlights.

As the summer after tenth grade started, Bianca and Darnell came up with a plan: They would run away to Jamaica. Bianca's passport was ready. She had a suitcase in her closet, and she'd chosen the clothes to pack. She had just started saving three hundred dollars for a one-way ticket when her father dashed her plans by hiring a husband-and-wife escort to take her to the wilderness program in North Carolina.

The counselors told Bianca that she was ready to start on her last project at base camp, writing her life story. She quickly wrote about the idyllic years: baking biscuits with her mom and singing in the car on the way to church. Describing her mother's death was surprisingly easy; it was as though the words had been corked up and needed to spill out.

As Bianca wrote, she forgot everything around her. That summer a severe drought had struck western Massachusetts, and by August it was so dry that the pine needles were turning yellow and russet and cascading from the trees. But in her mind Bianca was transported to the soaking humidity of Florida. She could see herself on a Monday at the start of seventh grade, wearing a T-shirt with her nickname, "Shorty," as she volunteered as a coach for first-grade girls. That fall, she became friends with an eighth grader named Raul. He always showed up at the soccer league, making funny faces and getting the girls to giggle. Raul had a serious side, too. He never wanted anyone to stop by his house, and he often looked for an excuse to delay going there himself. Bianca had heard that his father drank. Raul's grades were so poor that he had been held back, so the next year he and Bianca were in eighth grade together. When the first report cards came out, Raul, smiling and giddy, ran to Bianca. He had gotten all B's and A's, compared with four F's and a D in the marking period before summer vacation. Bianca hugged him.

A few days later, on October 30, Bianca was leaving school when she saw Raul. She asked about his plans for Halloween and Raul made a vague comment about needing to stay home. "I know my dad's going to do something."

"Like what?"

Raul just waved his hand. He said they'd see each other on Monday when Bianca coached the soccer league.

The next night, another friend called Bianca. "Did you hear about Raul?" he said. "He's dead." Bianca scolded him for joking. There was nothing funny about death. She hung up. She was doing homework at the kitchen table when she overheard Raul's name in a TV news bulletin. She watched numbly: Raul's father had shown up drunk holding a pistol. Raul, fearing for his mother's safety, tried to wrestle away the gun. During the tussle, he'd been fatally shot. By coincidence, Raul was buried a few feet from the grave of Bianca's mother.

When Bianca started writing about tenth grade, she paused. Something had happened then — something she'd kept secret for a year.

A counselor named Hannah stopped to see how she was doing with her life story. Bianca said she had a question. "What do you do if there's this thing you've never talked about and you really don't know how to deal with it?"

Hannah suggested that she write it — just jot it on the paper without trying to polish it into perfect pearls of prose — and see if that helped.

Bianca wrote. In the fall of sophomore year, she and Darnell had unprotected sex. She had been careful about using birth control most of the time, but in some ways she probably didn't care about anything. After her period didn't come, she went to her doctor and found out she was pregnant. She had just turned sixteen, and she was going to be a mother. An abortion was out of the question because of her religion. High school had been a breeze, so she was confident she could finish her diploma while raising a child. Her school even had a program for pregnant students. And then, in yet another cruel twist, she had a miscarriage at the end of her first trimester.

As she wrote, she tallied the losses:

Her mother
Her stepmother
Raul
Her child

The day after Bianca read her life story to the rest of the kids, the counselors assigned her to the toughest chore, the water haul. After hand-pumping water at the river, she had to walk up and down hills carrying containers weighing forty pounds each. She figured out a way to hold sticks with a partner and let the containers hang from the sticks. With the water sloshing around, a stick broke and one of the containers crashed down. As Bianca turned to look, another fell. She lost her composure for the first time in base camp. "I can't do it!" she wailed. "Oh my god, this sucks! I can't stand it." She sank to the ground and sobbed.

Five kids had gone on the water haul with Bianca. A counselor told them to put down their jugs and gather in a circle. It was obvious that Bianca needed help. They'd have a group right there. This time it didn't take any coaxing to get Bianca to talk. She said what she'd been thinking for a year. "I'm such a weak person. I lost my baby. I can't do anything right."

# 7

# Stoners, Wiggers, and Wanna-bes

Every few days, the kids heard branches snapping and boots crunching on the path to the campground. Someone was arriving to begin life as a shadow: another pissed-off kid dressed in generic cargo pants and a too-clean T-shirt. The boys kept watch for a hot girl. The girls wanted to see if a new guy was cute. Everybody enjoyed the guessing game: What had the shadows done that was awful enough to get them sent to the boonies?

At home, everyone had a look. For wanna-bes and wiggers — well-off white kids, or "white niggers," who imitated black gang members — it was Sean Jean or Phat Farm parachute pants draped over Air Jordan sneakers or untied Timberland boots with the tongues hanging out. For preps, it was Polo collared shirts, Seven jeans, or Abercrombie khakis; the girls wore Saucony sneakers, the boys New Balance 991s. Stoners prided themselves on not caring much about appearance, but they, too, had a uniform: Phish T-shirts, JNCO jeans or baggy Rocawears, slightly cuffed, over Birkenstock sandals.

As the newcomers peeled off their black concert shirts and Kikwear hoodies at the intake shed, they were discarding their images. These were no longer potheads or thugs or ghetto gang-bangers; they were young people embarking on a mission to find their core identities, their beautiful selves. Or so the Swift River staff claimed. Of course, being part of a clique meant much more than wearing the right brands. It meant walking with a certain beat or cocking one's head just so. Before a word was exchanged at base camp, before two pairs of eyes met in a split second of recognition, kids could peg each other. A stoner could pick out another stoner's loping gait and slow, screw-you grin. Preps could recognize each other's aloof, I'm-too-cool-for-this-place attitude. A girl with the last defiant streaks of purple in her hair, five holes in her ear lobe, and a world-weary slump was a Goth. A boy with an exaggerated bounce in his step — maybe even a fake limp — was unmistakably a wanna-be.

On a still, stifling August morning, Trevor, an English boy who had grown up in several countries, showed up to give Group 23 an international flavor. He had spent the past couple of years going to raves in London nightclubs and doing pot, mushrooms, acid, Special K, Ecstasy — you name it. He told the others matter-of-factly that he had overdosed while "snowballing" — mixing cocaine and heroin — and almost died. Trevor had a round face and a perpetual smile. The girls found him adorable. The boys liked him because he told wild stories about taverns with names like the Rat and Parrot. "Life's a permanent party," he'd say, and the others would answer with a hearty "*Ho!*"

Trevor was livid at his mother and father. They'd never mentioned that he was being sent to Swift River. Instead, they hired a pair of men to escort him to the edge of campus. His parents met him there and drove the last fifty yards to the entrance of base camp. Although they hadn't exactly disobeyed the school's rules against using escorts, they'd broken the spirit of the rules.

Trevor made no secret that he was just killing time at Swift River. In Britain, he said, kids were legally independent of their parents at age seventeen, a year younger than in America. In two months, on his seventeenth birthday, he'd pack up and return to the permanent party.

Not long after Trevor arrived, a stoop-shouldered boy named Phil slinked in. Although he was American, he'd grown up in Africa and Central America, with stints in Washington, D.C. His parents worked for the Peace Corps and nonprofit groups. Phil had been booted from four boarding schools in a year and a half. In one, he mentioned in an offhand way that he had once fantasized about a school shooting. Columbine was fresh on everyone's mind, so he was expelled even though he was raised as a Quaker and a pacifist; he abhorred violence and refused to kill insects. Three months later, he was kicked out of the next school when the staff caught him trying to get high from residue left over from someone else's bong. They also found forty sleeping pills, painkillers, and amphetamines in his room.

Phil didn't speak much, but when he held forth on meds, he exuded the authority of a wine connoisseur conversing about the latest Bordeaux.

Like most of the kids, he knew how to get high on Robitussin and other cough syrups by "Robotripping," taking five to seven times the normal dosage. Those who'd tried it said it had something to do with DXM, whatever that was. Phil, who regularly consulted drug sites on the Web, elaborated: "DXM is the cough suppressant Dextromethorphan. It's a synthetic drug, a replacement for codeine, that's similar to morphine. The lower doses are like a Ketamine high, but when you get above a couple hundred milligrams you get the whole mind-fuck that more traditional hallucinogens produce. I've never gone over a thousand milligrams, but it's supposed to be like a PCP high: You lose motor control and everything."

On the surface, Phil seemed like an American version of Trevor. Both had lived in several countries; both knew arcane details about all sorts of hallucinogens. But the resemblance ended there. Trevor played the piano and the guitar and memorized liner notes from hundreds of CDs and dreamed of spinning — working as a deejay. Phil spent his free time listening to political talk shows on National Public Radio. While Trevor kept discussions on the surface, Phil relished a hearty conversation that wove together strands of history, economics, and ethics. He was overjoyed if he could stir up an argument and draw on his theories about overpopulation, exploitation of workers, and the devastation of Brazil's rain forest. Trevor had theories about the optimum temperature for storing pot; Phil had theories about global warming.

Actually, there was another similarity: Both boys exasperated the staff. When one of the counselors asked Trevor how he was feeling, he ramped up his English accent and said, "Fine. How do *you* feel?" The counselors constantly rebuked Trevor for disguising his feelings by being too flip. They scolded Phil for covering up his feelings by intellectualizing. Asked about his feelings, Phil would look down at the ground and mumble something about Locke or Hobbes.

"Calvin and Hobbes?" someone ventured.

"No," Phil sighed. "John Hobbes, the eighteenth-century philosopher."

While the other kids weren't sure what they wanted to be when they were adults — they couldn't even envision being adults — Phil had it all figured out. He would be a philosopher, a physicist, and an environmentalist. He was a devout believer in a budding spiritual movement, Chillisism, which he described as a blend of Buddhism and absurdism stoked by drugs for chilling. He was the founder and leader of Chillisism. So far he was also its only member.

A tall, lean boy with muttonchops swaggered in. Andy came from a community on Long Island that was known for top-ranked public schools. Back home, he'd gone cruising with his buddies at ninety miles an hour on suburban roads while quaffing Johnnie Walker Red Label. He broke one rule after another at home. After his parents demanded that he reveal his AOL password, they read his e-mails and found that he had been regularly drinking, smoking pot, and skipping classes. Andy had a sincere way of talking to counselors, but several of the kids decided it was an act, and they didn't buy it.

With the departure of the watchtower girl, a spot had opened unexpectedly in Group 23. It was filled by the girl whose brother had written "fuck you" during an admissions office visit. She'd crashed the Volvo, stolen from her parents, and repeatedly snorted coke. Another girl, Ashley, had a pretty, freckled face and a cute button nose but said she felt ugly. She had been adopted at birth by a couple who lived in a Manhattan neighborhood of stately old apartment buildings where doormen stood sentry outside marble-lined lobbies. She'd attended a fancy private school and shown a lot of promise as a singer. By middle school, she was hanging out with a seedy crowd downtown. Ashley kept changing her story: She did acid, cocaine, or crack, or she just smoked pot and Marlboros. She'd had sex with guys she didn't know, or she'd almost had sex. It was hard to tell who she really was. She mused about running away from Swift River, but no one took her seriously: She was scared of bugs, scared of the woods, scared of the dark.

Everyone who arrived was infuriated at his or her parents, but no one's rage surpassed that of a girl who arrived from Ohio in September. She had gotten in trouble for drinking, shoplifting, and discussing sexual fantasies with a boy on-line. Then, three weeks before sending her to Swift River, her parents told her that she was adopted. Their newfound honesty was due less to a crisis of conscience than to practical considerations: Swift River's admissions office had said she couldn't be admitted until she knew about her identity. When she found out, she was stung and confused. Not only had she been living a lie for sixteen years, but she'd learned the truth only when her parents wanted to get rid of her.

The last girl to arrive had a tangled family situation; her father had left the family to marry her mother's best friend. That girl, too, was adopted;

she'd spent her first month of life in an orphanage. Like D.J. and Ashley, she changed her story so often that it was hard to know exactly what she'd done to get in trouble: She either did or didn't use a lot of drugs. One of the boys remarked that, rather than writing a truth list, as the counselors required, she should write a "quarter-truth list."

The kids had a sixth sense for figuring out who was gullible, and they went to town on the new girl. When she'd finished being a shadow, she joined Ashley, Andy, and D.J. as they stretched on the dew-covered PT field before a morning run. "Hey," D.J. asked hopefully, "are we going to do chakras today?" The frizzy-haired, den-mother counselor had promised to let the group do chakras — yoga relaxation exercises — if they were behaving well.

The new girl's eyes widened. "Shock? You get shock therapy here?"

Andy, the Long Island kid, didn't miss a beat. "Yeah, we have shock therapy. Every week."

D.J. nodded vigorously. "They didn't *tell* you?"

"That's why we have to keep our shirts tucked in," Ashley said. "So no one can see the scars."

Seeing the grave faces around her, the gullible girl began to cry. The kids laughed until Ashley explained that chakras had nothing to do with electricity.

❧

Group 23 was so easygoing that a counselor dubbed them the Brady Bunch. In many ways, Bianca set the tone. She came up with nicknames for almost everybody. She liked to stretch out their names, then add a vowel or two to the end. Trevor was Trevoria; Bianca gave it a singsong twist: *"Tre-VOE-ria."* Ashley was "Ash-LEE-yah."

When they carried water or firewood along the trails, the kids played geography — in fact, they played so often that the counselors put them on "geography bans." They resumed when the counselors couldn't hear: Mary Alice started with "Egypt," the place she was supposed to have visited on a family trip if she hadn't been sent away. The next in line, Ashley, needed a place that started with *t*.

"Tampa," she offered

It was Phil's turn. "Atakpame."

"At-a-*whaaat?*" the others said.

"Atakpame. It's a medium-sized village in Togo. I don't like it. Kind of a dump." He looked around, sensing confusion. "It ends in *e*."

Tyrone was next. When he was dragged into the game, he'd call out places that were no farther than a subway or a ferry ride from Queens. A minute passed. Phil prompted him. "The island where the immigrants came to. Starts with *e*."

"Ellis Island," Tyrone said triumphantly.

☙

The kids were all aware that the record for the shortest base camp stay, held by a girl, was sixteen days. The past winter, an especially defiant boy had endured the longest stay: ninety-nine days, through a stretch of snow and subzero temperatures. The kids put great stock in those numbers. Even though the counselors said there was no correlation between the length of a base camp stay and success or failure on campus, everyone figured that a quick tour of duty at base camp guaranteed an easy ride during the rest of Swift River.

Most of the kids in the group plowed steadily through their assignments, trying to get out of the woods quickly. Not D.J. With the grass glistening in the early morning sun, he could be seen dangling from a metal bar at the PT field, doing extra pull-ups. When the time came for reading and writing, though, he dawdled. The growth-book stuff was boring. Like "Self-Reliance" by Emerson: "Trust thyself: every heart vibrates to that iron string," it said. "Accept the place divine providence has found for you, the society of your contemporaries, the connection of events." What did that mean, you were supposed to give up the idea of going home and be thrilled about living with weirdos and druggies and pushy counselors for fourteen months? No way. Phil, who could read kids well, decided that D.J. wanted to mess up in base camp so that he could delay going to campus, where he'd probably be the only ninety-five-pound kid among the hundred students, including some pretty hard-core bullies. D.J. said that was stupid; he just wanted to go back to New Jersey, to his dog, Firecracker, and his friends and his normal life.

D.J. was hard to figure out. He was adopted, but he said he didn't care about that. Unlike the rest of the adopted kids, he showed no curiosity about his biological mother or father. He had run away from home once, but he hadn't gotten involved in drugs, drinking, and sex the way most of the kids had. Something fragile about D.J. made most of the girls want to treat him like a kid brother. Unless the subject was rock climbing or *The Simpsons,* he rarely uttered more than four words at a time. When he read letters from his parents, everyone listened raptly.

In one note, D.J.'s dad wrote about his own life. He had emigrated from Hungary in the 1950s as a small child with his mother, who was a widow. They lived in a crowded tenement in New York City, where his mother worked ten-hour shifts in a factory. Borrowing money from a relative, she sent D.J.'s father to a boarding school in Pennsylvania. He was six and barely spoke English. "I cried myself to sleep every night," D.J.'s dad wrote. "I vowed never to send my son to a boarding school. Sending you to Swift River has been the most agonizing thing I've ever done."

When someone asked how it felt to read those words, D.J. stared ahead blankly.

At base camp, the counselors prohibited "war-storying" — boasting of exploits involving drugs, alcohol, or sex. As soon as the counselors were out of range, of course, everyone war-storied. While others in base camp bantered casually about the drugs they did and the things they stole, D.J. seemed to try too hard. He reminisced about setting off bottle rockets in mailboxes with his buddies, who called themselves the Parkland Mafia, after the name of their school. Soon it became clear that the Parkland Mafia was hardly an elite group; it had just two other members who spent a lot of their time playing video games.

D.J. boasted about his heavy smoking: "Three packs a day."

"Wait, you're telling us you smoked three packs of Camels a day?" Phil countered. "The average pack of Camels is about four dollars, depending on the state tax. If you were to multiply four dollars by three packs by seven days, you'd get eighty-four dollars a week. Okay, let's say you bought them by the carton at twenty-five dollars: One carton would last you three point one days. You'd go through slightly over two and a third cartons a week, which still means fifty bucks a week on butts. You said your allowance was thirty-five dollars a month. It doesn't add up." He rested his case.

D.J. looked at him dumbfounded. Phil was probably his best friend in base camp — his only friend, really — but when it came to certain subjects like drugs, Phil hewed to his principles.

"Didn't you say you smoked reefers laced with acid?" Phil challenged.

D.J. nodded, but he already looked defeated.

"Dude, that's fuckin' physically impossible. You *cannot* get a trip by smoking acid. LSD — that's lysergic acid diethylamide — is inherently unstable. An open flame would degrade it. You might get a placebo effect, but you won't get stoned."

Phil wasn't finished. "That's if you believe in the placebo effect. I personally think the jury's still out."

D.J. backed off and left the war-storying to others. Phil, who was just fifteen, had his own war story: At his last boarding school, he'd tried smoking pot. After a month of that, he'd given a friend money to buy drugs, and the friend came back with a grainy brown-yellow substance. Phil tried it. In just one month, he'd gone from pot to heroin. Then there was Andy. He routinely ignored his parents' curfews and stayed out drinking. At one point, his parents were so enraged that they locked the house, changed the code of the burglar alarm, and left a note telling him to find another place to stay. At three in the morning, Andy smashed a window to get in. His parents called the cops, and Andy ended up in handcuffs on his own driveway.

Trevor was the undisputed champion of war-storying. In a dulcet voice, the voice of a dad telling a bedtime story, he reminisced about running away to Amsterdam for a month and spending all his money on marijuana so potent that it had a THC count of thirty-one. That elicited oohs of appreciation; ordinary marijuana has a THC count of seven. "One hit of that bud," Trevor said with a dreamy look, "and you were laid out."

If Phil was the *Encyclopaedia Britannica* of drugs — complete with histories, etymologies, and trivia — Trevor was the *Michelin Guide* to narcotic hot spots. He could hold forth on the best 4-20 celebrations around the world. (As everyone knew, April 20, or 4-20, was known as National Stoners' Day and International Smokeout Day. By some unwritten tradition, it had become a day when many kids skipped school to get high.) Kids debated the origins of 4-20, which supposedly had started in California. Some maintained that "420" was the police code for marijuana; others claimed it was the number of chemicals in cannabis; still others speculated that it was the time of day when students used to gather after school to smoke joints. Although 4-20 celebrations had been around since the 1970s, the Internet recently had helped popularize the phrase in even the most remote towns. It had taken on a sinister meaning in 1999 because the killings at Columbine High School had taken place on 4/20. For the Swift River staff, the phrase symbolized that adults and teenagers inhabited different worlds. While many of the kids had prattled on about "four-twenty" since seventh grade, most of their parents had no idea what they meant.

Lunch alternated between pita bread with peanut butter one day and pita with a hunk of cheese the next. Mondays and Thursdays they made couscous for dinner; Tuesdays and Fridays, beans and rice; Wednesdays and Saturdays, mashed potatoes. Sunday was pasta night. A boy named Tanner, the son of a major league baseball player, quickly became Trevor's best friend. Tanner, who looked like a teddy bear, had done hard drugs. He'd even been involved with a gang, and his upper arms bore mysterious tattoos. Rather than talking about that, Tanner got everybody debating the merits of Doritos versus Cheetos or rhapsodizing about Pizza Hut, KFC, TGI Friday's, and Taco Bell. Then, at mealtime, they returned to the reality of the rice-couscous-potatoes monotony. Luckily, Trevor provided relief. While he was reliving hallucinogenic highlights one morning, a counselor walked by. "Hey, no war-storying," he barked.

Trevor turned on his charm. "We're not war-storying," he said in the decorous voice of a member of Parliament. "We're talking about how we made mistakes."

No matter what the subject, Trevor had a good story. He inhabited a world of "mates" who lived in their own flats and supported themselves by spinning. He knew everything from Beethoven's sonatas to ska, from Tchaikovsky to techno. He was a self-taught computer geek, too. Once when he was bored, he said, he went on his school computer in London and hacked an American Web site that automatically answered questions. The logo featured a butler in a tuxedo. It reminded Trevor of a penguin. For several minutes, he said, viewers around the world noticed that the well-known site had been renamed "AskPenguin.com."

Trevor's passion for telling stories didn't extend to discussing his troubles. When Bianca and others tried to find out why he had almost killed himself while snowballing, he eluded them. Exasperated, the staff put him on "smile bans," ordering him to keep a somber face while looking at his past. Trevor nodded, but he couldn't hide his amusement at the overly sincere American counselors. *Smile* bans? Just the thought of it made him grin.

Bianca noticed a tinge of melancholy behind Trevor's jauntiness. His smile was wide, but his eyes were cheerless. Something was missing from his story. A boy didn't simply start doing Ecstasy at age fourteen, stop talking to his parents at fifteen, and move away at sixteen. After listening to Trevor for a few days, Bianca started to wonder about his rose-tinted reminiscences. Despite his sophisticated accent and his globe-trotting–deejaying–computer-hacking existence, Trevor was just a kid in pain. All of them were, Bianca realized. Even herself. They gloated about their lives at home; they war-storied about sex and drugs and hip-hop; they yearned for the halcyon times with their best, best friends. But if things had been so great — if life had truly been a permanent party — none of them would have needed to run away or get drunk and stoned day after day.

# 8

## "Y'ALL HAD NO CLUE"

BIANCA LIKED MALLS and burger restaurants. She liked microwaves and waterbeds, hair dryers and hoop earrings. She liked Florida's flat landscape and sweltering weather and the nonstop air conditioning that made it livable. She sped through the work at base camp, bent on breaking the sixteen-day record that she'd heard about. During her six weeks in the North Carolina wilderness program, she'd had enough un–air-conditioned wilderness to last a lifetime.

She'd arrived after Tyrone and Mary Alice, but she soon caught up to them in the growth book's reading and writing assignments. She was neck and neck with Mary Alice in the Turtle stage, then overtook her in Coyote, and shot ahead in Beaver. Not that it was a rivalry or anything.

Bianca was nice to Mary Alice, but she didn't trust the blond southerner with the whiny voice. Maybe it was because they both were intensely competitive in everything they did, from Wiffleball to wood hauling. Maybe because Mary Alice came across as a vapid rich bitch who would have regarded Bianca and her friends back home as ghetto trash. Or maybe because Mary Alice reminded her of a stuck-up girl on the varsity soccer team who had been mean to her. Whatever the reason, Bianca liked the idea of besting the spoiled girl from Dallas. If Mary Alice enjoyed the outdoors as much as she claimed, let *her* spend extra time communing with ants, fleas, poison ivy, and pee holes.

The time came to go on solo. The experience was meant to give a kid two days and nights in solitude. For years, researchers had said that American teenagers didn't have quiet time, a break from television and shops and friends to decelerate and reflect. A counselor told Bianca to take advantage of the silence and think about her life as she worked on two assignments.

One was the truth letter to her father, detailing every secret she'd kept from him over the years. The second was a truth list for the counselors, revealing any rule she'd broken since arriving at base camp. So long as she came clean, she wouldn't be punished.

Bianca packed her sleeping bag and tarp, some trail mix, a can of tuna, and a water jug. A counselor led her up to a ridge, then stopped at a clearing surrounded by a stand of birch trees and gave her a two-way radio to be used only in an emergency ("if a bear approaches, that's an emergency"). Someone would check on her once a day. Good luck.

Then she was alone.

Bianca sat with her back against a rock. The sun poured through thirty-foot-tall hemlocks and ash trees. She was enveloped by the sounds of nothingness — leaves rustling, a woodpecker pummeling a branch, a blue jay calling out a greeting. Writing a list of misdeeds at base camp was simple because she didn't have much to admit. Other than filching a few extra slices of cheese now and then, she'd stuck to the rules. The truth letter to her dad was far more difficult. She filled in her father on the details of the night she and Darnell had been caught nearly naked in the theater. They'd promised the manager they would wait for the police, but when he turned around they ran away. The cops tracked them down and found them at a restaurant. She also wrote about the time she sneaked home from school to fool around with Darnell. She could still remember her father opening her door and finding the two of them in bed. Her father already knew these things, but that didn't make detailing them in a letter any less humiliating.

Bianca had heard about other kids' truth letters. Boys revealed they'd hocked the family silverware or had blacked out from taking pills. Girls admitted having sex with older men they'd met on the Internet. Bianca didn't drink or use drugs; she didn't steal; she rarely went on-line. Still, she had other secrets. Was a truth letter like confession at church? When was it necessary to tell the complete truth, and when did a half-truth suffice?

In her letter, she described the nights she'd slipped out her window and walked over to Darnell's house. Her father knew that. But she revealed that even after he fastened her window shut, she often escaped through the window in her sister's room. She told him that she had been saving money to run away to Jamaica. Revealing part of the truth seemed better than none at all. She didn't tell her father about something that had happened in a locker room in eighth grade, and she didn't write a word about her miscarriage. Her dad would never understand.

A few days later, Tyrone packed up his gear and went off on his solo. "I am writing a letter about the things you probably don't no about me and my friends," he wrote his mother.

> One, you don't no when I stay out late at night. You know I hang out at Lance house. What you don't know is that he smokes pot. I still hang out with him though. Now Lance drinks. And Manny smokes weed. And he was scared that you would think less of him if you new. I never did drugs, even though I hang out with them.
>
> There were nights when I almost got arrested for throwin rocks at cars. One time Paco and I were about one block from our house and we were throwing rocks at taxis. And they called the cops and we almost got arrested but they let us go.
>
> The second time when I was with Paco and Manny we through rocks off a roof across the street from his house and someone called the cops. And they came up to me and they thought we were stealin a car, but after examinin the car they asked us if we did anythin and we lied to them and they let us go. I have also had sex with Anika. I was safe, though.
>
> Well, that's all I have kept from you, basically.
> Love,
> Your son. Tyrone B. Harriston
> PS, I hope this do not change anything with my friends and I hope your not mad at me.

Tyrone was on the verge of writing something else, but he didn't want to scare his mom.

Before Mary Alice went on her solo, a counselor told her it was time to stop pretending she'd just slipped up once or twice at home. She needed to tell her parents — and herself — what her life had been like. Mary Alice began writing as soon as she was alone. It took a few drafts, but eventually she owned up to some of what she'd done. "I started smoking pot my freshman year and smoked every day after I quit cheerleading," she wrote. "I tried acid for the first time my freshman year. I have tripped about 20 something times since then."

> I first tried Ecstasy last August at a rave. About 25 times I think I have done Ecstasy. I also would sell Adderall to my friends or snort it with them. I have also snorted cocaine a couple of times, whenever anyone I know had any.
>
> Usually every weekend when y'all would go to bed, I would have people over and we would drink and smoke or be on some other drug. We would usually all hang out in the basement or playroom and y'all had no clue.
>
> When I said I was studying for exams I would usually be getting high with friends.
>
> I started stealing cash from y'all about a couple of months ago when y'all started to notice all the times I would take the credit card. The most I ever stole was 200 dollars. I used this money to buy weed for the Lone Star Youth Ministry Western Tour.
>
> I love you both so much and hope you can forgive me for my dishonesty and poor behavior.

Signing off, Mary Alice felt like a changed person — she felt cleansed. Because she still had another day on solo, she wrote an extra letter to her parents. She told them she had tears in her eyes because she realized that in four months, for the first time, she wouldn't be able to wake up and run downstairs to see presents under the tree on a Christmas morning. Also, she wanted to be with her little sister, who was starting seventh grade, because middle school could be treacherous for girls.

"I have to say though I am learning a lot about myself and how I was so self-destructive," she wrote. "I'm beginning to realize how much drugs and sex hurt my life and my relationship with y'all, with friends and myself as well as God."

At the end, she added a note: "I made a list of everything I forgot. Mom, please send it. Also, I decided that it would be better if I had brought both my snowboards. This means my Burton Balance, the one with the stickers. It is black and has custom bindings. And my custom board. It has Salomon 3 bindings. Please send these. Also my boots."

After Mary Alice finished her solo, the counselors read her truth list. She had not been such a precious angel in base camp, after all. She'd been war-storying with Trevor. She'd had cravings for drugs. Most important, she had purged in the woods after a meal.

Mary Alice had been acting as though her eating disorder was cured. It wasn't. Girls weren't punished for being anorexics or bulimics, of course, but they did have to start talking about what memories and feelings were causing a relapse.

At night, after the kids had gone to sleep in their A-frames, the counselors compared notes on their progress. In writing page after page of her life story and other assignments, Bianca had the flat tone of someone filling out forms for the motor vehicle department. Even her summary of her mother's death had a just-the-facts tone. Bianca needed a different approach. Somewhere inside that sixteen-year-old mind, there surely was a flicker of passion. The question was how to release it.

"Write something creative," one of the counselors told Bianca the next morning. Creative? That was different. Bianca was bored with trying to recap her life. While others chattered among themselves after PT, she leaned against a rock and wrote a story:

> Once upon a time, there was a flamingo in the Everglades. Her name was Bianca. She was the pinkest flamingo, really fuchsia. Her brother was more white, their sister a pastel pink. Bianca was very content being fuchsia and her mom took care of her, telling her it's okay to be the color she is and be different. Her mom protected her from the alligators who taunted her. Bianca told her mom everything. On the other hand, her brother and sister were usually with their dad, talking about how the Everglades are shrinking because of the overpopulation of old people in Florida.
>
> One day while the two sisters and brother were eating minnows, their dad came through the saw grass crying. Their mom was caught by a trapper and taken to some far-off place. Bianca was devastated. Then she looked around and saw that her siblings and dad needed help.

Bianca thought that because she wasn't crying at the moment, she had to help, so she got shrimp for them and made sure they had family dinners every night.

Bianca started making friends and was staying up at all hours of the night. She wanted to be popular and accepted among the other flamingos on the wrong side of the saw grass. Her boyfriend didn't use any of the bad grass in the swamp and he made her feel really good about herself.

One night her dad heard a noise and went to check on his daughter. To his terror, she wasn't there. When Bianca came back, her dad started squawking and said a lot of hurtful things and grounded Bianca. She started thinking of ways to get around all the rules. She got the portable cattail so she could talk to her boyfriend.

The next morning her dad sat at the rock and asked Bianca what was going on and how she was feeling. Bianca yelled at her dad again and stormed out of the house, breaking the door.

Bianca went to her friends, and they all said that she should be able to do whatever she wanted. She agreed. She had constant fights with her brother, sister and dad. She stopped having family dinners and lived off of mangroves and other junk food. Her father decided to take drastic measures and send her to an island where troubled flamingos go and work on emotional stuff. She learned that she had never mourned for her mother's disappearance, and she always pushed her emotions aside to look strong, when inside she was probably one of the most torn flamingos in the Everglades.

As Bianca finished working on her story, her dad sent the final letter to base camp, the one the counselors called the "affirmation letter." It was meant to remind a kid that no matter what had happened, he or she was treasured. "We've been dwelling on negative things a lot, so it's time for me to tell you why I love you so much and what makes you special," he wrote. "You are tenacious, Bianca. I remember you running yourself into exhaustion playing soccer, driving yourself because you felt you were needed. When you volunteer at the hospital or help in other ways, you do so happily and enthusiastically."

Bianca shivered. "Remember just a few months ago, in the car you broke into song, pantomiming the radio? That streak of spontaneity and playfulness that I so loved and needed from Mom I find in you."

Bianca's flamingo allegory and her father's letter showed the staff that she was ready for the next step. Although she had arrived after the watchtower girl and Tyrone and Mary Alice, she would be the first one to head to main campus. It had taken her just twenty-four days. Again, she didn't want it to seem as if she was competing with Mary Alice or anyone . . .

The counselors kept saying that a quick stint in base camp was no guarantee that things would go smoothly on campus. But Bianca had never needed to put a lot of effort into school. Swift River was for kids who were more messed up than she'd ever been, so how difficult could it be?

# 9

## TYRONE: "LONELY ONCE AGAIN"

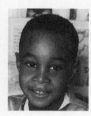

EVERY NIGHT, the kids in base camp elected a leader for the next day. Time after time, they voted for Tyrone. Just as he'd promised, he finished everything he started. He didn't whine or throw tantrums; he didn't alienate anyone by spreading gossip. Between breakfast and lunch, most kids went through the gamut of emotions — giddiness, dejection, outrage; cursing their parents and then missing their parents — but Tyrone remained reassuringly stoical. Once in a while he flashed a contagious smile after finishing PT or chores. He didn't admit it, but he found base camp relaxing. He felt a sense of accomplishment when he won a race, hauled the most logs, or checked off a box in his growth book after finishing a chapter of *Jonathan Livingston Seagull*. After three weeks, the counselors made him a hawk — the highest level at base camp. Just a few more days and he'd move to campus.

During group therapy, though, Tyrone faded into the tree trunks. Andy, the boy from Long Island, pointed out that whenever someone asked about Tyrone's father, Tyrone refused to say anything negative.

"That's because I don't have anything negative to say," Tyrone said.

"But what kind of things does your dad do with you?"

"He plays basketball with me."

"How often does he play?"

"Well, my mom usually won't let him come over."

"When you were little? How often did you play basketball with him?"

"Sometimes. A few times. He worked nights so he slept during the day."

Andy cocked his head and gave a don't-bullshit-a-bullshitter scowl. He asked why Tyrone's father barely even visited. Tyrone said that his mother had gotten an order from a judge. Some kind of protection order, because she didn't like his father.

The counselors said Tyrone needed to be a real part of the group. That meant talking honestly instead of ignoring others or feigning ignorance. They put him on spice bans and told him he had to shake hands every morning with each student and counselor while looking everyone in the eyes.

Ashley, the button-nosed girl from Manhattan, was a city kid through and through, and she made Tyrone laugh (one morning she let loose a blood-curdling scream when she awoke to find a chipmunk cuddled up in her sleeping bag). It was a short subway ride from Tyrone's block in Queens to Ashley's place on Park Avenue, but they might as well have been on different continents. Tyrone lived in a cramped house and went to a public school so large that he didn't know the names of most of his classmates; Ashley lived in a building with white-gloved elevator operators and went to an elite private academy where some kids got dropped off by limousine. Tyrone and his friends saved up money to go to video arcades; Ashley went to thirteen-year-olds' parties that featured singers who had been on MTV. Tyrone's most memorable vacation had been at Disney World; Ashley spoke with authority about the Louvre.

Still, Tyrone and Ashley connected when they talked about what food they missed the most. They both loved McDonald's. Not Burger King or Taco Bell. Just McDonald's.

"I always get number four," Ashley said.

"Me, too. Double Quarter Pounder and fries."

"*Ho!*" Ashley said. "With Coke."

"Sprite."

There in the woods, a two-hour hike from the nearest fast-food restaurant, they found a bond. Tyrone would have a friend when he made it to main campus. That was reassuring for someone who had felt alone for as long as he could remember.

In Tyrone's world, not much was reassuring. His mother, Natalie, had grown up in a Harlem railroad flat, sharing a bedroom with her two brothers. Money was so tight that they scrounged in garbage cans to find cardboard to insulate their shoes. Natalie's father worked in a plant that made amphetamines for pharmaceutical companies. The amphetamine dust seemed to affect him; after work he had extreme ups and downs. Natalie's stepmother was a bitter woman who ordered Natalie to shut up when she hummed while doing the dishes. Natalie wanted to go to college but went to work instead at age eighteen. She married Lerone, a college dropout who had studied computer programming. They had a daughter and then a son, Tyrone. Their firstborn was so accustomed to getting all the attention that she completed Tyrone's sentences. As a toddler, Tyrone simply stopped speaking for several months — a practice he resumed in adolescence.

Natalie cooked, cleaned, and worked full-time as a technician at the phone company. She had never relied on anyone, and she wasn't about to rely on her husband. It was she who found out about a Korean couple who had been burglarized and couldn't wait to leave Queens. Natalie paid $30,000 for their home, a tiny, two-story frame house. It faced the intersection of two busy avenues and looked squarely at the Projects. The view out back was even worse — a bus depot. But she owned it free and clear. Natalie took off the iron grills that covered the windows because she hated to feel she was imprisoned in her own home. If some junkies wanted to steal the family's meager possessions, then let them (someone did just that, breaking a back door and hauling away a stereo and jewelry).

Tyrone's childhood memories were a blur. His mother's account of those days contrasted so sharply with his father's that Tyrone no longer knew what was true. Most of what he'd heard came from his mother. She claimed that Lerone used heroin. When Tyrone was six, the family went to a Fourth of July party thrown by Natalie's relatives. Lerone huddled with a group of men in an alley the whole time. Strange things started to happen after that. Lerone removed himself even more from family life; he started working the overnight shift and spent the days in bed. His bank account, which had grown to $18,000, dwindled to zero. Natalie would come home with cash in her pocketbook and half of it would soon disappear. While doing the laundry, she emptied Lerone's pants pockets and found vials of powder that looked like Comet. Several times, Lerone locked himself in the bathroom and then emerged, leaving blood in the sink. Thinking back on the party, Natalie had a queasy feeling. A relative told her that one of her brothers-in-law had introduced Lerone to cocaine that day.

Lerone constantly announced his good intentions. He wanted to take Tyrone to the movies, to the zoo, to a ballgame. But he usually arrived late or didn't show up, and the plans rarely turned into reality. He had a friend who was an accountant, and they sat in the kitchen coming up with moneymaking schemes while Natalie bustled around them cooking and cleaning. She learned to tune them out — just as she tuned out a lot of other things that were going on around her. One night, she came into the bedroom and saw Lerone hunched over, snorting something. She walked downstairs without saying anything. Lerone followed her to the kitchen and said he was just using occasionally. Natalie turned on him. "You do what you want, but when you stop doing your job, which is providing for the children, you'll find skid marks on your butt from sliding down the street. That's how fast you're gonna be moving when I throw you out."

According to Natalie's version of events, Lerone was laid off and life got worse. After more money vanished, Natalie began tucking her cash in her bra and sleeping with it. Lerone withdrew money from the ATM, forgetting to tell Natalie, who tracked every cent in the household. Lerone signed up for one credit card after another and racked up $26,000 in debt. Then a letter arrived from the IRS: The Harristons were being audited. They needed to present proof of the medical expenses they'd deducted for treating Tyrone's sickle-cell anemia.

"Sickle-cell *anemia?*" Natalie sputtered. She had let Lerone and his friend do the taxes and she'd signed the 1040 without looking at the details. "You're so sick that you used your own son for tax fraud!"

The IRS slapped them with a $6,000 fine and another $8,000 in penalties. Because Lerone had no money, the government put a lien on Natalie's bank account. Signing a tax return without reading it was not an excuse, and she lost the money. In the middle of the financial mess, a woman called frequently, looking for Lerone. The woman sounded strung out on something or other. "I have two children but the BCW took them," she volunteered, referring to the Bureau of Child Welfare. Natalie didn't know what the woman wanted from Lerone, nor did she care. She likened herself to a subway-commuting, cooking, dishwashing zombie, dazed from one shock after another, such as the fire that consumed their house. Actually, there wasn't a fire — but Lerone and his accountant crony had invented a roof-melting, wall-buckling inferno for the IRS. They were audited again.

One day when Tyrone was nine, he looked up from television to see two cops handcuffing his father and dragging him out of the house. Natalie explained that she had filed for divorce and had gotten a judge's order of protection to ensure that Lerone kept his hands off her. "Don't you see what your father's been doing?" Natalie asked Tyrone. Natalie's brother-in-law had died of a seizure after drinking, and several of her relatives and neighbors had overdosed on drugs. She said Tyrone's dad had an illness called addiction. She took Tyrone to a Narcotics Anonymous meeting, but he was too young to understand.

Barricading himself in his little room, Tyrone refused to talk or eat. He could wait. After all, his father had sworn he'd return and straighten things out. Every month or two, he showed up to take Tyrone and his sister out for ice cream. He emphatically denied using drugs and said that Natalie was a bad mother. Tyrone, unsure of what to believe, became increasingly withdrawn. He was cranky in the mornings when it was time to walk to elementary school. It was an old brick building with hissing boilers and windows that didn't close all the way. After school, Tyrone would let himself in at home and watch television or play Nintendo. He wasn't allowed to have friends over without adult supervision, and he followed the rules. Parents want compliant children, but Tyrone was almost *too* compliant; he was listless all the time, and he showed no interest in anything other than video games. Natalie fretted about her son's long, lonely afternoons, but she had to pay the bills, and that meant keeping her job at the phone company. At night, she and her daughter would fix dinner and Tyrone would eat alone in front of the TV in his six-by-eight-foot bedroom.

Tyrone advanced from grade to grade mostly because he sat quietly in the back of the room without stirring up trouble. But when he reached eighth grade, New York City announced it would abolish the tradition of social promotion. To move to the next grade, students would have to pass their classes and standardized tests. Tyrone squeaked into ninth grade at a five-story high school that took up a city block. The school had 3,900 students; two-thirds of them were so poor that they got free or subsidized lunches. Tyrone hated passing through metal detectors every time he entered, he hated the catcalls that echoed through the halls, and he hated the fights that broke out over the smallest provocation. Before teachers could learn his name, Tyrone decided high school wasn't for him. He'd stay awake till four or five in the morning, take a nap, then wolf down breakfast and walk around the block. As soon as Natalie left for work, he'd sneak back home and go to sleep until five in the afternoon. Every day, a computer would call the house and announce that Tyrone had been absent from school. Tyrone let the answering machine take the call, then pressed the erase button.

Although Natalie suspected her son was cutting some classes, she didn't realize he was skipping entire weeks of school. No one showed an interest in him. Natalie went to see a truant officer who made it clear that he didn't care whether Tyrone showed up or not, though he explained that he wanted to keep Tyrone's name on an enrollment list so the school wouldn't lose several thousand dollars in per-pupil funding from the district. Natalie went to the Board of Education offices to argue that Tyrone needed to be moved to a special program with small classes because he had a learning disability or depression. The specialists rebuffed her. Tyrone wasn't disruptive or dangerous; he wasn't classified as "at-risk." They implied that he was just a shiftless teenager with a lazy mother.

Natalie eventually remarried, a man who had been drafted to Vietnam and had risen from private to corporal in the army, then finished his tour of duty on the brink of becoming a sergeant. After the war, he'd married and raised three daughters. Although his first marriage didn't last, he prided himself on being a father who was caring as well as strict. He tried to be a good influence on Tyrone, too. He took the boy bowling and shooting pool, things Tyrone had never done before. He took Tyrone to his first Yankees game. Tyrone went along but didn't exchange more than a few words with his stepfather. He was waiting for his dad to come home.

Natalie kept promising Tyrone that she'd make more time for him, but life got busier. Tyrone's sister, who wasn't married, had a baby. Natalie, still trying to raise Tyrone, found herself a grandmother at age forty-seven.

Tyrone had a small, loyal group of friends. There was Paco, his Puerto Rican friend from childhood, and Lance, who was getting ready to go into the army. And Black Manny — not to be confused with Fat Manny, who was Mexican, or Little Manny, an eight-year-old Italian boy who sometimes followed them around and imitated them. Little Manny cracked them up, bellowing "Yo, niggah!" as if he were the big man on the block. On the night before Tyrone had to leave for Massachusetts, the guys came over to the house. They hung out drinking Pepsi in the living room, which was so small that their knees bumped when they sat on the sofa and the two easy chairs that faced it. Tyrone had a few CDs, all featuring parody artist Weird Al Yankovich.

After a while, they left Tyrone's house and walked past the Projects and over the footbridge that connected Queens to Roosevelt Island. Roosevelt Island was a development in the East River between Queens and Manhattan that tried to have the flavor of an old-fashioned city, with apartments over stores and parks out back. Tyrone and his friends liked the south end, whose old, abandoned buildings were perfect for exploring. They walked through a crumbling structure emblazoned with gang graffiti. Tyrone didn't talk about the fact that he was being sent to a boarding school — a "go-away school," he called it. The other guys wondered how he would stand being stuck in the sticks with a lot of rich white kids. Paco said Swift River sounded like a military academy. Paco had credibility: He had gone to school every day in ninth and tenth grades, while Tyrone stayed in his bedroom.

"You never did homework," Tyrone countered.

"I didn't do nothing. But I passed, right?" Paco said. "Now look where they're making you go. See, you shoulda went to school."

☞

On a torrid afternoon in late August, with the drought well into its third month, the kids from Group 23 sat in a circle on the parched grass for a therapy session with the base camp counselors. Andy coughed and cleared his throat and said he had to come clear about something. Everyone waited. Had he tried to sneak a Heineken out to base camp? Was there a secret he had hidden from his parents, something horrible he'd done at home?

"I have to be honest," he said in his deep voice. "I took two apples at breakfast."

It was pure Andy. He'd confess to something almost for the sake of confessing. No one was very impressed by his newfound conscience. Stealing a piece of fruit or a hunk of cheese at base camp now and then was like smoking a joint at home; almost everyone did it. Still, Andy's confession led Ashley to say that she, too, needed to clear up something. Maybe she was inspired by Andy; they'd been watching each other and flirting in not-so-subtle ways. Something about Ashley's quivering voice caused everyone to stare. It was apparent that she was going to own up to something more serious than, say, ripping off an apple.

"I was going to run away tonight," she said.

"*Was?*" one of the counselors asked.

"I'm not. Not anymore."

The counselor asked if she was sure. Yes, she said, she'd decided to stick out base camp. Running wouldn't make things better. Anyway, Ashley conceded, her plan wasn't much of a plan; it involved walking on a path down the hill and listening for the sounds of cars. When she found a road, she'd have hitched a ride to New York.

The counselor asked her if she'd shared her plan with anyone. She hesitated.

"Who was it?"

Her eyes got teary.

"Who?"

She looked down. "Tyrone."

All eyes turned to Tyrone, who sat stone-faced.

Ashley explained that she had approached him while they were pumping water. She'd made sure no one else could hear. "Can you keep a secret?" she had whispered. "I'm going to run tonight."

"That's crazy," Tyrone had said. "You can get lost. What happens if you trip? Who's gonna find you?" Ashley had thought about it and promised she wouldn't run.

The counselors' attention switched to Tyrone. They asked if that was how it had happened. Yes, he said. "Do you realize what you did?" scolded a counselor. "You jeopardized the safety of the group. What's the most important thing here?"

Tyrone was silent.

"Safety," the counselor said. "You're about to finish up and go to campus. Hawks are supposed to set the example here. Why didn't you tell us that Ashley was planning to run away?"

"Because she promised me she wouldn't."

How did Tyrone know Ashley wouldn't run? Why didn't he alert a counselor? Hadn't he heard that other kids had taken off in the middle of the night and had to be rescued? Tyrone's face looked contorted. He held up his hands and started crying. It was the first time anyone at base camp had seen him cry. He said that he didn't want to tell on Ashley because she was a friend. He shook and wheezed as the tears fell. "I've only had three friends in my life," he sobbed. "I didn't want to lose a friend."

The counselors told Tyrone that he would have to spend an extra three days at base camp, working on writing assignments. Before moving to main campus, he needed to understand more about what had happened in his childhood that made him so fearful of being abandoned. Tyrone reacted by sitting stiffly and looking straight ahead, his arms crossed.

Before going to sleep, he wrote a poem in pencil. He titled it "Lonely Once Again."

> Where you going? Can I come?
> I want to follow. I cant. Why not?
> > Your voice is getting softer. You must speak up, you have to
> > tell me why.
> No not again. I am all alone.
> I hate this feeling. Why me? Always me.
> The people who left me are the only people who cared.

Tyrone didn't show the poem to anyone. During the first days in base camp, he'd resolved not to tell other kids about his life and his feelings. Now he'd learned a valuable lesson: He didn't even want to hear about their lives or their feelings. Somehow he'd keep his head down and get through this crazy school. Anyway, he was just here for the academics.

# 10

## BACK TO PATTERN

FOR SOMEONE who had just spent close to a month in a forest, the campus was a daunting sight. The volleyball net rustling in the breeze and the glistening blue water of the pool gave the place the look of a resort — a suddenly abandoned resort, because as Bianca headed down a trail and glimpsed the main building, all the students were in classes in the academic building across the way. She had so many questions — what were the kids like? would she make friends? would she like the teachers? — but they could wait. The only thing that mattered now was indoor plumbing. She had been dreaming of taking a long shower and shampoo to scrub away the dirt and sweat and the stench of too many campfires.

That night, Bianca had to stand in front of everyone in the great room and say her name, her age, her hometown, and one random fact about herself. "Hi, my name is Bianca," she said tentatively, her voice barely audible in the huge old hayloft. "I'm sixteen. I'm from West Palm Beach, Florida. I can twirl fire."

Kids cheered in welcome. A tall boy approached. "Can I have an appointment with you?" Bianca started to ask, "What the hell is an appointment?" but she stopped herself, not wanting to sound foolish. She quickly found that life at Swift River bore almost no resemblance to life at her old high school. The weekdays started with wakeup at 6:30 A.M. sharp, then breakfast and a half hour of campus cleanup. Students spent the next four hours in classes, went to lunch, then had another four hours of classes. On Tuesdays, Wednesdays, and Thursdays, group therapy lasted for two and a half hours. At five o'clock, kids had dorm time — a chance to hang out — followed by dinner and study hall. "Appointments," starting at 8:15 P.M., were supposed to be deep, hour-long conversations between two kids.

On the second floor, off the great room, was a nook with eight wooden carrels, each with a phone. Every student went there one night a week to call home. There were boxes of tissues for teary conversations. A counselor sat in the middle, listening to the cacophony of conversations, wagging a finger at a kid who was cursing, then telling someone else, "Talk to your dad about your feelings." At 9:15 P.M., everyone gathered in the great room for "closing," when two or three students read essays or spoke about something that had happened in their lives. At 9:30 P.M. kids hugged one another and said goodnight. Lights out was at 10 o'clock. No exceptions.

Sometimes, kids said, a bunch of boys and girls carried sacks of flour dressed in baby clothes, as part of a lesson on dating and sex.

Swift River was weird, Bianca decided. Very weird.

In base camp, Tyrone excelled at knots, chores, and PT. The writing was more difficult, but he'd soldiered through it. Then he'd gotten stuck in the woods for an extra three days as a consequence of not revealing Ashley's runaway plan. On his twenty-ninth and final day at base camp, he looked relieved. Everyone fell silent as he read his mom's affirmation letter.

> To me, you are amazing. I got all the things all the other moms want. A son who keeps himself and his room clean and orderly, who respects others, whose friends are acceptable, who doesn't drink or do drugs.
>
> You are able to see what most of us miss. For example, when you were three or four you were always exclaiming "Look at that — ." We always missed it. But one time I was able to get a glimpse of your ability. We were under an elevated train structure (remember how dark and dirty it is with stores and people all over the place?). You said, "Look at the yo-yo." There, where no one would expect it to be, was a blue yo-yo, suspended by its string.

She concluded: "Maybe it's your mind, open to all possibilities, that lets you see what most of us just don't believe is there." When Tyrone read the last sentence, he heard a sympathetic chorus of "*Awww*" from the other kids. The corner of his mouth turned up slightly, then he looked away.

After thirty-four days in base camp, Mary Alice was ready to leave. In her truth letter, she had told her parents a great deal about her drug use and her stealing. She reminded them — as if they needed reminding — that the summer after sophomore year started with a call from the police on a beach resort where the family was vacationing. After pulling Mary Alice over for running a stop sign, the cop had spotted pot in her car. He released her into her parents' custody with a warning: "You're on a dangerous course." The Chamblisses kicked Mary Alice out of the house for four days.

After reading the truth letter, Mary Alice's parents reacted as mildly as if she'd 'fessed up to having an overdue library book. "You are one of the most wonderful, talented, kind and loving people — you are so full of life, which shows in your beautiful sparkling eyes," her mother wrote. "I love you more than anything."

Mary Alice shook her head at that. It would've been easier if they'd been pissed.

*⁂*

On her first day out of base camp, before going to the predinner meeting of all students in the great room, Mary Alice leaned into a mirror to inspect herself. She took inventory of the flakiness, scratches, and uneven tan on her forehead, cheeks, nose, jaw, and neck. She brushed her hair for twenty minutes. She didn't take long to go back to pattern. Her posture changed; now, with an audience of several dozen boys, she arched her back, making sure that her breasts stuck out. Gennarose Pope, the new English teacher, said Mary Alice sashayed as if she were going down a runway.

As she shook hands and exchanged small talk, she sized up the social order. Swift River counselors talked about their grand goals — honesty, trust, deep friendships — but Mary Alice had already been through three middle schools and high schools. She knew about the intrigue and social land mines that flourished wherever groups of teenagers gathered. The campus had about sixty boys and forty girls — very good odds — but many of these girls were quite accomplished backstabbers and traitors; this wasn't the National Honor Society, after all. Having been the victim of hurtful gossip, Mary Alice saw other girls as either potential allies or potential traitors.

By lights-out time, she had met all the hot guys at Swift River. Her Southern accent, which had thinned out at base camp, was now as thick as molasses.

*⁂*

Toward the end of base camp, the staff had noticed Tyrone and Bianca spending a lot of time together. The wilderness counselors' summary warned the counselors on campus to watch out for flirting. When Tyrone arrived on campus, the pair began having breakfast together before walking over to the classroom building. "We're like two flakes of pepper in a mound of salt," Bianca said. They discussed the fact that, unlike almost everyone else in the school, they weren't white and they weren't rich. Bianca had considered herself part of the Latino crowd back home, and Tyrone was one of only three black kids on campus (the first was adopted by a white couple and the second was from a well-to-do African-American family).

One day in September, while sitting in the great room, Tyrone stammered, "I just wanted to tell you that I have feelings for you. More than a friend."

Bianca looked away.

"Once I told another girl that," Tyrone continued, "and she didn't feel that way about me. We never talked again."

"So if I say no, you're not ever going to speak to me again?"

"That's just how I am."

"I don't want to lie to you. I just want to be your friend. I don't think of you as any more than a friend."

"Fine. Don't tell anyone about this so I don't get in trouble. You might get in trouble too." He walked away.

Bianca confided in Ashley, the other New Yorker. Ashley told the counselors. They confronted Tyrone and Bianca in group. True to his word, as always, Tyrone finished what he started. He ceased speaking to Bianca.

On the morning of the second Monday in September, headmaster Rudy Bentz bought the *New York Times* at a grocery store north of the school. He smiled when he saw the front page. The paper had spent weeks researching a story on therapeutic boarding schools. DESPERATE MEASURES: EM-BATTLED PARENTS SEEK HELP, AT ANY COST, declared the headline. The article, which jumped to almost a full page inside, included a picture of Swift River and a profile of a boy who had graduated. It quoted Rudy on the subject of parents who fear their own children: "I refer to some of these kids as emotional terrorists . . . the home is a war zone."

A largely favorable story in the *New York Times?* The admissions office was thrilled. Corporate headquarters in California called to congratulate the team. The timing was fortunate because the corporate owners planned to expand Swift River's student population to take advantage of the demand from across the country. Although Rudy opposed the expansion, he figured that any publicity would help Swift River attract the right applicants — the kind of kids and parents who would take the program seriously.

Another front-page article noted that the economy was slowing. But the tenor of the *Times* suggested that it was a good moment in history. There was so little pressing news that the front page carried a light feature about a tennis player. The date was September 10, 2001.

The next morning, the Academy at Swift River — the bubble — seemed more remote than ever. No one knew about the attacks on the World Trade Center and the Pentagon until Gennarose ran in with breathless reports of the bulletins she'd heard while driving. In an emergency staff meeting, Rudy and others decided that the school should stick to the regular schedule until there was more information. But even as the meeting was breaking up, the campus was abuzz. It was impossible to keep a secret from a hundred teenagers. Every few minutes, parents from New York and Washington called to say they were safe. A girl named Eva had often said that she wished her father was dead. After she learned that he had been in the World Trade Center just an hour before the attacks, she felt racked by guilt. The staff waited for hours to hear from Tyrone's mother, who worked in a phone company power station in lower Manhattan. Tyrone paced the halls. She finally called in the afternoon to say she and others in the family were okay.

An eerie silence enveloped base camp, where seven of Group 23's twelve members remained. The counselors turned off their two-way radios to cut off the anxious chatter from campus. The kids figured that something was going on because the staff didn't enforce rules with the usual rigidity. Before telling the kids anything, the counselors wanted to make sure that the families and friends of the boys and girls in the wilderness were unharmed. The process showed how isolated base camp was. Masai tribesmen in Kenya knew what had happened on 9/11, fishermen in Borneo knew, but a handful of teenagers in the woods of western Massachusetts, a half-hour drive from the bustling college town of Northampton and four hours from Ground Zero, had no idea.

At midday on September 12, the counselors gathered the campers in a clearing in the forest and told them the news. Ashley cried as she thought about the times she'd hung out in lower Manhattan. Andy got teary because he'd spent the first years of his life in New York City before moving to Long Island. By coincidence, Phil and D.J., base camp's resident cynics, had spent several days making a case that humans were evil, with Phil citing Hobbes. The gullible girl — the one who had feared shock treatment — sobbed because maybe D.J. and Phil were right.

D.J., though, showed no emotion. "Why should I care?" he wondered. The people who died were a bunch of strangers.

As the final members of Group 23 trickled onto campus — including D.J., after forty-eight days in the woods — Rudy Bentz pulled Tanya Beecher aside to share some news. Group 23 was going to grow. The school was "adjusting" a girl named Willow, who argued frequently with counselors. In plain language, she was being dropped into the group so that she could spend several more months at Swift River. Willow had been adopted at birth by a couple in New England. They were quiet people who lived in a two-bedroom house. Willow was a rambunctious girl who found her home boring and couldn't concentrate in school. She had used speed and heroin and gotten into a relationship with an older man who hit her, cheated on her, then enticed her back. At one point, she had been homeless for a few weeks. Willow was wild.

The kids at Swift River knew all that, but they also saw a carefree side of Willow. She loved to mimic students, staff, movie stars — anyone. She'd scrunch up her face, lower her voice two octaves, and growl, "You're going on a restriction," as others howled at the depiction of a cantankerous white-haired counselor. As the kids sat in the great room waiting for a meeting, she'd cock her head and mimic lines from Austin Powers movies. "*Mini Me!* Stop humping the laser!"

With the addition of Willow, Group 23 was complete — nine girls and five boys. In many ways, they weren't much different from any random cross section of fourteen teenagers. The families came from a tony block in Manhattan and from a town in Vermont where cows roamed behind the houses, from booming Sun Belt subdivisions and staid Northeastern suburbs where couples endured long commutes and paid a premium for homes because of the superiority of the public schools.

The parents' incomes ranged from $40,000 a year — Tyrone's mother's earnings at the phone company — to the high six figures. The fathers' occupations included computer programmer, international development worker, electrician, toy maker, teacher, baseball player, architect, and lawyer (two lawyers, in fact). The mothers included a nurse, a real estate broker, an investment banker, an interior designer, a public relations executive, a doctor-turned-homemaker, a quilt maker, a part-time accountant, and a teacher.

On average, they were better off than most Americans. Three of the families had weekend lake houses, beach cottages, or ski chalets. But others lived middle-class lives, saving up for one-week vacations in Orlando or on Cape Cod. The kids attended private, parochial, and public schools — or, like Tyrone, they didn't.

The families were Catholic, Jewish, Protestant, and atheist. Of the fourteen sets of parents, three were divorced — not exceptional in a country where almost half of all marriages end in divorce. The kids came from families with one, two, three, and four children. They were firstborns, secondborns, and a twin. Only four of the kids said they had frequent contact with grandparents. Just two had aunts, uncles, and cousins who lived within ten miles. Most of their parents and grandparents had grown up around extended families, but this generation was isolated and adrift. The mothers and fathers remembered where they were on November 22, 1963, when John F. Kennedy was assassinated in Dallas. The kids remembered where they were on September 7, 1996, when Biggie Smalls, or somebody, killed Tupac Shakur in Las Vegas (their point of reference changed on 9/11).

As a seven-year-old, the gullible girl had blown up a neighbor's goose with a cherry bomb. But at the same age Willow ran in front of her father's lawn mower, trying to protect dandelions from decapitation. The students had played on soccer, basketball, and rugby teams; they'd excelled at gymnastics, ballet, and modern dance; they'd mastered piano and guitar — though most had dropped their after-school teams and classes by ninth or tenth grade.

Most of the kids didn't want to follow their parents' career choices; almost all wanted to work fewer hours than their mothers and fathers. The kids' plans changed constantly, but that fall, at least, their preferred occupations ranged from rap artist to stockbroker, jewelry designer to hotel manager. Bianca wanted to be an actress, Mary Alice a photographer, Tyrone a computer programmer, D.J. a blasting expert at construction sites or a pyrotechnician, setting up fireworks displays. "I'm going to smoke a corncob pipe and be known as the crazy man in town," Phil the Philosopher announced. Overhearing the plan, Willow quipped, "Believe me, Phil, you won't need the corncob pipe."

Four of the kids didn't drink or do any drugs. The other ten had used drugs, including pot, cocaine, heroin, mushrooms, methadone, Ecstasy, speed, acid, nitrous oxide, and tobacco; several of them had abused painkillers, tranquilizers, stimulants, mood stabilizers, and almost anything else that could be swallowed, snorted, smoked, or injected.

In some quantifiable ways, of course, Group 23 was distinctly different from the average bunch of teenagers hanging out at the mall. Five of the kids were adopted, including the Ohio girl who hadn't known about her adoption for most of her life. Four of the girls had eating disorders. And by middle school, ten of the kids had been labeled with at least one of the "D" diagnoses: attention deficit disorder; attention deficit–hyperactivity disorder; oppositional defiance disorder; nonverbal learning disorder; learning disabled; or depression.

The fourteen kids of Group 23 would continue going to group therapy three times a week. If they could keep up their Brady Bunch behavior, they would graduate on the first Friday in October 2002. That was a big "if." In Swift River's four-year history, no group had ever graduated intact. For every ten students who started, two or three inevitably got dropped to other groups or expelled. Sometimes hell-raisers who entered kicking and shrieking did well, while their charming, well-liked classmates got booted out for breaking rules. Other times, Swift River's consulting psychiatrists diagnosed severe conditions the school couldn't handle, and parents were asked to find a residential treatment center.

In reviewing the experiences of several hundred students, the admissions office hadn't been able to identify reliable indicators of success or failure. Nobody — not the psychiatrists, not the headmaster, not a well-trained counselor like Tanya or an empathetic teacher like Gennarose — could predict who would triumphantly stride across the stage for graduation in a year and who would end up in a lockdown facility, on the streets, or in jail.

# PART II

## SHAMES
## AND BLAMES

# 11

## Ph.D. in Manipulation

Swift river looked like a country club from the outside and a cage from the inside. That's how it seemed to Mary Alice. The place had a rule for everything, and that wasn't an exaggeration. The thick stack of official agreements started with students' appearance: no Mohawks, no dyed or bleached hair, no body piercing, no baseball caps worn backward, no sunglasses indoors. The school stressed that it wasn't trying to create docile automatons who looked and thought alike. Instead, the counselors wanted to continue what they'd started in base camp: to peel away the layers of images and artifice — of bullshit, really — and reach the true essence of each kid.

The list of prohibited clothing filled a page: No thongs or tank tops. No revealing spaghetti straps. No T-shirts with large brand names or logos. No tight pants or short shorts. No hoodies (the sweatshirts with hoods that stoners liked). No sleeveless cotton undershirts — what some kids insisted on calling "wife-beaters." Mary Alice was allowed three dresses, five pairs of pants, two pairs of shorts, three long-sleeved collared shirts, three short-sleeved collared shirts, four pairs of shoes, and a pair of boots. Mary Alice's mother had chosen her clothes. They were new, all top-selling brands — with a heavy emphasis on Abercrombie and J. Crew — but they were so preppy, so *middle* school. Mary Alice had gone through that phase at thirteen or fourteen: "This is what everyone else is going to wear so I'm going to wear it, too."

Somehow one of her most treasured pieces of clothing had made it to Swift River: her precious, hip-hugging black Bebe pants. As soon as Tanya saw the pants, she took them away.

At home, Mary Alice had her own suite — a bedroom, sitting room, bathroom, and walk-in closet lined with shoes, boots, sandals, and slippers, at least thirty pairs in all. Her bureau drawers were stuffed with silver and gold jewelry, costume jewelry, and funky jewelry. At Swift River, she shared a room with three other girls. Each girl was allowed a bed, a night table, a bureau, and a little armoire. Swift River even had rules about plant placement (number five: "One plant may be kept on top of the armoire and one may be placed on the dorm's table. Any other plants must be placed neatly on lower-level window ledges or nightstands").

New girls could wear only one piece of jewelry at a time: a necklace, bracelet, ring, or one pair of matching earrings. As they progressed through the program and earned trust, girls could wear up to four items. The rules remained exacting: "No jewelry made with hemp. No jewelry that portrays a sexual, violent, or drug culture image."

The counselors read faxes and letters to make sure parents and kids were being honest with each other. They opened packages to make sure that parents weren't sending unapproved clothes or other contraband (in Swift River's early days, a father mailed a son his favorite CD, not realizing that two joints were tucked inside the case). The staff checked dorms every morning to make sure beds were made, floors tidy, and sinks spotless.

Students weren't allowed to tape anything to the walls. Instead, each kid had a small bulletin board for mementos. These could be photos of relatives but not boyfriends or girlfriends. And nothing reflecting an obsession with body image or drugs; no pictures of supermodels, rock stars, or hip-hop artists. Mary Alice filled her bulletin board with approved memoirs, starting with photos of herself snowboarding and hanging out on the beach. Most days she looked admiringly at the skinny, platinum blond teenager in those pictures. Other days she thought the girl looked sick.

It took a while for Mary Alice to understand Swift River's ways. Nestled in the hills, an hour from the nearest mall, the school was so isolated that kids called it "the bubble." The closest supermarket was four towns away. The one television set was turned on only briefly, to show CNN Headline News for an hour on Sundays and an occasional game of football or basketball. Cell phones weren't allowed on campus. Not that it mattered; parents who showed up for admissions tours noticed that their phone displays said "no service" because there wasn't a cell tower nearby. There were several small therapeutic schools in the Berkshires, and some students came up with the idea of challenging them in basketball or baseball. But Rudy, the headmaster, insisted that the tight daily schedule didn't leave time for practices and travel. Besides, he worried about players from different therapeutic schools swapping joints or pills. That didn't stop a couple of the kids from musing about a league comprising Swift River, the John Dewey Academy, and the DeSisto School: How would the DeSisto Druggies do against their archrivals, the Dewey Dopers? Could the Swift River Snorting Ravers blow away the competition? Who would win the coveted Ecstasy Trophy?

Mary Alice saw that Swift River had its own customs, its own curriculum, even its own language. Technically speaking, the school didn't have rules, it had "agreements." They started with the three major agreements: no violence, no drugs, no sex. The description of the agreements and the consequences of breaking them filled loose-leaf books several inches thick. Opening a fire exit meant a day of work projects; walking around with a shirt untucked meant dishwashing duty; wrestling in the dorm meant the offenders had to do an interpretive dance during the nightly closing. The concept of agreements was important because after a few months the students themselves were supposed to enforce rules on campus. Swift River wanted them to see that for a community to run smoothly, everyone must pitch in.

Mary Alice could see why sex was forbidden, but dating and kissing? Hand-holding? During a meeting, Rudy explained that the rule was intended to make a kid focus on himself for fourteen months ("there can never be a 'we' without a clear understanding and acceptance of 'me,'" as he put it). The staff didn't want boys strutting to impress girls or girls preening to lure boys. Nor did they want gay kids sneaking off to the bathroom together, as sometimes happened; bathroom sex sent a message that sex was tawdry and shameful.

After mealtimes, the dining room was turned into a restriction room, a work area for students who had broken major rules. Those who ran away, cheated in class, or brought in drugs — those on a "self-study" — sat along the perimeter, staring into mirrors and writing in black folders. They were forbidden to talk to all but ten or so other students. Those caught lying or breaking the sex agreement in smaller ways, such as kissing, were on the next-highest restriction, a challenge. They sat alone with red folders. Self-studies and challenges lost privileges to buy goods at the school store and to go off campus for weekend trips.

Kids who wanted help thinking about adoption, sexual abuse, or other issues were put on reflections. They were given writing assignments and could work anywhere in the school. To help counselors and teachers keep track of everything, a board in the faculty mailroom listed students' names with any restrictions that applied to them. On a typical day, several had "B-LS" (bans with the lower school), while others had "C" (challenges) and another had "SS-TB" (self-study and touch bans).

One of two things happened to students who didn't straighten up after several warnings: They would be dropped to a lower peer group, as Willow had been, or they would be expelled.

Mary Alice greeted Tanya at the mailroom the same way every day: "Is there anything for me?"

"I don't know," Tanya answered. "But you can start by saying 'Good morning' before asking."

"Anything for me?" Mary Alice sang out after that, peering in for packages. "I mean, good morning, Tanya. Anything today?"

Within a week a three-foot by three-foot box arrived from Mary Alice's mother. Tanya opened it and found it stuffed with new clothes for the fall. Mary Alice gathered the booty and dashed back to her room, grinning all the way. When Mary Alice was excited about something, her eyes shone like jade. When she was in a funk, they faded to a dull gray. She hadn't looked so joyous since coming in from base camp. But the bliss didn't last long. Her mom still hadn't sent mascara and bronzer. Tanya frowned and shook her head. Swift River's rules were clear: no makeup, no exceptions. Mary Alice had to learn how to appreciate herself.

"I need it!" Mary Alice pouted. "It's not fair. I feel naked!"

A week later, a medium-sized box came, again from Dallas. Tanya pulled out some clothes for Mary Alice and mailed the excess back.

A third box arrived in the middle of October. It was full of clothes and jewelry. In her first two months on campus, Mary Alice had received more clothes than all the other members of her Group 23 combined. Tanya didn't finish going through it; she simply sealed it up and sent it back. She called Mary Alice's mother and told her not to send any more presents.

"But that's how I show her I love her," Lillian said.

Tanya suggested that she look for another way to express her love.

When Mary Alice heard that the flow of gifts had been cut off, she confronted Tanya in the hallway. "You're not letting me have my things!" she screamed, her face turning scarlet. "You can't tell me how many clothes I can have!"

Actually, Tanya said, she could. Mary Alice knew Swift River's agreements.

"I didn't agree to that shit!"

✍

Gennarose Pope, the new English teacher, was twenty-two but looked like one of the kids. She had a nervous habit of sweeping back her long silky hair every few minutes. She even had a swath of pimples on her forehead. Rudy Bentz approached as she carried a tray in the dining hall on her first day. "Where are you from?" he asked, posing the opening question he put to a student fresh from base camp.

"Columbia University," she said.

Gennarose was immediately taken by the sixteen-year-old from Dallas. Mary Alice loved art, and she wanted to know about the painters Gennarose had studied. Although some of the kids dismissed Mary Alice as a spoiled Southerner, Gennarose could tell she was much more complex. She was a natural athlete but she had avoided sports for a couple of years; she radiated confidence but she felt others were prettier and smarter; she missed the comforts of life in Dallas but she was starting to question the values of a place where people were judged by the cars they owned.

Mary Alice had an understated sense of humor. When people introduced themselves, they asked her the obvious question — "Why are you here?" — then waited for the reflexive response. Girls usually said "drugs," "drinking," "eating disorder," or "promiscuity."

Not Mary Alice. "E — all of the above," she'd answer.

Mary Alice could be blunt when something was on her mind. Not long after coming to campus, she studied Gennarose. Her eyes assessed Gennarose's skin blemishes, her teeth, her pelvis, her pinched waist, her long thin legs. "You're anorexic," she announced.

Gennarose swallowed. She didn't want to be analyzed by a sixteen-year-old. Without going into details, she told Mary Alice that she'd had a tough adolescence and developed an eating disorder at age fourteen. Back then, she could walk through a mall and pick out other anorexics. If gays had gaydar to detect fellow gays, she supposed anorexics could have "andar," or whatever it was called.

Mary Alice, too, had highly developed andar. Gennarose's boyfriend had never remarked on her anorexia during their four years together. She'd kept it in check for a while, but in the past couple of weeks she'd had a relapse — partly because she sat in group therapy with Mary Alice and other girls who were fixated on their weight.

Mary Alice could be disarmingly perceptive one minute and oddly out of touch the next. In group one afternoon, she mentioned that her parents were going to buy her a Mercedes after graduation. But, she added, wrinkling her nose in distaste, the model they had chosen was too small. She wanted an SUV. Gennarose wondered what Tyrone thought about that — Tyrone, whose clothes came from J.C. Penney. Gennarose, who had grown up in a working-class neighborhood, was on the verge of saying "Fuck you and your Mercedes," but she held her tongue.

And yet, just when Gennarose was exasperated, Mary Alice would shrug her shoulders and say, "You think I'm a little entitled, huh?" For one of her classes, she had to write an essay describing a photograph that captured a significant moment in her life. Writing assignments were often difficult for Mary Alice. She'd start, then lose interest. This time, she sat in the computer room looking at a snapshot of her family — all sinewy blonds, all grinning broadly — at an oceanside resort a couple of months before she was sent to Swift River. The words rushed to the keyboard.

> When you see the picture you think, "Wow, that looks like a really nice attractive family that has it all together." We are standing on the beach all dressed up right before dinner at the club, my mom, dad, sister, two brothers and myself. I'm 16 but I look about 21. I'm wearing black pants and a leopard halter-top, both from Wet Seal, and Steve Madden platforms. My hair is short and strawberry blonde, I have on makeup and am burned from laying out all day with baby oil and iodine rubbed all over my body.
>
> This is a great example of how my family can portray that we're all happy and having a grand old time, which is usually never the case. The vacation was, and I quote my mother, "a complete DISASTER." I got messed up, partied, hooked up with guys, stole money and just did not give a crap about anything.
>
> The night this picture was taken, I decided as usual to go out and

party instead of having dinner. I ended up getting arrested and got kicked out of the house.

✍

In October, several girls told a counseling supervisor that Mary Alice was restricting — severely limiting her food. At lunch, the supervisor stood a few feet away and watched Mary Alice stabbing at pieces of lettuce and inspecting a spoonful of cottage cheese as if it were radioactive. The supervisor brought her to an office for a private talk. "I'm worried about you," she said.

"I'm fine."

"You're barely eating,"

Every muscle in Mary Alice's face seemed to ripple. "I know about a balanced diet. I can have a salad and a scoop of cottage cheese. I'm not purging so it's okay!"

"Calm down, Mary Alice. Your reaction tells me more than my suspicion was telling me."

Mary Alice hesitated. Then she admitted that she had been trying to lose weight. "My eating disorder is a coping mechanism. I go from complete control to out-of-control behavior where I don't love myself."

"Hello, I'd like to talk to Mary Alice," the supervisor retorted. "I don't want to talk to your last ten therapists."

"But it's true, my eating disorder is about control and self-image."

"I know, I know. I've read about eating disorders. What else is it about, in plain language?"

"I'm a fuck-up."

✍

Next to the great room, in an office the counselors shared, a shelf full of books and pamphlets about adolescent health all noted an increase in anorexia and bulimia, especially among girls in wealthy communities. Anorexics have an obsessive fear of fat; anorexics are 15 percent or more below normal body weight. Anorexics often feel invisible and incompetent; they get a high off of starving themselves and having power over their own appetites. Bulimics make furious efforts to get rid of weight, by vomiting, fasting, taking laxatives, or exercising excessively. Research shows that the overwhelming majority of bulimics have normal body weight; only 15 percent are overweight. Many teenage bulimics have been abused, or feel ignored by their fathers or slighted by their mothers. Some live in permanent domestic chaos, with parents battling alcoholism, depression, or anxiety. Bulimia is their way of satisfying a hunger for connections or establishing order amid the chaos.

Some of Mary Alice's earliest memories had to do with food. There was the housekeeper, Bea, who cooed at Mary Alice's baby sister and grew exasperated with Mary Alice's ploys to get attention. "You're gonna be fat like me." In elementary school, Mary Alice was known as the muscular girl — and it paid off because each side in a tug of war and other games clamored for her. By middle school, though, there was hardly anything worse than being a brawny girl. Classmates taunted her, calling her a boy or "Free Willy" — a blubbery whale. Mary Alice put on a few pounds at puberty, and even though her doctor said the weight gain was normal, she felt gross. Mary Alice's gymnastics coach observed that she was "getting thick around the middle." He merely put into words what Mary Alice had already sensed: Every other girl she knew — every mom, actually — was skinny. At one private school, girls formed a "cracker club," nibbling Saltines for lunch. Girls traded tips about weight loss the way their grandmothers exchanged recipes for roast beef. Some girls looked at "pro-ana" Web sites that advocated anorexia. There were all kinds of tricks, such as taking big gulps of water in between bites of food to feel full faster, or swallowing vinegar before eating — supposedly to suck the fat out of the food.

Rather than talking about her obsession, Mary Alice read diet magazines and came up with her own concoctions. She ate lunches of lettuce (zero calories) topped with mustard (zero again). She learned to love Special K with water; she drizzled lemon juice on everything else, because lemon is a diuretic. She sliced grapes in half to slow down her eating. She tried diet pills. Cigarettes killed her appetite. She jogged in the shower. She did two hundred stomach crunches in the middle of the night, then five hundred, so many that her parents complained that their bedroom ceiling shook when she was supposed to be sleeping in the room above them.

Mary Alice felt alone and unloved. She thought her mom was too busy socializing with friends or taking care of the younger children. Her father was building his company or hunting with his buddies — "pleasurizing," as he called it. Once, when her parents were traveling in Asia, Mary Alice stayed up late with a baby-sitter watching a movie about a girl with an eating disorder. Mary Alice tried what she saw: jamming her fingers down her throat and throwing up everything in her stomach. She had found a way to have the satisfaction of eating but still lose weight. She, and only she, could control everything. She decided she wanted to be able to lock her thumbs and forefingers around her thigh. Her weight dropped from 120 pounds to 96. Her thumbs and forefingers fit snugly, but she decided to lose a few more pounds.

Mary Alice's father remained dubious — "these girls with eating disorders ought to go to Africa to appreciate what they have," he liked to say — but her mother fretted. One afternoon, several other girls from seventh grade asked to meet with Mary Alice's parents. They said she was purging at school daily. A doctor concurred; Mary Alice was starving herself. She had so little body fat that she got bruises on her skin just from sleeping.

She weighed only eighty-five pounds by the time her parents took her to a hospital, where a cardiologist warned that she was on the verge of doing lasting damage to her heart. Her parents flew her to a clinic and ranch in Arizona for girls and women with eating disorders. Some of the patients had feeding tubes strapped to their bodies; others were so weak that they were confined to walkers or wheelchairs. Mary Alice was so obsessed that, rather than being repulsed, she was jealous of some of the super-thin girls. In four months of self-esteem lessons, nutrition classes, and equine therapy she gained back fourteen pounds. The clinic urged her to stay for another couple of months of therapy, but she insisted she was over her eating disorder. Her parents took her home.

She wasn't over it. As she entered high school, she felt more pressure to fit in. She never felt thin enough, blond enough, or pretty enough. Her mother weighed less than she did, her friends sat at restaurants discussing body fat, her favorite music videos featured stick-thin singers and dancers. When she ate, she heard her old housekeeper's voice admonishing: *You're gonna be fat . . . fat . . . fat.*

A counselor at Swift River once asked Mary Alice to give her eating disorder a name. "Bea's voice," she replied.

In the fall, the staff noticed an epidemic of entitlement on campus, a host of students who thought they were exempt from the rules. Kids who wanted to listen to music in the great room or weasel out of dishwashing duty kept asking teachers and counselors until they found someone distracted enough to say yes absentmindedly. Rudy Bentz warned that the students were playing one staff member against another, just as they'd played one parent against another. "These kids," Rudy said, "have Ph.D's in manipulation."

Mary Alice, though, found that manipulation didn't work nearly as well as it had at home, especially with hard-ass sticklers like Tanya. The day came when Mary Alice was to go on her first field trip. It was a Saturday in October, and the crisp air smelled like apples. Twelve students were taking a van with Gennarose to the Massachusetts Museum of Contemporary Art, which had opened in a former textile factory an hour west of Swift River. Mary Alice had been cooped up in base camp and campus for three months, and she had eagerly waited for this trip. Wearing her best clothes, a white top and tight blue pants, she breezed through the hallway past Jason, a counselor who helped Tanya with Group 23. "Wait a minute!" Jason demanded in his gravelly voice. "Where do you think you're going?"

"The field trip. I signed up."

"With *those* pants?"

"They're baggy in the legs. They're sweatpants."

"Put on something else, Mary Alice."

"You don't decide what I wear."

"Go change!"

"No way. Stop fucking telling me what to do!"

"You're off the trip!" Jason barked. Mary Alice ran to her room, crying and letting loose every curse she could think of. She pulled off a shoe and hurled it so forcefully that it punched a hole in the wall. "Fuck you, Jason!" she yelled just as he strode in. Jason announced that Mary Alice was being put on a challenge. She could start right away by going to the restriction room and writing about why she was so obsessed with her appearance.

While her friends were partying in Dallas, she was stuck in a cage, with everyone observing and analyzing her. She couldn't be herself for fourteen damn months.

# 12

## D.J.: "THE BAD THING THAT HAPPENED TO GOOD PEOPLE"

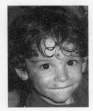

GROUP THERAPY SUCKED. Classes were boring. The dining hall meals, which used to taste awesome compared with the monotonous diet of base camp, seemed bland after a couple of weeks. D.J. didn't find much to recommend about Swift River.

During classes, his fingers itched for his PlayStation console, especially for Grand Theft Auto 2. GTA was mad fun. You started by stealing a car, cruising around for a while, beating up a prostitute, and ripping off her money. You hijacked helicopters, speedboats, and tanks and killed people with AK-47s, M-16s, Uzis, and rocket launchers. You could do anything — have sex with the prostitute, go to a strip club, fight with a Cuban gang, deal drugs, join the Mob, move into a mansion.

The only thing worthwhile about Swift River was Tyrone. D.J. hadn't known what to make of Tyrone in base camp because during the two days they'd overlapped, D.J. had been a shadow, barred from contact with the others. Out there in the woods, Tyrone seemed like a tall, brooding inner-city boy — unlike anyone D.J. had known at his private school or anywhere in his New Jersey neighborhood of curving streets and cul-de-sacs. They'd had their first real conversation after D.J. finished up base camp and went to main campus in late September. Tyrone had asked if D.J. liked video games. *Like* them?

D.J. and Tyrone were in a second-period class, Ancient History, with ten other kids. The teacher, whose glasses were smeared and crooked, was the kind of guy who couldn't tell whether people were laughing at him or with him. While he blathered on about Herodotus's accounts of the Persian Wars or Hindu burial rites or something, Tyrone and D.J. whispered about

Final Fantasy, where a loner has to find clues about his mysterious past. If you couldn't play video games at Swift River, at least you could talk about them.

One of the worst things about Swift River was appointment time. After a whole day of classes, meetings, therapy, and more meetings, you were supposed to sit down and tell your life story to another kid. You couldn't just go through the highlights, either; you had to talk about how you felt about the things that had happened. The next night, you were supposed to swap life stories with somebody else, and then someone else, so that eventually you knew all of the hundred kids on campus.

That was how you earned trips to the gym, mini-golf, or the movie theater on weekends. But it never ended. Every two months a peer group graduated; every couple of days new kids hiked in from base camp, so you had to start all over. D.J. made an appointment with Tyrone for one night, then the next, and the next. They didn't get around to telling their life stories because they were too busy playing Magic, a strategy game with collectible cards.

At first glance, D.J. and Tyrone seemed unlikely friends: the wiry, hyperkinetic white kid from the suburbs and the taciturn, muscular black kid from the city. Yet at Swift River, they clung to each other. Tanya thought that D.J. liked the idea of a strong male friend, someone he could look up to. And Tyrone liked having an alter ego who didn't push him to talk about the past — other than video games he'd played in the past, of course. The kids in the group sensed that Tyrone and D.J. had much more in common than they wanted to admit: D.J. felt abandoned by his biological mother, Tyrone by his father.

If Tyrone was quiet during group, D.J. seemed nonexistent. By November, the counselors had made a rule: D.J. had to talk for at least five minutes in every group. It didn't really matter what he said, so long as he contributed. D.J. lucked out, though, because the Ohio girl who had recently found out about her adoption kept getting in trouble. She irritated the counselors by saying wacky things, then contradicting herself. It was as if she were trying on personalities. She'd been raped. No, she was a virgin. She'd given oral sex to five guys in a mall parking lot. Well, not really, she'd just fantasized about a blowjob while sending e-mail to one guy. She'd done a lot of drugs on April 20, National Stoners' Day. Actually, she'd pretended to do drugs on 4-20.

Truth was, D.J. had been thinking about the twists and turns in his life, but he didn't want to talk on command, like a poodle doing tricks. Once in a while he tried to imagine his birth mother. He knew only two things: She was fifteen — the same age he was now — and she did drugs. He had a theory, and it had to do with 4-20. The way he figured it, his mom was doing drugs to celebrate 4-20 back in 1986, when she was less than eight months pregnant. Her body had a bad reaction to the drugs, and she went into labor. D.J., after all, was born premature the very next day, April 21.

From time to time, he tried to summon an image of her. Was she pretty? Was she tall? Did she have red hair like he had when he was little, or coffee-colored hair like his now?

What was she doing today?

Did she have other kids? Did she keep them?

D.J. and Tyrone had plenty of important things to talk about during appointment time, Tanya said. D.J. could start by sharing his questions about his birth mother. For his part, Tyrone could talk about his dad. He'd written a letter to his father and was awaiting a response. He had spent much of his life waiting for his dad — how did that make him feel? Tanya and the other counselors said that these kinds of conversation made friendship deeper. D.J. nodded in agreement. He would get to his birth mom and all that stuff soon enough.

After one more game of Magic.

In the spring of 1986, after dealing with infertility for seven years, Theodor and Janice Pandowski received an answer to their prayers. An adoption agency called to say that a baby boy had been born to an unmarried teenager. She had decided she wasn't ready to be a mother. The baby, six weeks premature, weighed only five pounds. The Pandowskis didn't know much about the baby's biological mother, and they knew nothing about the father. They didn't care. They would be his real parents.

He was so tiny and delicate they nicknamed him Peanut.

D.J. went from crawling to running without bothering to walk. His red hair flying, he opened cabinets, spread jelly on walls, and toppled vases. Everything was a negotiation — from getting dressed in the morning to staying in bed at night. And yet he had a beguiling charm. He'd hug his dog, Firecracker, as soon as he woke up. He'd squirt a juice box over the kitchen, flashing a rapturous look as if he'd just painted the Sistine Chapel. On vacation in Florida, he trudged along a beach with a fishing pole, carrying on intensive conversations with retirees he'd never seen before. A family friend who, like D.J., enjoyed bird watching dubbed him the "red-headed jibby jabber."

One day, Theodor was talking to a coach during the halftime of a high school lacrosse game. As they watched, a six-foot defense stick seemed to march back and forth by itself behind the bench. The stick was taller than the chipper four-year-old brandishing it. At a kindergarten back-to-school night, Janice glanced at laminated self-portraits the children had attached to calendars. Her eyes went immediately to one with chaotic lines in a rough semblance of a face, with a huge smile in the middle. There was no mistaking D.J. Theodor and Janice had talked to D.J. about his adoption since he was a toddler, but he never seemed very interested. It was just another story in his life. At night, D.J. prayed, "God bless Grandma and Grandpa, Mom and Dad, Firecracker, my gerbils, my cousins, my birth mother and birth father, wherever they are. I pray for peace."

D.J. couldn't stay out of trouble for long. In kindergarten, the principal sent home a report saying he kept running up and down the aisles on the bus. Janice, who had spent her career as a teacher, worried: Elementary-school kids get written up for breaking the rules on the bus, not kindergarteners. She took D.J. to a psychologist, and he diagnosed attention deficit–hyperactivity disorder. At age five, D.J. started taking Ritalin. The Pandowskis mentioned to the psychologist that fire fascinated their son. The psychologist told them to give him a safe way to act on his urges. All D.J. needed to do was say, "I feel like lighting something," and his parents would let him light candles while they watched.

Living with D.J. was like living with two completely different kids.

The first D.J. horsed around at the shore and zipped down ski slopes on weekends and vacations. When he was eleven, Theodor took him deep-sea fishing in Hawaii, and D.J. landed a thirty-four-pound, fifty-two-inch mahimahi (it was exactly half his weight and almost his height). Sitting in the fighting chair on the starboard of the boat, reeling in the fish, he almost cried with joy. Theodor splurged on a taxidermist and they flew across the country with the giant stuffed dolphinfish.

The second D.J. materialized, tense and morose, on school days. Theodor or Janice would ask an innocuous question about homework and he'd punch walls and throw things. For a while, Janice had to take D.J. to LensCrafters at the mall every couple of weeks for new glasses. He walked around the house lost in his headphones, drumming in the air to Slipknot:

I am in a buried kennel. I have never felt so final.
Someone find me please. Losing all reserve, I am fucking gone, I
    think I'm fucking dying.

In sixth grade, Theodor and Janice switched D.J. from his public school to a private school a couple of miles from their house. Theodor took a job teaching math and coaching at the school. It meant leaving another teaching job he loved and taking a pay cut, but he would save a two-hour roundtrip commute. They could spend more time together. The day D.J. heard the news, he wrapped his arms around his father.

When D.J. was in eighth grade, Janice spent one evening cleaning out documents on her home computer and found photos of naked women with whips and chains. She opened other files, files with innocuous names like "Homework," and found pictures of women wearing only stiletto heels and handcuffs. She confronted D.J. He turned his back on her and stormed into his room — the one with the BEWARE OF ATTACK GHEKO sign on the door and the shiny, four-foot-long mahimahi hanging over the bed.

Soon after that, the Pandowskis received various bills amounting to $200 from a mail-order CD club and a clothing company. Among other treasures, D.J. had bought a black T-shirt that said *I'm the Bad Thing That Happened to Good People.* He wore it often. Then Janice and Theodor noticed long-distance charges on their phone bill. D.J. muttered something about how he'd gotten to know a girl at a party. When his parents pressed for details, he admitted that they'd connected on an AOL chat room, then called each other, but had never met in person.

Before Janice became a teacher or a mother, she had written her master's thesis on the alternate teaching styles that worked for different learning styles. Some kids, she'd argued, learned better from reading, others from hearing, and others from hands-on activities. In nearly two decades as a teacher, she'd seen an increasing number of students, especially boys, diagnosed with ADHD. Colleagues griped that it seemed like a convenient label for kids who didn't pay attention. But Janice believed that some kids were so active and distractible that they needed help. She read books about teaching hyperactive children, medicating hyperactive children, and understanding hyperactive children. At a seminar she learned that ADHD was often "comorbid" with other psychological issues; a teen with ADHD had a higher-than-average probability of being bipolar or obsessive-compulsive, suffering depression or having learning disabilities. Kids with ADHD, in need of constant stimulation, were especially prone to smoking and drug use. She got the shivers. This wasn't abstract pedagogy — it was her son.

When he started high school, D.J. went for psychological testing. There was a significant gap in the results between his verbal ability and his performance, which could indicate ADD or learning disabilities. "His brain races ahead of his hands," the psychologist said. He recommended that Janice and Theodor buy D.J. a day planner and help him organize his time. By the end of the week, D.J. lost the day planner.

It was one thing to know all about ADHD — and to make accommodations for her students' needs — but it was another to deal with a son who constantly pushed the limits. Even vacations started to lose their appeal. Theodor and Janice chaperoned a school skiing trip to Italy during D.J.'s winter break in ninth grade. Both Theodor and Janice had had hip replacements, so they couldn't join him on the slopes, but they reveled in the way he'd come home from a day of snowboarding with scarlet cheeks and tales of the moguls he'd taken on. On the last day, an American tourist spotted Janice on the elevator. "You probably want to know this," she said. "Your son is walking up and down the street smoking with a group of kids."

D.J. wasn't remorseful. Actually, he said, he'd been smoking a pack a day for a while. Janice didn't know whether he was trying to shock her or confide in her. She flushed his Marlboros down the toilet — so that it clogged and the hotel had to send up a plumber.

Shortly before D.J. finished ninth grade, Janice noticed an acrid smell coming from his room. She walked past the Nine Inch Nails poster on the door to find him lying on his bed flicking a Zippo. Lighter fluid had leaked out. Janice told D.J. to put the lighter away immediately.

"You supervise me even if I'm lighting an incense stick!" D.J. complained. He flicked the Zippo for punctuation, and a ball of fire erupted in the air. "*Cooool!*" D.J. exulted.

Janice scolded him for putting the family in danger. "I know what I'm doing," D.J. retorted. Janice ordered him to wash the fluid off his hands. He walked into the bathroom and slammed the door. They'd had other arguments that spring, but this one seemed different. Something told Janice that D.J. shouldn't be alone. She sat on a chair in his room. "You're gonna stay there all night and guard me?" D.J. asked when he came back. She was thinking about doing just that, but after a while she left.

D.J. turned on his fan and closed his door. Janice slept fitfully. Early the next morning she poked into D.J.'s room. The bed was empty and the window was open. There was only one way out: leaping to the garage roof, then climbing down a tree. Janice realized that he'd turned on the fan to drown out the sounds of his escape.

Theodor cruised the neighborhood while Janice canvassed friends. No one had seen D.J. They were about to call the police at 7:00 A.M., when D.J. phoned. "Hey, Mom," he said casually, as if nothing had happened. He'd hitchhiked with truck drivers to find the high school of the girl from the AOL chat room. Instead he got lost in a city an hour and a half away, standing on a street with an elementary school on one side and boarded-up tenements on the other. He had no food, no money, and no way to get home. D.J. ran away the way he did everything else — ADD-style, without planning or considering the consequences.

✍

In October, a few weeks after D.J. got to main campus, he passed by the logistics coordinator of base camp, who complimented him for filling out and standing taller.

"I still don't see why I need to be here," D.J. grumbled.

"Listen, pal. You weren't out there stealin' cars or selling pot on school grounds, but I'll give you another year and you would've gotten into real trouble." He explained as soon as D.J. was out of earshot: From the day he saw the baby-faced boy crying in base camp, he sensed this was a sweet kid. A sweet, misguided kid. "I worry about him because he'll do anything to fit in. He's a rudderless boat, just bouncing around on a very stormy sea."

It seemed as if every time Tanya saw D.J., he was trailing Tyrone. She and the other counselors discussed it during a staff meeting. Friendships were fine, but it was clear that when D.J. found someone he felt safe with, he didn't want to let go. Both D.J. and Tyrone had isolated too much at home. Now they'd actually found a way to isolate together, if that was possible. They were sixteen going on twelve. They needed to stop living in a fantasy world of Magic cards and video games, and to learn to connect with other people.

Tanya and her colleagues debated what to do about the D.J.-Tyrone alliance. Soon after that, Tanya and Jason got D.J.'s attention. "You and Tyrone are on bans."

D.J.'s face went pale. "But we're friends. We help each —"

Starting immediately they couldn't talk to each other, except during group. If D.J. had a problem with that, he could bring it up in the next group. It would be refreshing to hear his voice. Tanya made sure she didn't threaten D.J.; this was about pushing him to open up, not about scaring him. But the other kids didn't see the distinction. When they talked among themselves, they decided that Tanya had thrown down the gauntlet: If D.J. didn't get with the program, he could forget about graduating in October.

# 13

## STORMING, NORMING, AND FORMING

THE "I'M DIFFERENT" discussion started with Tyrone. The kids had circled up for group in a science classroom decorated with posters of suspension bridges and skyscrapers. Tyrone, wearing a black shirt, black pants, and black boots, sat silently, staring ahead. As the others talked, he leaned back in his chair with his arms crossed, shrinking into folds of black fabric.

Tanya asked Tyrone why he refused to participate in the group. He said everyone talked about things that didn't apply to him; he didn't drink or do drugs.

Jason, the gravel-voiced counselor, interrupted. "Then talk about what you *do*. Why can't you be part of this group?"

Usually, Tyrone just shrugged when confronted. This time he shrugged and said, "I'm different."

Jason pushed him to explain. Everyone else was white, Tyrone said. They had more money. They didn't even speak the same way he did. Everyone here said "dude," but no one said that in Queens. He hoped he'd never hear the word *dude* again.

Tanya didn't buy it. In the next few months, she wanted Tyrone to see that losing his dad made him afraid to connect with people. He'd come to associate trusting others with disappointment. "You *are* different from everyone else, but you won't look past those differences. You use your differences as an excuse, just another reason to continue isolating yourself from the world, just another reason to stay disconnected from other people."

Tyrone's complaint prompted an outpouring from the others. D.J., too, felt different. He was short, and everyone treated him like a little kid because he was fifteen and looked younger. He hadn't gotten in big trouble: He didn't skip school, he didn't do drugs or drink, he didn't steal. He longed to be back home skateboarding with his friends, the Parkland Mafia. They didn't stand around analyzing their feelings.

Bianca was next. If anyone was different, *she* was. She was the only one of the fourteen kids who understood what it was like to lose a parent. Besides, she was used to being with regular people, not those who had nannies, maids, and ski chalets. She didn't look at Mary Alice when she spoke, but it was clear whom she meant. At home, she said, she hung out with blacks and Hispanics, but she couldn't do that here. Everyone knew about Tyrone; he still hadn't spoken with her.

When Mary Alice had a chance to speak, she said she was *really* different. She couldn't explain it, but . . . she just came from a certain kind of family. She had nothing in common with the kids from Group 23. She felt like she belonged with another group, one that was more mature (although she didn't state it, everyone knew that group included a certain tall, preppy boy with azure eyes).

Others jumped into the discussion. Phil, the resident philosopher, didn't go for niceties. He lamented that he was stuck with "a bunch of two-faced perfectionist control freaks." The kids didn't agree on much, but they decided that Phil truly *was* different. Since base camp, everyone had carped about missing the same things: fast food, drugs, beer, television. Not Phil, though. He had his own quirky withdrawal pangs, which were worse on weekday afternoons. "It hits me at four o'clock, when it's time for ATC," he said wistfully.

"You mean THC," Mary Alice corrected.

"ATC," Phil said dismissively. *"All Things Considered.* On NPR. It's pretty informative. So is *Morning Edition,* but I never woke up in time for that."

Tanya let everyone air their frustrations. "We're not asking you to be the same," she said, "just to listen." If they listened, they might learn from one another. Who could tell? They might even like one another.

From her studies, Tanya knew that people in a small group pass through several phases. Some Swift River counselors described the phases with terms identified by a psychologist in the 1960s: "storming, norming, and forming." First, in the storming phase, the kids insist they don't want to be together and want nothing to do with one another. The kids in Group 23 were slowly developing norms — codes they could live by. If a group took on a whining, manipulative, rule-breaking character, then fence-sitters like D.J. would make trouble. If it was a positive group, D.J. and the others would fall in line. Tanya was glad her group included Bianca, who not only had a strong sense of right and wrong, but also spoke up.

After a few weeks together, a cohesive bond usually formed. *Group Work with Adolescents,* the textbook used by many Swift River counselors, put it this way: "As members draw closer to one another and to the situation, it is not uncommon for them to associate . . . as if in a family-like gathering." Tanya, Gennarose, and other staff members could give them structure. But ultimately, Bianca and the others would set the tone.

Bianca was unusual because she asked Tanya for extra work. She wanted to be put on a reflection in order to rewrite her life story. Night after night, after finishing her homework, she sat on her bed with loose-leaf paper. She started again with her happy childhood. She described cruising in the car with her mom, belting out pop songs. She recounted the rivalry with her big sister. She wrote about an aunt who broke her back in a fluke elevator accident and, of course, she wrote about her mother's death. When she reached the next section, about middle school, she was ready to write the truth, the real truth. She included something that happened in eighth grade, when she had her first boyfriend, Lester. She was fifteen; he was seventeen. She didn't tell her father about Lester. Her father was always talking about how getting into a good college could determine the rest of your life. Lester got C's, and he didn't care about college. And Bianca thought her father wouldn't like her going out with a black guy. She and Lester had kissed a few times. His hands always dropped down, trying to feel her. "No," she'd say curtly, moving away.

One night, while training for soccer, Bianca was working out at the gym. She ducked into the girls' locker room, hoisted her gym bag, and looked up to see Lester. No one else was around.

"Give me head," he growled.

Bianca refused. She said her grandmother was waiting outside and she had to go, which was true. She swerved around Lester. He jerked her back, smashed her against the lockers, and pushed her down on her knees. He pulled down his pants and forced her to perform oral sex. As he left, he slapped her and warned, "Don't tell anyone, bitch."

When Bianca's father came home from work that evening, his face was scarlet. "What's going on with you? Grandma waits to pick you up for twenty minutes, then you can't be bothered to say hello —"

"Get the hell out of here!" Bianca snapped. She ran to her room and slammed her door. She called her best friend, but even as Bianca started to talk she changed the story and said that she'd initiated oral sex. Her friend was suspicious; she said it just didn't sound like Bianca. "That's what happened, I swear," Bianca protested. When she started crying in English class the next day, the teacher sent her to the guidance counselor. She repeated the story that she'd told her friend. The counselor drove her to a police station, but she wouldn't budge from her story. Bianca's dad arrived. All he knew was that she had kept her grandmother sitting in the car while she had some kind of sexual adventure.

"Don't you have any respect for yourself?" he demanded as they drove home. Bianca stared out the window. How the fuck could she respect herself when no one else did?

Soon after, Bianca started skipping geometry. It had been one of her favorite classes. Her father was exasperated when a report card showed she'd been absent two dozen times in three months. Bianca said the class had become dull, the teacher was stupid. The truth was actually much more complicated, and much simpler: Lester was in the class. He sat right behind her.

For years, she had blamed herself for what had happened in the locker room. Maybe she had come off as slutty . . . or maybe she should have screamed . . . As she wrote about it and talked it out with Tanya, though, Bianca could see that it wasn't her fault.

She told Tanya that something worse had happened in ninth grade. She didn't want to go into the details. Tanya said she could talk about it when she was ready.

From time to time, Tyrone talked to Gennarose. She was from an Italian family, she'd lived in New York, and she was twenty-two, the same age as his sister. Tyrone had never had a real conversation with a teacher; you couldn't really do that with thirty-five kids packed in a chaotic classroom in a Queens school. Gennarose invited him to sit next to her during dinner on a Wednesday when she worked the late shift. He got his food — with four glasses full of red Powerade standing at the front of the tray like sentries —

and ate in silence. Gennarose asked why he closed up in group as if he were wearing armor.

"I'm just here for the academics."

"So you're going to spend fourteen months being a mummy? And not making friends?"

"I don't need anybody."

"Tyrone, excuse me, but what the fuck are you talking about?"

"I don't trust people."

"Why not?"

"Because I know they're going to hurt me."

"Do you know I'm going to hurt you?"

Tyrone didn't answer.

"I can promise you, Tyrone, I'm not going to hurt you."

Tyrone thought it over as he finished his meal.

Everyone wanted to know about Tyrone's life. Why didn't he talk about his dad? What had happened? Time after time, Tyrone had insisted that he had good memories of his father. They hung out together; they played basketball. His dad really understood him. One day in group, Tyrone surprised everyone by volunteering to talk. He said he couldn't remember doing a lot with his dad. When he was younger, his father worked nights and slept during the day. Then, after his mom got a court order to kick him out, his father rarely came around. The other kids asked about the court order. Why couldn't his dad visit? Tyrone's dad said his mom just decided she didn't want to be married anymore. Tyrone was waiting for his father to answer his letter and clear things up.

He reminisced about a day that his father forgot to pick him up from kindergarten. He sat in the principal's office and watched the second hand sweep around the clock. The other kids drifted out, then the teachers and the secretaries. Finally it was just Tyrone and the custodian. Tyrone's mother ran in. When they got home, Tyrone's father was sleeping.

"It happened just once?" Andy asked.

"No, more."

"Five times?"

"More."

"Ten times?"

He didn't answer.

And then it happened. A letter arrived for Tyrone. It wasn't one of his mother's letters, filled with inspirational sayings. It was a birthday letter from his father. It arrived late, but that wasn't important. "Since your mother and I went our separate ways she has been trying to keep us apart," the tightly packed script said. "SHE CANNOT."

It continued:

One reason you are in boarding school is because your mother does not want to deal with the responsibility of dealing with your education and teaching you about life.

I always knew you had questions. I even told you to ask me, but for whatever reason you did not until now.

You ask about the police being at the house. We will talk about that over the phone or in person. I did not leave you at a young age. I was forced to go, by your mother. At the time, I asked her but she would not tell me why. I know she was trying to hurt me by trying to keep you guys from me. It still hurts that I am not able to communicate with you on a regular basis.

Tyrone, I know you don't like it there. Remember I told you that you can adjust to any situation. Please tell me more about the program. Tell me if I can come and see you. Let me know if I can send you money, clothes, books or anything.

The letter raised as many questions as it answered. Tyrone had asked for an explanation of the divorce. Rather than explaining why she kept them apart, his father wrote, "You have to ask her why." Still, his father wanted to visit. It was right there: *Tell me if I can come and see you.*

The other kids had their doubts about the sincerity of that remark. But they were so happy to see Tyrone's smiling face that they high-fived him, and no one said "dude."

On an October morning, with a clear blue sky etched by a jet trail and the sun bathing the trees in gold, Tanya led the kids to the woods. In a clearing they gathered rocks and sticks and built a sweat lodge, a tepee insulated by leaves and thick blankets. Then, while a couple of student volunteers heated stones in a campfire, Tanya and the kids walked a half-mile away, to a ledge overlooking a pond shrouded in dried cattails. Tanya, who had barely said a complete sentence about her life, opened up. She reminisced about her childhood as a faculty brat at boarding school, where she always felt like an outcast surrounded by wealthy kids. She spoke fondly of her father, who had hung out with Beat poets in the 1950s.

Once a group got settled on campus, the counselors were supposed to talk about perseverance. To get through day after day of classes and therapy, to endure a long New England winter and a grueling Costa Rica trip, the kids would need to persevere. Tanya did an exercise with the kids, sitting them in a circle and asking them to think about the times they had stuck with something and overcome difficulties. She gave an example from her own life. A year earlier, as graduation day approached at the Smith College School of Social Work, she and five friends agreed to celebrate by going skydiving. They showed up at the airport one day and watched a training film, but the dive was canceled because of high winds. Tanya was relieved. They returned again, only to hear that again the wind was too strong. The third time, only one other classmate showed up. Tanya considered backing out but kept her promise to herself. She described the experience of standing in the doorway of a prop plane, tethered to an instructor, with the cold air slapping her face. Jumping into the clouds, they felt the yank of the parachute, and floated past the green slopes of the Connecticut River valley. When they landed in a field, Tanya had screamed with joy.

The kids listened raptly because she spoke so infrequently about herself. The fourteen of them had grown protective of Tanya. Mary Alice described her as a giant goose; she'd half-walk and half-waddle through the great room. Tanya may have been graceful while dancing or skydiving, but she was a klutz everywhere else. More than once she'd tried to bound over a couch and gotten her foot caught in the cushions. As she tumbled to the carpet, she let loose a giddy "Ooops!" She seemed to have a mysterious life of rock climbing and tango competitions. Of course, even as she appeared to talk spontaneously, Tanya was editing her story. She didn't mention that she had recently persevered in other ways, as her father was diagnosed with cancer twice in the past ten years. Tanya had watched him turn from a swarthy, politically active artist and teacher to an emaciated patient defeated by the rounds of surgery and tests. At one point the year before, a doctor had told the family, "It would be a miracle if he lived till tomorrow." He had not only lived, he'd rebuilt his strength. But Tanya was still raw from all the uncertainty and the emotional ups and downs.

After group, everyone crammed into the sweat lodge. Including Tanya,

Gennarose, and other counselors, twenty grimy, smelly adults and kids sat shoulder to shoulder. Although a thin beam of sunlight slanted in through a tiny hole, it was too dark to see more than anyone's profile. The kids took turns discussing what they had been thinking during the day. Bianca thought she should get to know her father better. Mary Alice felt terrible because she'd been a brat at home. D.J. resolved to speak up more.

Every fifteen minutes, the two volunteers rolled in hot stones from the campfire. The temperature kept rising inside the sweat lodge. One of the counselors estimated it was 140 degrees and rising.

After close to an hour, D.J. moaned, "I can't make it." Tyrone told him to breathe slowly.

"I have to get out."

Just ten more minutes, the others said.

"I'm gonna throw up."

Tyrone spoke soothingly, assuring D.J. that he would make it.

Gennarose was nauseated. She felt overwhelmed by the heat, the perspiration, the memories of her own rocky adolescence. Mary Alice, sitting nearby, could sense it. "C'mon, Gennarose, you're doing well. You're so great." Gennarose put her head down on the ground, which was cooler.

Seven minutes, six . . .

"I'm going to faint."

"Come on D.J., you can do it!"

Mary Alice spoke up. "I love y'all," she said. "I'm sorry I said I didn't want to be part of this group. "

Four, three . . .

"I'm so lucky to be with you guys," Bianca said.

"Yeah," an English accent piped up. "You're the best friends I've ever had."

Tanya praised everyone for persevering through the sweat. Although she didn't say it, they had broken a barrier. They had survived the storming and norming.

Then they broke into a song from their parents' era. "*Some times in our lives, we all have pain, we all have sorrow . . .*" D.J. still sprawled motionless on the ground moaning, his mouth gaping. "*So just call on me brother, when you need a hand.*" All around him the others raised their voices. "*We all need somebody to lean on.*"

# 14

## "I'm Angry at Myself for Being Born"

THE KIDS FELL APART in early November — right on schedule.

Teachers complained that D.J. couldn't stay in his seat for more than fifteen minutes at a time, not to mention a fifty-minute period. He had a nervous habit of pulling the sleeves of his turtlenecks over his hands, then making holes for his thumbs to pop out of. He chewed on pen caps, fidgeted with string, or kicked a hacky-sack. Trevor admitted that he'd "cheeked" his meds — pretended to swallow pills but instead kept them hidden in his mouth so that later he could crush them and snort them for a high.

Tanya knew that whenever a milestone in the program neared, the students would go back to pattern. Group 23 was about to go through two significant events. On a Tuesday in mid-November, they'd have their first all-day workshop, a sort of marathon group session. Then, three weeks later, the parents were coming for their first visit. After a session of family therapy, the kids would have three days to tell their life stories to their parents and to hear their parents' life stories. During any visit, the experienced counselors warned, emotions whipsawed up and down.

The weather didn't help. The clouds would spit out snow, but then it would get just warm enough to melt into slush. Swift River was on a ridge, and biting winds whistled across campus. Once daylight saving time was over and the clocks were set back, the sun set by 4:40 P.M. A long New England winter was just starting, and the kids already had cabin fever. Mary Alice got into another shouting match with a supervisor about a tight outfit she wanted to wear. Bianca couldn't contain her frustration. "What the hell are you doing, arguing about clothes?" she said. "You can't be serious. Not everyone is looking at you 24/7." As Mary Alice walked away, Bianca muttered, "You can ignore me, but I know you hear me."

Bianca regressed to her "mothering mode," making sure everyone else was okay. She stayed up late talking things out with a roommate who despised Swift River and consoling kids in her group who were anxious about seeing their parents. Before group, Bianca arranged the chairs in a tidy circle, then snapped at anyone who moved them. "You're such a perfectionist," Mary Alice shot back. Tanya told them to relax, but it was useless.

✑

Two weeks before Thanksgiving, Tanya and three other counselors dimmed the lights in the library, arranged logs in the massive stone fireplace, and hung sheets over the tall windows to keep out the morning light and ensure privacy. It was time for Group 23's first all-day workshop.

The kids entered in single file, in the order that they'd come down from base camp. Flames flickered in the massive stone fireplace. The kids' childhood nicknames — provided by the parents — had been written on labels on the back of chairs set in a semicircle facing the fire. D.J. smiled as he went to a chair that said Peanut; Mary Alice laughed as she spotted Precious Angel. Other chairs had names like Munchkin, Pie-Pie, Bumper, and Benito.

Many of the kids at Swift River had grown up in chaotic families. They were scared of separation and surprises. They loved rituals, meaningful activities that provided a sense of consistency and order. In a smoothly functioning family, rituals helped connect parents and children. In a group, rituals built a sense of trust and team spirit. The workshops were filled with rituals. They started with guided meditations or breathing exercises. Pop songs by Mike and the Mechanics, Enigma, and REM, chosen for their lyrics about love, friendship, or sorrow, played on the stereo. During a break, everybody silently ate a simple dinner of cold cuts. Then, with darkness settling in and the kids' guards down, the counselors ramped up the emotional intensity with a new activity. The rituals continued on the morning after a workshop, when the kids were allowed to sleep late. As they walked into a schoolwide meeting, they were greeted with hugs. Then they spent several weeks processing, mulling over what they'd learned before parents came to Swift River for discussions and family therapy.

Certain workshops touched different kids to different degrees, but months or years after a workshop, quite a few graduates of therapeutic schools would hear one of the Enigma or Mike and the Mechanics songs on the radio and start sobbing.

✍

Swift River, like many therapeutic schools, started with a workshop on anger. It was anger, after all, that blocked resolution and understanding with their families. Many of the kids used drugs to anesthetize themselves from their pain and anger. They couldn't get anything meaningful from therapy as long as they were mad. And yet most of the time they couldn't even remember why they were so pissed off, or who was responsible. "We need to show the kids that they have the right and responsibility to express their rage," Rudy Bentz said. At the same time, they needed to understand their anger. He liked to paraphrase a scene from Marlon Brando playing a hellraiser in *The Wild One*. The way Rudy told it, someone asked Brando what he was so angry about. "Whaddya got?" Brando sneered.

To uncork the kids' rage, the first workshop featured "dyads." The counselors divided them into pairs, making sure that each kid was with someone he or she trusted. The counselors called out, "I'm angry at you, Mom, for . . ." and told the kids to finish the sentence. They had to keep finishing the sentence, and they needed to let everything come out.

Bianca was in one corner. She clutched the hands of the girl who had stolen her parents' Volvo. She started softly, tentatively:

"I'm angry at you, Mom, for getting sick.
"I'm angry at you, Mom, for telling me God was going to take care of everything."

The other girl encouraged her to keep going. Bianca raised her voice.

"I'm angry at you, Mom, for not protecting me.
"I'm angry at you, Mom, for dying when I was ten.
"I'm angry at you, Mom, for leaving me all alone."

A few feet away, Mary Alice's voice trembled.

"I'm angry at you, Mom, for paying attention to everyone but me.
"I'm angry at you, Mom, for always telling everybody I'm just fine.
"I'm angry at you, Mom, for being so busy with your friends.
"I'm angry at you, Mom, for comparing me to the Sanderson sisters."

Tyrone started out so quietly that no one could hear him, but soon his voice was echoing through the room.

"I'm angry at you, Mom, for being mean to dad.
"I'm angry at you, Mom, for kicking out dad.
"I'm angry at you, Mom, for trying to be everything.
"I'm angry at you, Mom, for leaving me alone in the house."

D.J. started with his jaded, this-is-dumb face, looking around at everyone else. But after a minute he was quavering as he held Andy's hands.

"I'm angry at you, Mom, for pushing me.
"I'm angry at you, Mom, for trying to fix me all the time.
"I'm angry at you, my real mother, for getting pregnant.
"I'm angry at you, my real mother, for doing drugs.
"I'm angry at you for giving me up."

That round had lasted just three minutes, but it seemed like half an hour. The room felt hot. The counselors said it was time for the next round. The cue was "I'm angry at you, Dad." With her partner telling her to go for broke, Bianca launched in at high volume:

"I'm angry at you, Dad, for loving my sister so much.
"I'm angry at you, Dad, for not loving me enough.
"I'm angry at you, Dad, for not helping me after mom died.
"I'm angry at you, Dad, for remarrying.
"I'm angry at you, Dad, for divorcing.
"I'm angry at you, Dad, for saying everything was going to be fine.
"I'm angry at you, Dad, for trying to be my friend instead of my
     father.
"I'm angry at you, Dad, for not trusting me.
"I'm angry at you, Dad, for yelling at me.
"I'm angry at you, Dad, for bolting my window shut.
"I'm angry at you, Dad, for sending me here."

Mary Alice's face was crimson and the veins of her forehead were visible.

"I'm angry at you, Dad, for reading my diary.
"I'm angry at you, Dad, for putting pressure on me.
"I'm angry at you, Dad, for going away on business trips.

"I'm angry at you, Dad, for going away on hunting trips.
"I'm angry at you, Dad, for trying to make everything seem all right.
"I'm angry at you, Dad, for wanting me to be your perfect little angel.
"I'm angry at you, Dad, for pretending my eating disorder is cured."

Tyrone's eyes were closed.

"I'm angry at you, Dad, for forgetting me at school.
"I'm angry at you, Dad, for leaving.
"I'm angry at you, Dad, for caring more about my sister.
"I'm angry at you, Dad, for missing my birthday party.
"I'm angry at you, Dad, for missing everything in my life.
"I'm angry at you, Dad, for not answering my questions.
"I'm angry at you, Dad, for not knowing me."

D.J. was lost in the past.

"I'm angry at you, Dad, for yelling at me in the morning.
"I'm angry at you, Dad, for yelling at me for wetting my bed.
"I'm angry at you, Dad, for letting me wrestle big guys.
"I'm angry at you, Dad, for wanting me to be stronger.
"I'm angry at you, Dad, for wanting me to be smarter.
"I'm angry at you, Dad, for saying I can't sit still.
"I'm angry at you, birth father, for not knowing me."

The combination of the fire and the emotional energy made the room stifling. That round, too, lasted a long three minutes. Tanya walked around, patting the kids on the back and exhorting them to "Go for it! Let everything out!" Bianca didn't need any encouragement.

"I'm angry at myself for not taking care of Mom.
"I'm angry at myself for not crying.
"I'm angry at myself for getting fat.
"I'm angry at myself for getting molested.
"I'm angry at myself for having sex before marriage.
"I'm angry at myself for not letting myself be a kid.
"I'm angry at myself for getting pregnant.
"I'm angry at myself for losing my baby.
"I'm angry at myself for being a bad daughter.
"I'm angry at myself for not being good enough."

Mary Alice's hair flew in the air, a blond fury. "That's it!" Gennarose cheered, pumping her hands.

"I'm angry at myself for being such a slut.
"I'm angry at myself for using coke.
"I'm angry at myself for sticking my finger down my throat.
"I'm angry at myself for being such a fuck-up."

Tyrone, oozing sweat, cried out:

"I'm angry at myself for not going to school.
"I'm angry at myself for not having more friends.
"I'm angry at myself for losing friends.
"I'm angry at myself for being stupid.
"I'm angry at myself for being quiet.
"I'm angry at myself for being lazy."

D.J. gripped Andy's hands and bellowed:

"I'm angry at myself for being hyper.
"I'm angry at myself for running away.
"I'm angry at myself for being the kid no one wants to be around.
"I'm angry at myself for being born."

The last round lasted six minutes; not including breaks, the dyads had taken all of twelve minutes. The fourteen kids collapsed into a heap on the floor and breathed heavily. "The Living Years," a moody 1980s pop song by Mike and the Mechanics, filled the library.

It's too late when we die
To admit we don't see eye to eye . . .
I wasn't there that morning
When my father passed away
I didn't get to tell him
All the things I had to say . . .

The Ohio girl gently rubbed D.J.'s head while D.J. rubbed Willow's shoulders. Bianca gave a neck rub to Ashley, the New Yorker whom she had briefly considered her best friend. Tyrone seemed to fall into a deep sleep. Bianca covered her eyes and cried as the closing refrain hung in the air:

I'm sure I heard his echo
In my baby's newborn tears
I just wish I could have told him
In the living years.

It was nearly one in the morning. Tanya and Gennarose placed envelopes next to each kid. The embers of the fire glowed. Slowly, one by one, the kids opened their eyes and read cards from their mothers and fathers. D.J. passed his father's card to the others.

Dear Peanut:
I'm sitting here in your room looking at the picture of you after you caught the mahimahi. I remember the way your face lit up when the line signaled a hit on your pole and we strapped you into the charter boat's fighting chair. Your face reflected all sorts of things — happiness, courage, determination, joy, excitement, awe and wonder.
Taking you fishing has opened new horizons for me and I look forward to fishing with you (and learning from you) in the future. You are a capable, caring and lovable boy whom I love very much.
I am very proud and very happy to call you my son.
All my love, Dad

D.J. had been impassive since his early days at base camp. Not even 9/11 had shaken him. But sitting in front of the fireplace on this cold night in November, with the wind whistling through the bare trees outside, he shivered and cried.

# 15

# FALLING IN LOVE AGAIN

> I haven't seen my dad in five months. I'm nervous about his reaction
> to my disclosures. My dad tends to think that he can change the past
> and make everything fine. I want him to know that I'm telling him this
> stuff so we can have a better relationship. I don't want him to try to
> change the past. I just want him to be understanding.
>
> — Bianca's journal, December 10, 2001

BIANCA'S FATHER, Alan, walked into the great room for Group 23's first
parents' visit, or "family resolution," in Swift River's jargon. He didn't know
what to expect during the long weekend. For that matter, he didn't really
know *whom* to expect. He might find the preadolescent Bianca — the cud-
dly little girl whose hair he used to comb in the mornings before elementary school, the girl whose descriptions of books and band practice and
friends came out in torrents. Or he might find the Bianca of the last few
years, the teenager who sneaked out the window late at night and lied to his
face the next day.

Six months had passed since Alan had hired the husband-and-wife escort team to whisk Bianca away to a wilderness intervention program in
North Carolina. Alan had gotten a glimpse of that familiar Bianca — the
tempestuous teenager — when he'd picked her up in North Carolina halfway through the summer to take her to Massachusetts. She'd spent most of
the trip seething under her Walkman headphones.

This time the day was overcast and chilly. Tattered brown leaves
swirled outside. Swift River's buildings didn't glow in the sun the way they
had when Alan had dropped off Bianca in July; they looked like they were
hunkered down, bracing for a mean winter. In the great room, Rudy Bentz
faced the parents. "When did you lose your child?" he asked, his voice
bouncing off the rafters. "When you saw his red eyes walking through the
front door and smelled that sour mix of beer and cigarettes and dope on
his breath?"

Mary Alice's parents nodded.

It wasn't hard to tell that Rudy had started his career as a drama teacher. He paced in front of the room. "When did you lose your daughter? When you stopped in her room that night to say 'I love you, honey' and saw an empty bed?"

Alan, too, nodded.

"When was it? When you signed the admissions papers here? When you opened your arms for one last hug and your child said 'Fuck you' and walked away, leaving you hugging nothing but air?"

Another couple of heads bobbed. Someone sniffled.

"When did you lose your son? When you drove away from the base camp parking lot and looked for his goofy grin in the rearview mirror, and instead saw that he'd turned his back on you?" Rudy waited. "For a while, you've been feeling as if you buried your child."

He asked the parents what their lives had been like before they sent their children away. Hands shot up.

"A war zone."

"Hopeless."

"No social life."

"Scared, worried sick."

"A living hell."

Alan uttered a nervous, one-syllable laugh, the parental equivalent of "*Ho!*" "Bianca was out of control," he said. "I was always on guard, always worried that something was going to happen." The others nodded sympathetically. "Always wondering what kind of phone call I was going to get next."

Rudy cautioned the parents that Swift River would be a gradual process, and along the way every kid would falter now and then. But it wasn't just about the kids. The parents needed to stand back and take a hard look at their own weaknesses and problems, just as their children had been doing since base camp. "I say this with all respect: If you are not now engaged in therapy or other work to grow personally, or if you are not willing to take apart your thinking, your feelings, your motivations, please take your bags, get your kid, and leave."

No one left. They never did.

"The students are here doing hard emotional work, and they think mom and dad have been home for a few months lazing around playing golf, or sitting around smoking cigars and drinking beer."

"A hundred and seven days," said D.J.'s dad, Theodor.

The other parents looked over quizzically.

"That's how long D.J.'s been here," Theodor said. As a wrestling coach, he'd gotten in the habit of counting the days that remained until a season began. Now he was counting time at Swift River. D.J. had 296 days to go.

While the parents craned their necks and looked at the stairs, waiting to catch sight of their children, Rudy explained the schedule. They would soon split into groups of a dozen kids and parents, each with a couple of counselors, to start family therapy. Then the parents and kids would have three days for conversations — three days without the phone calls, e-mails, office reading, stock updates, errands, housecleaning, cable news, sitcoms, and other distractions that interrupted them at home. Small talk was fine, but each family needed to set aside time to go to a quiet place and share life stories. Each kid needed to open up to his or her parents, and parents needed to open up to their child. Rudy gave a hard stare. As difficult as it might sound, the parents should be honest about their own struggles with booze and drugs.

During the weekend, he warned, the parents and kids would be tempted to play games of "ping-ponging blame." By that he meant that adults and children often had wildly varying recollections of events. A boy might have a searing memory of his mom humiliating him for spilling paint on the floor, for example, while the mother thought she'd used restraint. Rudy explained that the dyads were meant to make students see that they'd often blamed parents, teachers, and others — the ubiquitous "them" — for everything. The kids were beginning to understand that they themselves bore plenty of responsibility for running away or taking drugs or arguing at home. But they still had different perceptions from their parents, and often the truth was somewhere in the middle.

"We're not here today to decide who's right," Rudy said. "We're here to assist you with the next step, which is falling in love again."

"The Living Years," the song from the ten-hour workshop on anger, reverberated in the great room with its somber warning: "It's too late . . ."

Rudy gave a thumbs-up signal to a counselor. A door opened and Group 23 stampeded up the stairs. Bianca fell into her father's arms. Mary Alice lunged into a bear hug from her mom, then her dad. Tyrone towered over his mother and clutched her, then briefly shook his stepfather's hand.

Gennarose, the English teacher, draped her arm over Tyrone's shoulder and grinned. "Watching him has been like watching a flower blooming," she told Tyrone's mother.

D.J. allowed his mother to embrace him. He let his father hug him briefly before pulling away.

"There's so much going on in Dallas," Mary Alice's mother, Lillian, told her as they waited for lunch. "Did you hear about Luke? He got caught bringing Ecstasy to a dance."

"He did?"

"The homecoming dance," her father said.

"And he was such a goodie-goodie," her mother said. "Did you hear about Robert?"

"Mom, I don't hear *anything* here."

"He wrote his brother and his parents a farewell letter and killed himself."

"Omigod."

"And Melissa? She got caught doing cocaine —"

"Mom, she's like a fucking cokehead," Mary Alice said.

"She was doing it at school."

"I used to get high with her and Gordie."

"Gordie went to Dr. Thompson's house and stole a car and video equipment," her father said.

"The problem is," her mother added, "that so many parents are so naive. They don't want to know what's going on."

An hour later, Mary Alice and her parents met with two other families and two counselors in a classroom for family therapy. The kids set up the chairs in a circle and explained the rules to their parents: to avoid physically intimidating someone, you needed to be at least two seats away before speaking. Everyone had to tell the "hard truth." The counselors explained that in this first family group, kids and parents both needed to discuss the anger that had built up for years. Mary Alice started. Looking at her parents, she talked about feeling isolated from the family. Even as she spoke, she noticed that they happened to sit together and she ended up on the opposite side of the room. She complained about having three younger siblings by the time she was four, including her baby sister, who needed extra care when she was born prematurely.

"It wasn't a great situation," her mother admitted. "It was tough for Mary Alice to be the first of four and feel like she was having to compete with the other ones."

"We didn't realize how hard things were for Mary Alice," her father said. But he added that he didn't see that as an excuse for what had happened in high school. "She just stopped listening to us. We were worried our daughter was going to kill herself."

One of the counselors raised a hand. "Don't talk to everyone else; talk to your daughter. She's right here."

Mary Alice continued. "You left me with like six different nannies."

"Mary Alice, I loved being a dermatologist. I thought I could be a mother and a doctor. I tried it for a few years, and I thought you were in good hands with the nannies."

Mary Alice talked about the housekeeper she despised. "Bea hated me, she was always yelling at me."

"Honey, you made me realize that something had to give," her mother said. "I stopped working and we let Bea go."

"It wasn't just the nannies and housekeepers, mom. You put so much pressure on me to play the right sport and have the right friends. You just wanted me to be like the Sanderson sisters. You wanted me to pretend that everything was fine. That's how we were raised, to say that everything is under fucking control!"

Mary Alice's mom spoke to the other parents in the circle as if addressing a jury. "We wanted to do the very best for Mary Alice, to do the right thing for our daughter, even though we might have been misguided and meeting our own needs."

The next day, a Friday, Mary Alice didn't mention her outburst. She pulled three easy chairs together in the great room so she and her parents could share their life stories. Lillian spoke about growing up poor, the only child of divorced parents. Her small house had mismatched furniture, so she was embarrassed to invite other kids over. Feelings of inferiority had pushed her, too. Lillian had put herself through medical school on a scholarship.

She pointed out that she hadn't been perfect; she had tried several kinds of drugs herself in her teens, and she had to admit, without getting too detailed, that she had sex before she started dating Burns. She winced as she said it, but Mary Alice didn't seem surprised.

Burns came from a Dallas family with money, but his childhood had been far from ideal. His father worked all the time, even on vacation. No one talked about emotions. (Burns jokingly dismissed therapy at Swift River and elsewhere as "namby-pamby, feel-good stuff.") Burns's father had been wild as a boy, and Burns himself had been such a handful that his parents sent him away to boarding school at age eight. Looking back, Burns realized he must have had ADD, but in those days kids weren't diagnosed; they were just considered hell-raisers. "Mary Alice," he sighed, "it's in your genes to challenge the rules."

When Mary Alice's turn came, she talked about feeling unimportant amid her parents' whirl of business trips, European vacations, and quail-hunting jaunts. "Dad, you spent so much time at your job."

"Honey, I worked so you could enjoy life, and I left the office early to coach your basketball team. I did my best to have evenings free for you."

"You made a fuss over the baby and you scolded me all the time."

"I loved you equally if not more than the other kids."

Mary Alice tried to prepare her parents before telling her life story. She explained that her truth letter from base camp had merely touched on the low points. She started by talking about the times she'd ripped off her parents. Several times, for example, she'd used her Chevron credit card, which her parents had given her for gas, to buy cigarettes. Then there was the time she went to Home Depot and bought four $300 gift certificates. Without even leaving the store, she redeemed them for items worth a few dollars and used the leftover cash for drugs. Mary Alice went through the litany of drugs she'd used: pot, coke, Ecstasy, acid, Adderall, painkillers that a friend had been prescribed for a broken arm. From her diary, her parents already knew that she'd tried crack. Since she was coming clean, she admitted that she'd used it more than once. Probably five times.

Burns and Lillian listened, their faces ashen. "It takes a lot of courage for you to . . . to face all these issues," Lillian stammered. "But still, it pains my heart to see how my little girl has hurt herself so much."

"What is so sad is that all I really wanted was to be a good father," Burns said wistfully.

Lillian added, "It's not like you wake up one morning and say, 'I'm going to screw up my kid's life today.'"

On the other side of the great room, D.J. and his parents leaned back on a couch. While telling her story, Janice wanted D.J. to see that she, too, had struggled with school. "I felt very stressed, very lonely. I had a hard time learning math by rote because I had to understand it first. That's why I became a teacher. I figured if it didn't work for me, it didn't work for other people." Janice also hoped that D.J. would understand the pain she'd felt when one pregnancy after another failed. She tried to catch his gaze while she spoke, but D.J. kept craning his neck, looking for Tyrone and the other kids. Theodor suggested they go to a place with fewer distractions. They continued the discussions in D.J.'s dorm room. There, Janice told about how, finally, a baby boy — Peanut — had been the answer to their prayers.

When Theodor told his life story, he remembered the day they drove home from the adoption agency with D.J., who was one month old. A light rain was falling. Normally, they'd pull around to the side of the house, into the garage, then walk through a door into the kitchen. But not today, Theodor announced. The rain be damned. "This is D.J.'s home, and he's coming in through the front door!"

Before telling his own life story, D.J. walked up a dirt path with his parents to show them a base camp site where he'd stayed during the summer. "Okay, I've been procrastinating," he said as they approached the main campus. "Time to tell my story." He whipped through it: He was born; he was a hyper kid; he wet his bed; he went from specialist to specialist; he hated writing; he got together with his buddies in the Parkland Mafia . . .

"Slow down, D.J.," Theodor urged, but D.J. careened along, covering each year in about forty seconds: He joined the wrestling team; he learned to rock climb; he climbed out of his window and ran away; his parents sent him off to Swift River so he couldn't be near his friends, his school, his dog.

During breaks from talks with their children, the parents commiserated. Two fathers who were lawyers agreed that all the demands of meetings and billable hours had made them miss dinners more than they wanted to. Several parents lamented that by the time they cut down their workloads, their children had reached middle school and wanted nothing to do with them. One father said he'd always thought that only aloof, uninvolved parents had problems with their kids; on the contrary, he'd always stepped in to help his daughter in a pinch. Seeing that she was overwhelmed by a report for a seventh-grade English class, for example, he'd told her to go to sleep and had done the report himself.

"The platypus!" the father from Ohio exulted. "It was her eighth-grade paper. I stayed up writing till three o'clock." He added, proudly, "The teacher gave it an A."

The first father wondered if he'd done too much for his daughter. Not long before, she'd sneaked home from school and taken the family Volvo for a spin — and she'd spun it right into an expensive sports car. Because she didn't have a license, her parents took the blame so the insurance company would cover the damage. In just a couple of years they'd gone from writing reports for their daughter to lying on her police reports.

D.J.'s parents kept asking themselves whether they had done too much or too little. His mother started every school year by briefing D.J.'s teachers on his ADHD, encouraging them to take advantage of his overflowing energy and to help him with organization. When D.J. had trouble writing his homework assignments, his mother took dictation. Now she blamed herself for undermining his confidence. "I was trying to help him, but I made him feel I didn't love him the way he was."

Tyrone's mother and stepfather stayed apart from the rest. Natalie couldn't get over the Ohio mother and father who had hidden the news of their daughter's adoption. "You can't lie like that to children because they know something's missing," she said. "And when they know something's missing, the shit they make up is even worse." Natalie felt passionately about that. For years, she had wondered why her mother seemed to despise her. Then, at thirteen, she accidentally found out that the woman in her house wasn't really her mother — she was a stepmother. There was more: When Natalie was two, her real mother, who was pregnant, had been murdered on a rooftop in Harlem. Natalie never found out why.

Natalie shook her head, too, as she watched Mary Alice's mother and father. "The more the child tries to show that she's in pain, the more the parents try to put on a happy face and act like everything is hunky-dory. If their house is burning down, if things are crumbling around them, they'd say, 'We can do this, it's under control.'" But she had little sympathy for kids like Mary Alice, who had the nerve to curse out their own parents. "It's like the children set the rules and the parents cower and follow them," she said in wonder, "Nobody knows their roles any more." Tyrone had had his troubles, but at least he understood who was the child and who was the adult in the family. He had cursed at her in first grade, but just once — washing his mouth with soap took care of that.

Tyrone's stepfather, who had developed a no-nonsense attitude in the army, raised three daughters of his own. All three had gone on to college. He attributed their achievement to a mixture of love and discipline. His motto about parenting was simple: "This is not Burger King and you can't have it your way."

✑

A mother from California kept peppering Rudy with questions, anecdotes, and advice: Couldn't the work crews scrape and paint the exteriors of the buildings? Why didn't Swift River have movement therapy? What about deep-breathing exercises? During a break, the mother sat on the floor of the great room and did her breathing exercises as the other parents walked around her to get coffee. After the break, she started in again on the headmaster and other staff members, grilling them about the rate of college acceptance for Swift River graduates. Natalie grimaced. The girls and boys had barely scraped the base-camp dirt from their fingernails, barely started figuring out how everything had gone to hell, and this woman was agonizing about whether she'd be able to put a UCLA bumper sticker on her car?

"Some of these parents," Natalie whispered to her husband, "should be taken out and flogged."

✑

Looking at the mothers and fathers before him, Rudy said, "It's not that you're bad parents, but you probably did some bad parenting."

He explained that Americans' notions about the right way to raise children have swung back and forth between strict and indulgent. Even the notion of proper parenting was a twentieth-century concept; before that, parents' foremost concern was getting children through infancy and childhood unscarred by disease and malnutrition. "Parents today are incompetent," John Watson, a behaviorist, wrote in 1928, arguing that mothers and fathers needed to be disciplinarians. "Most of them should be indicted for psychological murder." Watson was hardly alone. A booklet called *What You Ought to Know About Your Baby*, distributed free by a company that made sewing patterns, included H. L. Mencken's diatribe against a woman who was seen in public playing with and kissing her child.

By the middle of the twentieth century, child labor laws and women's suffrage helped shape the notion that there must be a more humane way to parent. When Dr. Benjamin Spock published *Baby and Child Care* in 1946, his emphasis on giving children freedom of choice and encouraging self-expression resonated with Americans, who had been shaken by the rise of Fascism and a world war. The book sold three quarters of a million copies in its first year. In the 1960s, parenting theory had become more concrete. Diana Baumrind, a research psychologist at the Institute of Human Development at the University of California, Berkeley, delineated three distinct varieties of parent. The first, permissive parents, are responsive to their child's desires and impulses and don't establish rules. Children of permissive parents are likely to show poor emotion regulation, to be defiant when desires are challenged, have low persistence to challenging tasks, and exhibit antisocial behaviors. At the other extreme are authoritarian parents, who are very demanding but not responsive. These parents are more likely to raise children who are anxious and withdrawn, but who do well in school and avoid delinquent, antisocial activities.

In the middle are authoritative parents, who are both demanding and responsive. They set rules and expect their children to use self-control and work toward goals, but they also explain the reasoning behind their actions. At the same time, they show warmth and affection and willingness to compromise. As a result, their children are likely to be lively and confident.

The 1970s brought a backlash from those who complained about children who had been "Spocked rather than spanked." One authoritarian approach, called Tough Love, argued that children responded best to unwavering rules and swift punishment. Later, John Rosemond, a psychologist and director of the Center for Affirmative Parenting in North Carolina, derided baby boomers for spoiling their children and abdicating their roles as parents.

Still others argued that all the emphasis on parents' psyches and styles was overdone. In 1998, in *The Nurture Assumption,* a psychologist named Judith Rich Harris argued that by the age of three or four, a child's behavior begins to be more influenced by peers than by family. Harris was inspired by vastly different experiences with her biological daughter, who helped around the house and excelled at school, and her adopted daughter, who couldn't abide by rules anywhere.

The proliferation of theories added to the confusion. In *Raising America: Experts, Parents and a Century of Advice about Children,* Ann Hulbert summarized the twentieth century's contradictory messages to parents: "Trust your instincts and train your insight, follow your baby's nature and spare no effort on her nurture — relax and enjoy those first years and don't forget for a minute that your child's future is at stake."

The problem with the experts — including self-taught healers such as Rudy — was that they often made parenting sound more rational than it was. Many of the Group 23 parents said they were trying to make up for their own aloof or absent parents. Mary Alice's and D.J.'s fathers talked about their painful memories of being sent away to boarding school. Bianca's dad said his own father was a functioning alcoholic who kept his job but lost his temper and withdrew from the family. Teresa had been the disciplinarian. The kids knew that if she said no, she meant it. Alan was looser. He wanted the children to like him. As the years passed, he decided that had a lot to do with growing up with a distant father who drank too much.

After Teresa died, Alan became increasingly permissive: "I felt it was even more important that the kids see me as their friend, so I didn't hold them to rules." If Bianca wanted to play, he pushed back her bedtime. Alan's "no" came to mean maybe. As Bianca entered adolescence, late bedtimes gave way to more extreme liberties. But setting rules was just part of the challenge. Teresa, the outgoing one, had been good at getting Bianca and Claudia to open up and talk about their feelings. Growing up, Alan had one brother, who was eleven years older, and no female siblings or cousins. He was shy and didn't spend a lot of time with girls, so he didn't know how to talk to his own daughters. He kept putting off discussions of boyfriends and sex, and by the time he was ready, his daughters shrugged him off. They'd already learned from friends.

On the third day of the visit, Alan Bittman sat on the worn brick steps of the classroom building with his daughter. It was drizzling, and the visibility was so poor that students passing a few feet away could barely see them. Bianca shivered. She talked about the years after her mother's death — how she lived in a family with three other survivors, but felt all alone. She talked quickly, the words jamming together, as she always did when she was nervous. Then she took a breath.

"Dad, I have to tell you some things, and I just need you to listen."

"I promise."

"And not judge me."

"You have my word."

"And not want to go out and do something about what I tell you."

"Okay, Bianca."

Bianca started by telling him about the day in eighth grade when her grandmother was waiting in the car outside the gym. She told him that Lester, her boyfriend at the time, had forced her to perform oral sex.

Alan draped his arm over her shoulder. He breathed deeply. "Okay, honey, that explains the way you treated Grandma and me that day. There's more?"

She nodded and told him about the pregnancy and miscarriage a year earlier, in the middle of tenth grade.

"You were *pregnant?* Why didn't you say something?"

"You couldn't have dealt with it. Dad, I didn't even feel comfortable talking to you when I got my period."

"You're right." He shook his head. His face went ashen.

"There's something else." She had been raped. She didn't want to go into details yet, but it had happened in ninth grade, and it was a boy her father had met. "I know what you're thinking. You want to find out who it was and call the police."

"Actually, you're right."

"I want you not to do anything yet. I just need you to hold me."

Alan pulled her into his arms and shielded her from the rain.

On Sunday, the temperature dropped to the low forties and a downpour turned the campus muddy. Winter was settling in. A couple of hours before the parents had to leave, D.J. played foosball with his dad in the great room. A few feet away, Andy and his father jammed on their Fender guitars. Next to a rain-streaked window, Tyrone hunched over an old guitar with his stepfather, learning how to play a C chord.

Tyrone's stepfather took a walk so Tyrone and his mother could talk things over in private. Tyrone said he felt as if no one cared about him when he was growing up. Natalie said she'd been pulled in two directions — she needed to work to keep her family going, yet she also needed to be at home. No matter which one she was doing, she felt that she was sloughing off at the other one. Tyrone finally got around to the subject he'd been side-stepping. He wanted to know why his mother had kicked out his dad.

"Tyrone, the plain fact is your father was doing drugs. He was stealing money that I earned. That's how he supported his habit, with money that was meant to buy you food and clothes. Besides that, some woman started calling the house. She'd talk to me — she'd *confide* in me — as if I wanted to hear any of it. Your father was bringing our family down with him and I could not let that happen."

Tyrone looked down silently.

"Do you remember what happened the day before I called the cops on your father?"

He shook his head.

"I was taking a shower. I'd hid my money from him and he was raging mad. He came into the shower and hit me. He smacked me so hard that I screamed. You were there — you and your sister were in the next room. You knew it. You *heard* it, Tyrone. It's just that you somehow blocked it out of your memory. You've been living in a dark cave because you weren't able to deal with some things in your life. Your father had to leave. I'm sorry if you want to blame me, but that's God's truth."

In the girl's dorm, Mary Alice lay on her bed, peering into the two-inch screen of a video camera as she snuggled up with her dad. Her mom perched on the side of the bed. The three of them chuckled as they watched videos of Mary Alice as a toddler blowing bubbles, Mary Alice kicking a soccer ball, and Mary Alice at four clobbering her little brother on the head. They listened to a tinny recording of voices from twelve years before: "Now, tell him you're sorry, Mary Alice," Burns was saying.

"Okay. *Sorry*," the little girl chirped, flashing an impish smile.

Alan Bittman said farewell to his daughter in the front hall. He couldn't get over how far Bianca had come since he'd had her taken from home six months before. For once, Bianca seemed introspective and honest. "I love you and I'm proud of what you're doing here," Alan said.

Bianca gave him a perfunctory hug, then stepped back. "Yeah," she said. "Well, see you around."

He puzzled over that as he drove to the airport. See you around? He'd hoped for something more expressive, more emotional. But he sensed that after all Bianca had been through, she didn't know how to say good-bye.

# 16

## WINTER OF THE UNDERGROUND

THE SCHOOL that had seemed so safe and welcoming when Tanya applied for a job was now beset by insolence. As Thanksgiving neared, boys walked around with low-riding pants and shirttails flapping. Girls hiked up their skirts to show a lot more thigh and calf than was allowed. The logos on kids' jackets seemed to morph and swell, starting from a discreet, quarter-inch-tall name here and there to three or four garish inches of TOMMY and RALPH and ABERCROMBIE screaming from the sleeves. Those signals indicated a breakdown of order. While making the rounds at the end of dorm time one afternoon, Tanya knocked on the door of a boys' room. Swift River had strict rules about women counselors entering boys' rooms, so she stood outside. "Where's Mike?" she asked, when one of the roommates didn't appear.

"In the bathroom."

"Well, tell him everybody has to go to the meeting now."

"He can't — he's jerking off," a boy said, as the others broke into laughter.

Tanya wasn't the only one to sense the difference. Gennarose noticed one of her students doodling in class. She had no problem with innocuous doodling. She spent her free time painting and quite a few of her works had started out as sketches during professors' lectures. But this boy was drawing realistic revolvers. "No way," she declared. "That's not going to happen here."

The kid was miffed. He wasn't just sitting around drawing guns, he explained. He was also drawing bongs.

150

Soon after the last kids in Group 23 arrived on main campus, the next group started trickling in from base camp. One of its members was a slouching, spacey boy. He had done drugs since he was eleven, graduating from pot to ecstasy, acid, and cocaine. Now, at age fourteen, he had a way of sauntering through rooms, oblivious to everyone around him. A counselor scolded him for being out of dress code. He shrugged. The nurses caught him cheeking meds. He shrugged.

One day, the boy sat down for lunch with a couple of anxious parents who were in the middle of an admissions tour. Kids tended to turn on their charm with other people's parents. But not him. "This place is a fuckin' nuthouse," the boy told them. "You don't want your son going here."

The staff put the boy on "admissions tours bans." Convinced that he was doing more than scaring visitors, counselors demanded that he write a truth list. He blithely confessed to stealing food from the dining hall and breaking a toilet so that a geyser shot up every time it was flushed. And by the way, he had masturbated on the toothbrushes of all four of his roommates for three weeks in a row. He did it because he was mad at one of the guys but didn't remember who used which toothbrush. The boy showed no remorse, and the staff figured he had a serious psychiatric disorder.

A second boy who had arrived in the fall meticulously stuffed paper clips and plastic in a drain in the chemistry laboratory day after day until it overflowed. He also thrust a pen at a supervisor as if it were a weapon. A third boy liberated a bottle of air spray from a photography classroom and snorted the inhalant. A fourth sniffed a can of after-shave hoping to get high (instead he got nauseated).

Several students were afraid of a new arrival from base camp who had smuggled opium in his deodorant and gone to the woods to smoke it with three other students. After the counselors confronted him, he slammed his fist through a window. Another boy spent weeks debating whether to stay or go when he turned eighteen. Finally, on the eve of his birthday, he simply skateboarded out of Swift River's driveway and down a hill. He met a friend who was waiting with a car and never came back.

Gennarose was teaching her second-period class when Tyrone barged in, saying he needed to talk. Tyrone? Silent Tyrone? Gennarose stepped outside the classroom to calm him. "What, Tyrone?"

"I can't take those kids anymore!"

Several boys had been acting up in the hallway, he said. They wouldn't keep quiet. And now the kids in his chemistry class were throwing things and taunting the teacher.

"Speak up, Tyrone. Tell them."

"I can't."

"They'll listen to you."

"No."

Gennarose didn't push it. She let him vent, then walked him back to his chemistry class.

During a call home, Tyrone told his mother that Swift River was falling apart; the disrespect and disruptions reminded him of his old high school. Natalie figured it was just Tyrone being hypercritical of others. Hadn't he complained, only a couple of months before, that he couldn't stand the kids in his peer group? And then she had visited and seen him joking around with D.J. and reminiscing about cramming into the sweat lodge with everyone.

Others in the peer group sensed the change on campus. Calculators and pens, sweaters and pants disappeared from dorms. Someone ripped off Mary Alice's camera. Andy picked up his guitar in his room and found the strings busted. D.J. had trouble writing by hand, so the special education consultant arranged for him to use a small laptop. One day he left the laptop in a hallway and never saw it again.

After more than two decades working at therapeutic schools, Rudy and Jill Bentz often said that the programs are cyclical. There are magical moments when the staff and the kids are clicking, when the students are honest and decide to make the most of their time away from home. There are also quiet periods when everyone seems to be just marking time. But a campus with a hundred defiant, depressed, and angry teenagers is always verging on chaos. Sometimes, when too many small things are out of whack, chaos erupts. "It's the perfect storm," said Rudy, sitting at a desk piled with incident reports, the forms that counselors filled out for rule breakers. He corrected himself. "It's the perfect emotional storm. We have a hundred kids dealing with all sorts of issues, and once in a while everything churns to the surface at the same time. It's not necessarily one particular problem that sets it off; it's just the accumulation."

Normally, ten or fifteen students sat in the restriction room talking with counselors and writing out challenge or self-study assignments in loose-leaf notebooks while the rest of the school had free time or study halls. But that winter, the number reached forty-four, a record. Almost every seat was filled. So many boys and girls were ordered to look into mirrors and write about themselves that the staff ran out of mirrors.

While he stood in front of the students and staff to lead the Wednesday morning schoolwide meetings, Rudy liked telling anecdotes about a student's success or reading inspirational letters from graduates of Swift River and other programs where he'd worked. His favorite stories had to do with kids who had broken agreements and been on the verge of expulsion, only to find their "beautiful selves" after graduation. Increasingly, though, Rudy spent the Wednesday meeting bemoaning the decline of civility on the campus: "What's happening is way beyond disrespect, it's an invasion, an attack. It's emotional blackmail." (After 9/11, he had dropped references to emotional terrorism.) He scanned the room for the boy who had masturbated on toothbrushes, and his friend, the drain clogger. "Why do you two feel so weak that you have to do this disgusting crap? What are you so afraid of that makes you take away somebody's education by stuffing the drain in a lab? Do you screw everyone else because you don't know to deal with your own fear and your own pain?" Another counselor stood in front of the students and said that, for the first time in four years at Swift River, he had to lock his car doors because he didn't trust the students. He had tears in his eyes as he spoke.

One by one, the offenders were expelled — eleven in three months. One boy's sketchbook, found after he left, showed women in chains, their hands and feet cut off. And an ornery girl gave the school a special fuck-you gesture on her way out: While running away, she broke into a car and stole a cell phone. Amid the turmoil, Group 23 emerged as the most dependable one on campus. Tanya's kids didn't break toilets, smash windows, or stab anyone with pens. The counselors chose Bianca to serve as a dorm head, which meant she ensured that the girls kept their rooms neat. She and several of Tanya's other kids became work crew bosses, supervising the morning cleaning. Bianca was a benevolent boss; she often scrubbed toilets herself because she didn't like the halfhearted way her work crews did the job. Tanner, now known to everyone as "teddy bear," was so even-handed and trustworthy that the counselors put him in charge of scheduling all work crews. Trevor befriended kids who had pangs for drugs and in his suave accent encouraged them to hang in. (Some kids admired Trevor less for his powers to inspire than for his pharmacological expertise. One boy, desperate to get high on crushed Adderall, asked for tips on how to fake ADD to get a prescription. Trevor turned him in to the counselors.) On his seventeenth birthday, shortly before Christmas, Trevor didn't leave, as he had often threatened to do. Instead, looking past the lighted candles on a foot-long cake at the sea of faces singing to him, he remarked that it was the best birthday he'd ever had. It also marked the first time in four years that he'd been sober on his birthday.

Tyrone made the most dramatic turnaround. For one thing, he looked cheerier. That might have been because the counselors had put him on "black clothes bans." He'd stormed off, but a few hours later he wore a shirt with a dash of color (he kept wearing his black slacks and black boots). The kids chose him to run the school store, which opened for a couple of hours every Sunday. His body was in constant motion, filling bags with shampoo, pivoting to restock toothpaste, then checking a list to tally the purchases so that Swift River could bill the parents. His grades for the winter term reflected his new confidence. He got A's and a couple of B's, enough to put him in the top 20 percent of students. Tyrone — the kid who had barely shown up for school in ninth and tenth grades — made the honor roll. He'd never come close to that. When his mother heard the news, she danced around the kitchen.

Christmas week was difficult for everybody in Tanya's group. Mary Alice missed dashing down the stairs with her three younger siblings to open presents. D.J. missed having hot chocolate in the living room. Tyrone missed the way New York became even more frenetic than usual. Bianca missed Darnell, who had promised to marry her when she was done with Swift River. She didn't talk about her marriage plans because she was surrounded by girls like Mary Alice who liked to hook up with guys for a day or two; they didn't understand long-term commitments. While the kids sorted out their feelings of homesickness, they learned that another girl was going to be dropped into the group. She'd be the fifteenth member. She was short and so shy that she barely spoke. Her dark hair fell over her face as if to protect her from something. Her father lived in one country and her mother, who was crippled by severe depression, lived in another. When kids asked where her home was, the girl said she didn't know.

On Christmas Eve, the rest of the students leaped in the air and shrieked while lobbing giant helium balloons across the great room. They hugged as they opened cards and presents from their parents. Then they squeezed together on the couches, arm in arm, as a counselor read *The Night Before Christmas*. The dark-haired girl sat alone, knees drawn up to her chin, staring at the carpet.

Some of the others snidely referred to Group 23 as the "guru group." A guru was always volunteering to help out or passing incriminating information to counselors. The kids in Group 23 bristled at the teasing. During a school-wide meeting in the great room, Bianca said she had heard enough sneering. She stared down one of the hard cases. "You know, we're struggling with our own stuff, too. It's just that we don't take it out on everyone else."

To be sure, Group 23 was far from perfect. The Ohio girl who hadn't known about her adoption kept "borrowing" clothes from others, then hiding them in her room. In Swift River's rule book, that was akin to stealing. She also was caught in the computer room typing in *Cummington, Mass.*, and other destinations on MapQuest. A teacher realized she was plotting an escape route. And Mary Alice was still struggling. One Saturday she would enjoy an off-campus trip to the movies, chatting in the van with Bianca and a couple of other girls. They agreed that their fathers were overprotective and didn't trust them. They recognized that they'd taken a lot for granted at home — like the ability to leave with friends at a moment's notice. They ate candy and checked out guys at the refreshment stand. Then, just like that, the old Mary Alice would resurface. She spent so much time looking at the models in a copy of *Vogue* — someone had sneaked the magazine onto campus — that a supervisor had to remind her: "Real people do not look like that. Those are starving models." Although her tantrums were less frequent, she was so thin that one of the women on the dining hall staff dubbed her "the skeleton." Tanya made her keep a meal journal, with staff signatures showing that she ate a nutritious breakfast, lunch, and dinner. She was to be weighed daily in the nurse's office — but she wasn't allowed to see her weight. And, most humiliating, Mary Alice needed escorts when she went to the bathroom — girls in good standing who would ensure that she didn't purge.

At this point in the program, the staff was consoled by small victories. For Mary Alice, something seemed to click in mid-January, during

Group 23's two-hour Social Skills Seminar about risk-taking. The counselors talked about why an adolescent is compelled to take risks. They touched on theories of Freud, Erikson, and others about young adults' need for autonomy, affiliation, and identity. At one point the fifteen kids in the group had to examine their own behavior by writing a list. Mary Alice scribbled:

RISKS I TOOK
Sexual: unprotected sex, a lot of different partners
Social: doing things for people's acceptance
Substances: drugs, alcohol, cigarettes
Physical: sneaking out, skipping school, being defiant, having an
    eating disorder
Mental: being very unbalanced
Life risks: everything I did was a life risk.

⁂

Every week or so, several of the counselors drove to a bar in Northampton after work to listen to music and drink beer. Most of the nights out started with the same pledge: no shoptalk. Soon, though, they'd be leaning over a table, heatedly deconstructing the problems at school. They came up with three reasons for the upheaval: corporate pressure to make money, a shrinking pool of applicants who could afford Swift River, and increased competition from other therapeutic programs.

The corporate pressure was in many ways the most jarring. The word had come from headquarters in California announcing that Warburg Pincus, an investment firm, had invested millions of dollars to fund acquisitions and expansions by Swift River's parent company. Several of the counselors had a sinking feeling when they heard about the money: Investors wouldn't care about an overcrowded restriction room; they'd care about lowering the payroll and cramming in extra students. In 1998, Swift River had struggled to hold on to twenty students. It took another three years for enrollment to reach eighty, which many on the staff considered the limit. Now, construction crews were blasting holes in the ground and getting ready to put up two prefabricated dorms, bringing the total capacity on main campus to 145 kids, not counting others in base camp and Costa Rica. A regular school could easily handle 145 students, but this was hardly a regular school.

Just as Swift River was increasing its capacity, the number of applications had declined by close to 30 percent. That was the fallout of September 11: Middle-class parents, reeling from the stock market crash, balked at a $70,000 program. Even families in the South and West who did have the money were chary of committing to a half-dozen round-trip flights for admissions interviews, family seminars, and graduation at a time when security measures made flying onerous. The counselors felt the admissions office was becoming less selective. Several of the new students seemed to have severe problems, from cutting to Asperger's syndrome, that would have disqualified them in the past.

The third factor was, in many ways, a tribute to Swift River. The school had spawned imitators that poached its counseling talent and heightened the competition for applicants. Two of the original faculty members had recently opened a therapeutic boarding school in rural Virginia, and Swift River administrators worried that it would siphon off prospective students from the mid-Atlantic states. Another therapeutic program was starting in New Hampshire and a third in Costa Rica. And Swift River's executive director was busy scouting for property as the company considered opening more residential programs for adolescents.

All this left the staff short-tempered. "The key people are too tired," the special education consultant lamented as she surveyed the packed restriction tables. "The whole place is suffering from internal fatigue." Swift River, like most other therapeutic schools, normally had fairly high turnover, with young staff members burning out after a couple of years and quitting the $30,000-per-year jobs. But now there seemed to be a case of institutional ADHD. In just four months, eight counselors and teachers had left, forcing administrators to scramble to replace them. The new hires weren't always suitable for an unusual school. When Gennarose drove one of the new teachers across campus during a break, he put his head between his knees and shuddered. That was during his third day of work. He didn't return.

Rudy once wrote a grad-school paper comparing therapy to a new business. Just as exponential growth in the start-up phase of a business usually was followed by a plateau, early successes in therapy leveled off. Rudy didn't have a chance to caution Tanya to expect a plateau in the kids' emotional

growth, though. Instead, he called her into his office because he had a surprise: A talkative blond girl named Eva was about to be dropped into
Group 23. That would make Tanya's the biggest group on campus, with sixteen kids.

Eva had been caught flirting, lying, and planning to run away. She had
recently written a thirty-nine-page truth list that was rumored to be the
longest ever at Swift River. If her life could be represented on Rudy's white
board, it would resemble a Kandinsky painting — groups of concentric
circles for rape, divorce, anorexia, school changes, a father who screamed
and threw pans across the kitchen. One of the counselors called her "Eva
the everything kid." He added, "The only thing she hasn't had to deal with
is adoption."

When Tanya stopped a group to announce the news, the nine girls and
six boys reacted by crying and cursing. Just when they had gotten used to
each other, another kid was going to be added to the mix. And not just any
kid — Eva, the one who flirted with boys, infuriated girls, and stirred up
turmoil wherever she went.

# 17

## Disclosures

Amid the outbursts, expulsions, and staff changes that seemed to jolt the campus every day, Tanya needed to maintain the emotional safety of the group. If kids could feel comfortable with one another, if they knew they could speak up without being mocked or sullied by gossip, that would encourage them to be honest about what had gone wrong in their lives. And if they could look at the past with clarity and candor, they could start figuring out how to change. As one counselor often said, "You need to go backward to go forward."

Tanya liked to open group by reading a poem she'd come across or talking about a graceful tango dancer she'd watched. Then she had to call on the right kid. If she went to D.J. first, he'd go mute and start playing with his sleeves. The rest was predictable: One of the girls would chastise him for not contributing to the group. Someone else would jump in and defend D.J., arguing that if everyone kept ganging up on the kid for not talking, then of course he wouldn't bother to talk. That would provoke a confrontation that would leave the others agitated for the remaining two and a half hours. Tanya wouldn't get a lot of therapy done.

It was best to start with Bianca. Sometimes Tanya could simply look at her and say, "What's going on with you?" and Bianca would talk earnestly about missing her boyfriend or feeling like a pariah among the many rich kids at Swift River. She had so much to deal with — layer after layer of tragedies. It took Bianca several months to tell the others about the day when her favorite aunt had been crushed by an elevator while going to the laundry room of her apartment complex. The accident had damaged her spinal cord and left her a paraplegic. Bianca often approached Tanya before group and volunteered to go first. In February, Bianca got news from her father. She asked to discuss it in group.

The kids were chattering about scandals at the school, drawing on the blackboard, adjusting the blinds. Tanya told them to take deep breaths, close their eyes, and make sure their minds returned to the room, to the here and now. She nodded at Bianca and asked why she wanted to talk.

"It's my grandmother — she found a lump in her breast."

Some counselors liked to lead kids to a conclusion, but Tanya preferred open questions, which allowed students to make sense of things. "What does that mean to you?"

"I can't believe this. It's like everyone I know gets sick."

"What else?"

"I know that will happen to me, cancer. It runs in families."

The room was still. Tanya noticed several students leaning forward, ready to offer support. She looked at Bianca, letting everybody know it was her time. No one could rescue her.

"What's going on? It's right there, Bianca."

Bianca spoke in the tiny voice of a frightened girl. "I don't want to love anyone . . . I just get hurt . . . I can't lose anybody again."

It was tougher to get through to the boys. Especially Trevor. Although he talked glibly in group about his London raves and computer hacking, he rarely went below the surface to reveal what he was feeling. Tanya sensed that he was waiting for a chance to open up.

"What about you, Trevor?" Tanya said one day, after Bianca had checked in with the group.

"I'm fine, Tanya. What about you?" He flashed his big grin — the one that had prompted smile bans in base camp. The kids knew that when Trevor fobbed off a question, he was hiding something. Tanya pinned her gaze on him. Everyone waited.

Trevor said he had been thinking about something that happened years ago, but he wasn't ready to talk about it. "Come on," Tanner urged. He and Trevor had been inseparable for the first few weeks on campus, but then they'd found other friends.

Trevor slouched and looked at his black Vans sneakers. The other kids shifted their feet and cleared their throats. They listened to the clinking of flatware as the dining hall staff set up lunch across the way.

"It's okay, Trevor," Bianca said.

Trevor started talking without looking up. It began when he was eight and living in Spain, where his parents had been transferred. He used to go swimming with the twelve-year-old boy next door. Trevor, who felt as if he was rattling around the house while his parents were working, liked the attention. Trevor's parents were glad that he had a healthy activity.

He paused, as if weighing whether to say more.

"Take your time," Tanya said.

After swimming, Trevor said, they'd go to the boy's house to watch TV or just to hang out. One day, the boy touched Trevor while they were changing. It soon got worse. Trevor talked in a vague way, but he let everyone know that the boy molested him regularly — and threatened to kill him if he breathed a word of it. When he was finished, Tanner asked how long the abuse had lasted. About two years, Trevor said. He was crying.

As the group ended, Tanya asked Trevor to stand and look at the faces of the group as the kids said what they loved or admired about him.

"You're so fun to be with," said Mary Alice.

"You're cool," said Tyrone.

"You're so brave," said Bianca.

Trevor's disclosure encouraged other kids to open up in the weeks that followed. Phil, the founder of the Chillisism movement, was struggling with his sexual identity; for a while, he thought he might be bisexual. Andy, the boy with the muttonchops, talked about the times he'd get drunk and race through Long Island towns at ninety miles per hour with his best friend. The previous Christmas Eve, they'd gone out to breakfast. A few hours later, the friend had sped through town, crashed into a telephone pole, and died. Andy felt guilty for not speaking up about the drinking and driving, guilty for not being in the car with him, guilty for being alive. And he felt guilty for continuing to drive recklessly — even when he left the boy's funeral, he'd torn away at ninety.

On a bitter cold day, the kids sat in group making small talk. A counselor named Candice asked Tanner how things were going. He rambled about the work crews he was supervising. Other kids' eyes drifted to the window. Specks of snow had started to shimmy in the gusts outside.

Opening a folder, Candice urged Tanner to focus on his struggles back home. He looked at Candice, then Tanya, as if trying to guess what they were up to. Candice pulled out a half dozen folded loose-leaf pages. As she straightened them out, Tanner's oversized half-cursive, half-block handwriting was visible.

They had his suicide notes.

Tanner spoke haltingly about his low point, in eleventh grade. His grandmother had died, followed by his grandfather. His girlfriend had dumped him because he was drinking. His friends were dealing drugs. He went to his room, opened a suitcase stuffed with autographed baseballs and other memorabilia his dad had given him, and withdrew a Browning .22 semiautomatic that he'd bought from another kid for seventy-five dollars. He wrote good-bye notes to his best friends, his favorite teacher, and his former girlfriend. Then he put the pistol in his mouth and waited to squeeze the trigger but lost his nerve.

The candor inspired even Tyrone and D.J. Tyrone talked about how he'd lost interest in everything after his father left. He had daydreamed about killing himself, and one day he called a friend and said he was thinking about stabbing himself with a letter opener. In a strange way, he was lucky that the inertia that kept him from going to school and doing anything else also kept him from figuring out how to commit suicide.

D.J. was more reflective than he had been for months. He mentioned that he once broke a Christmas ornament in a pique and used it to scratch the surface of a grand piano that had been handed down in the family for three generations. Then there was the time his parents brought a punching bag to let him work out his aggression. He chopped it to shreds with an ax. Without prompting, D.J. brought up his childhood bed-wetting. Although he'd alluded to it before, he'd glossed over the details. This time he admitted that he'd worn disposable pull-ups till second grade. He couldn't go to sleepovers at friends' houses. His mother took him to psychologists, pediatricians, and urologists. Finally one said that his bladder had developed slowly and he would outgrow the problem — which turned out to be true. It was called nocturnal enuresis, and the doctor said it wasn't a big deal (enuresis sometimes appeared to be a big deal because fathers and mothers got frustrated and angry with bed-wetting kids, whose self-esteem was then shaken). Still, the whole fiasco made him feel defective — like merchandise his parents would decide to return to the adoption agency.

The girls revealed sexual secrets. Ashley, the New Yorker, talked about how her abusive boyfriend would charm her one day and force her to have sex the next. He was a rich, preppy guy and no one suspected he had a violent side. Once he'd pushed her down a flight of stairs. She'd invented an excuse when her parents noticed her bruises. Ashley said she took long showers whenever she remembered the abuse, trying to wash away the feeling that she was dirty. "*Ho!*" Bianca chimed in. She also took showers all the time, trying to cleanse herself of the memories of abuse in the locker room.

Mary Alice recounted one night when she was in tenth grade. She had been cruising in an SUV with two handsome seniors — guys whom every girl at school noticed. They pulled into a cul-de-sac and drank. One of the boys started fondling Mary Alice in the backseat. Soon they were having sex. When the boy got off her, the other pushed her back in the seat and had sex with her. Mary Alice wanted to stop him, but she was drunk and scared. A suspicious neighbor called the police. When the cops showed up, the boys said they were just hanging out. Mary Alice was so flustered she simply agreed with them. Within twenty-four hours, it seemed every high school student in a twenty-mile range knew the details of the incident. One boy left a message on the family's answering machine: "Hey, Mary Alice, I heard what you and those two guys did, you slut." Mary Alice's father listened to the message. He wasn't sure what had gone on, but he screamed at her for disgracing the family. After that, Mary Alice was so humiliated that she couldn't concentrate in school.

"I felt like a whore," she told the group. Tanya asked how she'd dealt with it, but she had already guessed the answer: Mary Alice locked herself in her bathroom and vomited.

Bianca seemed ready to deal with the memories she had suppressed. Tanya told her to take her time. When someone is violated, her control is taken away, so the last thing Tanya wanted to do was force her to talk — to violate her again. "I'll help you sort it through, but only when you are ready."

Bianca found it easier to write her disclosures before discussing them. She included this one in her revised, unabridged life story. It happened in ninth grade. Kenneth was a good-looking guy, a football player, who lived with his mom a few blocks from the park where Bianca used to hang out as a kid. Kenneth had a blustery way — he'd say anything that was on his mind. One thing he said was that he wanted to take Bianca's virginity, but she waved him off. She had just turned fifteen; she was going to wait till she got married.

One afternoon they were watching a movie in his living room. His mom wasn't home. They kissed.

Bianca wrote:

> He started taking off my clothes and I said I didn't want to have sex and pushed away from him. Then he started again and said we wouldn't have sex. I naively believed him and he picked me up and we went into his room, here he threw me on the bed and held my ankles to my wrists. The whole time I was yelling and screaming for him to stop and that he was hurting me. He raped me. He didn't stop until he came and then he just left me in his room and told me to hurry up and leave.
>
> I got dressed and walked home; no one was there but my brother. I took a shower, went to my room and cried.
>
> I never told anyone about this.

The winter took a toll on Tanya. While putting in longer hours than she had at Harvard, the group home for the mentally ill, and the inner-city schools where she'd interned, she couldn't tell whether she was doing any good. At night, just as Tanya was preparing to leave, D.J. would feel homesick or one of the girls would vent about a phone conversation with her mother. Tanya brought her job home with her: teachers' notes, forms summarizing calls with parents, monthly progress reports on the kids, bulletins on adolescent mental health, and so on.

A concerned supervisor ordered her not to take on any more work at night. Tanya promised to obey. But less than a week later, she was back on her living room couch, scouring a book about bulimia. In her free time, she visited her mentor, an expert on eating disorders, to discuss the best way to treat Mary Alice.

Tanya and Gennarose made each other laugh, and that was no small comfort after a day of dealing with everyone's emotional detritus. They skipped most of the noisy gatherings of counselors at the Northampton bar. Instead, they went out for coffee. They, too, tried to talk about anything other than the job: guys, dancing, music. Tanya admitted that she'd lost all perspective. She'd worked with a couple of co-counselors, and she couldn't tell how effective they'd been with Group 23. "It's such a whirlwind," she said. "There's never any time to reflect."

"You've got the best group on campus," Gennarose said. "You get some credit for that."

As Tanya felt more comfortable about the group's progress, she tried to figure out how much to talk about herself. Until now, she had tried to listen to the kids without telling them more than surface details about herself, just as she'd been taught. Once she had worked for a year with a young woman who had an eating disorder; on the last day, the client asked Tanya if she, too, had an eating disorder. Tanya's training kicked in as she made a quick judgment call. She wasn't a friend or a big sister or a parent; she was a counselor. If Tanya said she did have an eating disorder, the client might see her as a troubled therapist who had no business giving advice. If she said she did not have an eating disorder, the client might see her as a therapist who couldn't possibly relate. Rather than answering, Tanya turned the question back on the young woman: "What would it mean to you if I have an eating disorder? What would it mean to you if I didn't?" By the end of the discussion, the client didn't want to find out. (The answer was no).

At a program like Swift River, however, Tanya found it hard to be a blank slate. She ate with the kids, counseled them, and hiked with them. While on the late shift, she even tucked the girls into bed. Before group started, as the counselors stood in the hall planning their strategy, the kids would sit in a circle discussing which counselors smoked cigarettes (they smelled it on counselors' clothing), and who had broken up with a boyfriend or girlfriend (they read it on the counselors' faces). Kids like Bianca were especially good at sensing when a counselor was going through trying times. And Tanya was going through a trying time. She'd learned that her father's cancer had returned. In March the doctor said he had two years, at most, to live.

As group wrapped up one morning, Tanya said she needed to let everyone know something. She knew she had been distracted — walking by kids without acknowledging them. She didn't want anybody to feel slighted or misinterpret her moods. "I've told you that my father is sick. We found out the cancer is definitely terminal."

"What's 'terminal?'" D.J. asked.

"That means he'll die," Tanya answered. She tried so hard to use a matter-of-fact tone that her voice seemed unnatural.

"You're always saying you're here for us," said Ashley. "We're here for you, too."

"*Ho!*" Mary Alice and Bianca said.

Afterward, when Tanya couldn't hear, several of the kids speculated about what this news meant for them. It didn't sound good. One group after another had lost counselors during the riotous winter — they'd burned out or left to travel or followed a fiancé to a distant place. Tanya, meanwhile, had become a mainstay of the school: She spoke up at meetings when she objected to rude behavior, especially when the boys were treating girls as objects. The more forceful she was, the more controversial she became. Girls from other groups said she was too damn picky about the dress code. Boys from other groups griped that she was a feminist — often expressed as "fuckin' feminist." But the sixteen kids in Group 23 had closed ranks around her. After tussling with Tanya for months, Mary Alice now saw her as an example of a strong, principled woman.

One night, after Tanya returned from a weekend visiting her father in the hospital in upstate New York, she was sitting in the phone room, trying to keep tabs on five kids' conversations at the same time. Bianca stopped by.

"How'd it go?" Bianca asked.

It wasn't easy, Tanya said. Her dad was sick of being sick.

"I'm sorry. I know what it's like." Bianca used one of Tanya's phrases: "Let me know if you ever want to talk about it."

Tanya said she'd tried to cheer her dad by reading some of his old poems out loud and reminiscing about the days when she was a kid and they'd built houses for gnomes in the woods. But it was hard to be cheery with someone who was in pain, and tired of being probed by doctors.

"I remember scrubbing my arms and hands and going into my mom's hospital room," Bianca said. "I dreaded going because I didn't want to stand by and watch my mom die. You want to do something so bad, but you have no control, and feel guilty for not wanting to go."

Bianca recalled some good times, too. There was the day that she and her sister and brother smuggled their two cats into the hospital. Her mom was ecstatic. Another time, when her mother despaired of eating more hospital food, they sneaked in hot dogs and hamburgers and had a picnic. Bianca shared her seventeen-year-old-therapist-in-training take on terminal illness: "You want the end to come, you don't want the person to suffer any longer, but then you don't want the end to come."

Tanya was the first adult Bianca could talk openly to since her stepmother had left. If Tanya quit to care for her dad — if she couldn't go with the group to Costa Rica — then Bianca would once again watch someone walk out of her life. But this was larger than Bianca. She was sure that if Tanya left, the guru group would fall apart.

# 18

## MAKING CONNECTIONS

IN ALL HIS YEARS of attending classes and avoiding classes, Tyrone couldn't remember having a conversation with a teacher. The schools in Queens had been like factories: teachers showed up, punched the clock, and glumly waited for their shifts to end. Then there was Gennarose. She cried as she read poetry out loud, but she also spoke in a no-bull, New York way, cracking jokes and exploding with expressions like "Oh, my god, I shit in my pants!" Tyrone liked the way she didn't take crap from the rich kids who acted like they owned the place. Daddy and mommy's money didn't impress her; if a boy threw a book across the room or a girl said something vulgar, she'd sign them up to wash dishes for a week.

As they were walking across campus one day, Gennarose said she'd noticed that Tyrone avoided eye contact with Ashley, who had gotten him in trouble with her runaway plan in base camp, and Tanya, who constantly challenged him. And everyone could tell that he acted as if Bianca were invisible — even though she once had been his closest confidant at Swift River.

"Do you have a problem with women?" Gennarose asked.

"I don't want to talk about it."

"Go ahead. I can take it."

"I don't think women are as strong or as smart as men."

"Do you have a problem with me?"

"I don't want to hurt your feelings."

Gennarose stopped and looked at him. "But you think I'm a feminist and you don't like that, right? I've got news, Tyrone: feminists aren't all smelly, hairy-arm-pitted, organic lesbians."

"Well, you're sort of different, but that doesn't change my opinion."

"Believe me, by the time you leave here, your opinion will be changed."

Gennarose had a healthy smattering of oppositional defiance disorder, the kind of ODD that prompted her to grouse once in a while about Swift River's push to increase revenues by increasing the student population. Leaning against a wall, she'd roll her big eyes and run her hand through her long dark hair as she told the kids of her unease with profit-making companies insinuating themselves into education and mental health. She refused to kowtow to the school administration. She developed a course on existentialism for twelfth graders. The kids read Kafka, Camus, and Conrad. They spoke up about *Metamorphosis*, they debated *The Stranger* in the dining hall; it was as if they'd been waiting for someone to challenge their intellects. When Rudy Bentz heard that Gennarose was teaching *Heart of Darkness* over in the academic building, he sent word that she should drop it immediately. He reasoned that a teacher couldn't simply have a bunch of Swift River kids, many of whom had endured their own heart of darkness for years, read such a gruesome, upsetting book without the guidance of a trained counselor.

Gennarose considered Rudy a control freak, and she didn't have a lot of time for his therapeutic-boarding-school-style metaphors about hearts of darkness. She wrote a two-thousand-word note defending her assignment, but she didn't bother waiting for a response. She kept teaching the book, and Rudy never brought it up again.

Gennarose couldn't get over the fact that bright students who had attended schools in some of the country's fanciest zip codes were missing big chunks of their education. Although they could describe every character in reality TV shows, they had never read the classics. She'd ask if they'd ever encountered *The Scarlet Letter*. No. *To Kill a Mockingbird?* Nope. Did they remember who wrote *Romeo and Juliet?* What's-his-name. Writing in longhand, without a spell-check program, the kids didn't know how to spell or punctuate. And yet they could produce raw, poignant essays. They wrote with haunting details about disappointing their parents or watching their lives fall apart and feeling like losers among kids who used to be their closest friends in middle school.

During sixth period, Gennarose taught eleventh graders. She used the lecture notes she'd kept from the year before, when she'd taken a course called Foundations in American Literature with her favorite professor at Columbia, Andrew del Banco. "I'm not going to dumb down my vocabulary," she told her students. "I'm teaching you the kind of class you'll get in college because no one has done you any good by underestimating you." She had expected that Bianca would be the standout of the nine students. Bianca did her homework dutifully and acted polite. But that was about it. She sat in the back of the class and spoke up just enough to show that she was paying attention. Gennarose rearranged the seats in a circle, but somehow Bianca managed to disappear behind her notebook.

During that bleak winter they slogged through what Gennarose called the Dead White Male Triumvirate: Emerson, Thoreau, and Whitman. Bianca perked up a bit in the next phase of the class, when they read Emily Dickinson's poems. Each student in English 11 was required to keep a daily journal. Bianca wrote tepid entries that seemed to focus on how many pages of a book she'd finished. The readings, she allowed, were pretty interesting.

Gennarose realized that several of Swift River's teachers regarded the talk of holistic education as so much babble. They made it clear that they were busy putting together lesson plans, grading papers, and keeping order in the classroom; they didn't have time to be counselors or Ultimate Frisbee coaches on top of that. Gennarose, though, made a point of inviting each member of the peer group to chat in the great room or to sit down to dinner on Wednesdays, when she worked the late shift. Bianca seemed happy enough to meet, but she talked about herself in a distant way. She rattled off the litany of tragedies she'd known: death, divorce, rape. It wasn't a conversation so much as a recitation — an obligatory response to a school assignment, to be graded, discarded, and forgotten.

At last, Gennarose reached her favorite part of English 11, leaving behind the Dead White Males. She started with a book that had been a favorite of hers in high school, *The Autobiography of Frederick Douglass*. "You guys take so many things for granted," she told the class. "Douglass didn't know where he was born, how old he was, or who his mother and father were. Think about how awesome it was for Douglass when he learned to read." A few hours later, Gennarose saw Bianca in the hall, engrossed in the book. "It's great, Gennarose. Thanks for picking it." Suddenly, Bianca's journal was packed with observations about race. She filled page after page with descriptions of plantation life. She wrote about the struggles of those who look different or act different from the majority.

Gennarose told the class that the slave songs were like the 1800s version of hip-hop and rap; the slaves were mixing vernacular with mainstream English to come up with their own language. Bianca loved that. She went back to her dorm and dashed out rap lyrics. It was Frederick Douglass meets Tupac Shakur:

> What's this I hear you saying my life's easy?
> Boy, you don't know half the shit I go through just to be me.
> Like maybe what it's like to have someone hold you down and rape
>    you
> Or what it's like to have your mother die.

Now Bianca wasn't just an enthusiastic student, she was practically a co-teacher. When Gennarose asked if prejudice still existed, the other students shook their heads. Bianca, though, riffed on the subjects of segregation in neighborhoods and the scarcity of good roles for Hispanics in television shows. When they had lunch together, Bianca was brimming with questions about Gennarose's travels, her music, her interest in Spanish. Gennarose wondered how many times adults had given up on Bianca and the other kids at Swift River before taking the time to find their passions.

Several things happened that seemed to help Mary Alice, including a new diagnosis, new meds, and a couple of reminders of how much she'd matured. The first was the most controversial: The consulting psychiatrist had diagnosed bipolar disorder and given her mood stabilizers. Some of the counselors were dubious about the latest twist — bipolar seemed to be emerging as the catchall label for moody teenagers, and weren't teenagers supposed to be moody? But to other counselors, the diagnosis helped explain Mary Alice's behavior. One book in the headmaster's office, *Understanding Teenage Depression,* noted that bipolar disorder involves cycles of depression and mania — from insomnia and reduced appetite to irrational elation. The book seemed to offer a thumbnail profile of Mary Alice. "She may do her schoolwork enthusiastically and quickly, but in a disorganized way," it said. "Teenagers who are manic may start numerous projects with great enthusiasm but carry none of them to a conclusion, act fresh and talk too fast and too loudly, become overconfident of their abilities, have difficulty sleeping but nevertheless do not feel tired . . . Promiscuity can also be a problem."

Tanya knew that Mary Alice needed an adult she could trust. Who had ever listened to her or accepted the fact that everything wasn't fine? So Tanya listened in the dining hall, and in the dorm, and in the great room. Mary Alice stopped demanding facial creams and clothes. She got back into photography, walking the campus alone in the late afternoon and shooting close-up photos of trees from angles that made them look like sculptures. The images had such an impact that her art teacher displayed them in the hall of the classroom building. Mary Alice's weight gradually climbed to 126 — close enough to the goal of 135 Tanya had set, and in the normal range for a muscular girl of five foot ten.

Mary Alice needed resilience to deal with the latest package her parents had sent. It was the Garfield diary she'd kept the previous summer. She reread it with fascination and horror, like a voyeur peeping into someone's sordid affairs. Amid the descriptions of sex with random boys in her travels, she stepped back and made poignant observations. "Why is it that everywhere I go," she had written, "I always meet some kick-ass guy and fall in love with him and then I have to go back to the real world where no guys from Dallas will touch me because I'm such a slut, and I am." The diary was interesting, too, for what was missing. Mary Alice had been so self-centered that she rarely mentioned her siblings. The only reference to her mother and father read, "My parents basically told me I was ruining the family and that they just didn't care anymore."

At one point, she had scrawled, "I pray to God that nobody opens this or that would suck big time." Looking back, though, she was fairly certain she'd left the diary out on her night table so that someone *would* read it and pay attention to her.

Mary Alice was also jolted by a letter from a girl back home. "Dallas sucks!" the friend wrote. "There's nothing to do on the weekend and all we do is drive around and smoke bowls. Ha ha. I kind of need to stop." The friend mentioned that her parents were trying to thwart her drinking and drug use by giving her nightly Breathalyzer tests and frequent urine tests. The letter detailed girls' feuds and their sexual adventures, often both at the same time: "I was going to call Paige and say, *Hey, just wanted to remind you: Every time you kiss Rus, just know that he ate me out, bitch!"* Mary Alice read the letter over and over. Her friend sounded so callow, so superficial. Something else upset her. The casual allusions to drugs, sex, and vicious gossip sounded frighteningly familiar. "That stuff," she said one day in group, "that could have been me if I'd stayed home."

Tanya realized that whenever Mary Alice remembered her middle school and high school years, she used the words that others had called her, starting with "slut" and "free willy." She needed a chance to go beyond the labels, to redefine herself and recognize her strengths. It was time to put aside the past for a while and think about the future, Tanya said. What would Mary Alice be doing in five years?

Mary Alice eagerly took to it. She wrote a newspaper article that she hoped to see printed in her hometown newspaper in five years:

> Mary Alice Chambliss, a former Dallasite, just received the photographer of the year award along with winning the championship in the women's snowboard free-ride competition.
>
> Chambliss, who is 22, is one of the youngest ever to receive the two awards. She also has started EDA (Eating Disorders of America), helping thousands of girls and young women fight the battle of anorexia and bulimia.
>
> A former anorexic and bulimic, she struggled with her eating disorder for five grueling years. Her parents decided to send her to a therapeutic boarding school during her junior year of high school. She spent 14 months getting to the root of her disorder along with her drug problems and promiscuity. After several months of starving herself and relapsing, Mary Alice graduated the program loving and respecting herself truly for the first time in her life.
>
> She was able to go off to college and study photography and psychology and was the captain of the snowboarding team. She lived in Europe for two years. Mary Alice says, "I have never felt better about myself and where I am headed." Although she still has her struggles, she wants to get more involved with acting and singing and helping out her community . . .

Tanya nodded when she read the piece a day later. This wasn't the I'm-just-fine Mary Alice she had tangled with in the fall. Nor was it the I'm-a-slut girl who had flirted with death back home. It was someone trying to find a middle ground, to achieve balance, instead of living in extremes. That was progress.

✍

In many ways, D.J. made the most dramatic turnaround of Group 23. He befriended a gym teacher, a six foot two, 260-pound former Marine known as "Big Mike," who led a wilderness survival course. For fun, Big Mike entered strongman competitions on weekends. He threw telephone poles, lifted boulders, and strapped himself in a harness to pull his pickup truck. D.J. liked to talk about cars and exercise regimes with him. D.J. was most relaxed on Fridays, when kids took a field trip to a gym that had a forty-foot climbing wall. He'd strap on safety ropes and scurry to the top, grabbing the artificial rocks and contorting his body; for a few moments he was almost horizontal. Then he'd dangle in the air like a spider before scuttling down. In a classroom, D.J. had a nervous habit of stretching his long sleeves and poking holes in them with his fingers, but on field trips he stopped mutilating his shirts and even laughed. Gennarose thought of Huckleberry Finn, who despaired of sitting still in school when there was so much to explore outdoors. Huck said it best, "It was deadly dull and I was fidgety."

What if Huck had grown up in the New Jersey suburbs of perfect lawns and high-achieving parents and storefront SAT prep centers? The Widow Douglas and Miss Watson would have given him Ritalin — assuming they had health insurance. And what if Huck had tried to light out for the territory? They would have committed him to an institution — a therapeutic boarding school or, more likely, a lockdown facility.

D.J. gradually came alive in classes. One day when the kids were discussing "Bartleby the Scrivener," Gennarose asked D.J. what he thought. She expected a yawn. Instead, D.J. launched into a soliloquy. Bartleby, he explained, was a metaphor for the typical person who goes through adulthood in a state of hibernation, avoiding taking action, like a bear in winter. D.J. continued with the metaphor: Melville, as the narrator, was trying to wake Bartleby from his slumber, to make him stand up and do something. "Holy shit!" Gennarose blurted out. "Why don't you speak up more often?" D.J. blushed.

Kate Simmons, a science teacher, would start writing on the board in class and hear D.J. riffling through the drawers in the lab, pulling out a rabbit pelt to make static electricity or a rubber stopper to roll in his hands. "Do you really have to do that?" she'd ask, even as she realized he *did* need to. D.J. disliked reading from textbooks and he froze during tests, but as soon as the class did hands-on experiments, he perked up. In the fall term, when Kate taught biology, the class spent a couple of weeks studying water. Kate started by bringing in samples of tap water tainted with oil and coffee grounds. Lining up flasks and beakers, D.J. analyzed the samples, separating the layers of gunk. He invented filters made of charcoal, paper, and cotton. He came to class brimming with questions.

Other students flagged in the winter term, when the class segued to chemistry, but not D.J. Kate gave the students toothpicks and gumdrops to make structural models of chemicals. Whoever made them correctly got to eat the project. D.J. pieced together a naphthalene model in seconds, and while others were still toiling he was already munching on the gumdrops and cleaning his teeth with the toothpicks. A week later, D.J. was riveted when Kate opened class by producing a roll of pennies and teasing, "We are going to do something illegal. Don't try this at home. We're going to destroy U.S. currency." D.J. volunteered to lead the experiment. He filled small beakers with hydrochloric acid, dropped in pennies that he'd scratched, and left them overnight. The next day, he rushed in to class. The pennies made before 1982 were unharmed, while the acid chewed out the insides of the newer pennies. Kate asked if anyone had a theory. "The old pennies are almost pure copper," D.J. explained triumphantly, "but starting in 1982 they added a zinc alloy."

Later, in another experiment, D.J. volunteered to drop pennies into nitric acid. The pennies bubbled up in an Alka Seltzer–like fugue of red-orange. "Awesome!" D.J. said. Kate asked for a more scientific observation. "It's copper turning to copper ions," he reported. He was so excited about chemistry that he volunteered to do extra-credit projects. In his first two terms of science, he earned a B-plus and an A. Kate, like all teachers, had to send comments to the counselors. "D.J.," she wrote, "is a joy to have in class."

∽

On a raw Thursday in March, the Group 23 parents whisked their kids off for a three-day weekend at hotels across New England. The weekend, the kids' first away from Swift River, was a step toward preparing them to go home. The rules were simple: The hotel had to be within three hours of campus, and the parents and kids had to continue to discuss the issues that had divided them. And, of course, no drugs or drinking.

Mary Alice and her family set off for a historic inn next to snowboarding trails (and near some cute clothing stores). As they left, Tanya reminded Mary Alice and her parents of a special agreement they'd made: no shopping. All three started to protest, but Tanya cut them off: "No shopping. You need to find other ways to relate to each other." D.J. drove to an old speakeasy that had been turned into a hotel; it was next to ski slopes he'd loved when he was little. Bianca went to a Vermont ski lodge with her brother, sister, and father. As a Floridian, she knew nothing about snow skiing, so she'd relax in the indoor pool.

Tyrone didn't say much except that he'd sleep late and watch TV. No one asked for details, so he didn't add that while the others stayed in mountainside hotels with spas and four-star restaurants, he and his mother were going to a $45-a-night motel next to a bar in a dying factory town near Swift River.

During the weekend, D.J. played pool with his father, skied with his mother, and avoided talking about group therapy as much as possible. Over breakfast, he and his parents caught up on the gossip at D.J.'s old school, where Theodor taught. Things were going well until D.J. looked for a book of matches with the hotel's logo that had caught his eye. It had disappeared from their room. He looked at his parents accusingly.

"You thought I'd do something, didn't you?"

Theodor said he didn't want D.J. to be tempted. D.J. said he'd planned on saving the matchbook for his collection; he wasn't going to ignite anything. He stared at his father in stony silence, as if weighing whether to have an outburst.

"Okay," D.J. said finally. "What if you bring the matchbook home so I can have it when I come back?"

Theodor agreed. In many other families, the conversation wouldn't have been memorable, but Theodor kept replaying it to himself. D.J. hadn't lost his temper; instead, he'd found a way to defuse a conflict.

At the ski lodge, Bianca went swimming with her sister, her brother, and her father. As they splashed around, she talked about the last few years of her life. She started by telling them about the North Carolina wilderness program. At first, she despised it, but then she almost came to relish the simplicity of it — she found she was good at busting fires and cooking dinner with just a few ingredients. Finding a dead bee in her peanut butter was a bit too much, though. As she floated in the pool, she realized it was the first time she could remember her family swimming together since her mom died.

The conversation continued through dinner. Bianca talked about how she had felt when she lived at home. She couldn't confide in anyone, not even her own family, about everything she'd been through. Darnell, her boyfriend, was the only one who was there for her, listening and not judging. Bruno, Bianca's twin, didn't say much. He'd always been like that, but Bianca knew he was taking it in.

Bianca and Bruno went walking on snowshoes for the first time. They threw chunks of snow at each other and laughed. Then they sat in the lodge and Bianca grew serious. She told Bruno about the rape. It had happened a year and a half before. Bruno remembered Bianca coming home that day. He'd sensed that something terrible had occurred, but Bianca had barricaded herself in her room.

Several times during the weekend, Bianca had an urge to filch her father's cell phone and call Darnell. Her father wouldn't notice. But Tanya had made it clear: The hotel trip was about reconnecting with her family, not her boyfriend. Instead, Bianca called her grandmother in Florida to ask about her cancer. Her grandmother said she had started chemotherapy but she was feeling okay.

"I want to be with you," Bianca said.

"The best thing for you to do is to stay up there at that school and take care of yourself."

Afterward, Bianca and her older sister, Claudia, sat alone in a sauna. Bianca had decided to be honest. She said she'd always resented Claudia; everyone knew Claudia was their father's favorite. Claudia said it didn't seem that way to her; as the firstborn, she felt pushed by her father. Bianca explained to Claudia what she'd learned in group about perceptions; in some cases the truth wasn't as important as how people perceived things.

Bianca told her sister in detail about the rape. Claudia listened quietly, then revealed that a drunk guy had once attacked her at a party; she'd managed to slip away.

"It was what normal sisters do, sisters who get along: sit up all night and talk to each other," Bianca wrote in her journal. "It made me really happy that we could have that conversation and not be at each other's necks half the time and I didn't have to act fake. It also made me feel really sad, because I wish we could have had this type of relationship before."

Late that night, Claudia got a call from Florida. Her cat was dying. The cat had been a favorite pet of their mother's and had even visited her in the hospital. Claudia decided to cut short her visit and fly back. She got up before dawn on Saturday to pack. On her way out, Claudia bent over Bianca's bed and kissed her on the cheek. "I'm glad you're my sister," Claudia whispered. Bianca lay in bed, pretending to be asleep.

# 19

## DATING, DUMPING,
## AND DRY-HUMPING

IN EARLY APRIL, Alan Bittman received a letter from Bianca. She explained that the kids in her group had been doing an exercise to describe the kind of relationship they wanted with their parents. She had decided on an "honest, comfortable" one, even when it came to conversations about sex. "But I have to tell you it does feel awkward talking to you about some of this stuff," she wrote. "Because 1st you're my dad! And 2nd no one (I'm exaggerating) talks about this stuff!" At the end of the letter, she asked a favor. After months of being limited to writing to relatives, she had reached the part of the program where she was allowed to exchange letters with friends. She'd written to her boyfriend, Darnell, who had moved, and she hadn't heard a peep. She wondered if her father could get in touch with Darnell and remind him to respond.

Darnell? Alan grimaced. Why couldn't Bianca forget about him? She was a gifted actress and soccer player; she was going somewhere. Darnell, though, was a hapless dropout. Worse, really. As Bianca had reluctantly revealed when she told her life story, Darnell had been expelled from high school for carrying a knife. How could she have come so far at Swift River and still be thinking about that loser?

In his weekly call to Tanya, Alan Bittman asked for advice. What could he do to push Bianca to dump Darnell?

"Nothing," Tanya said.

"But she deserves so much better."

"Let her decide that. You can unload on me when we talk, but when you speak to Bianca, don't be judgmental."

That wasn't what Alan wanted to hear. He'd been too lenient with Bianca in the past. She needed help understanding that she'd soon be in college, surrounded by guys with ambition. Who better to explain that than her father? After all, he and Teresa had met at the University of South Florida when they were both sophomores, and they'd ended up getting married. Teresa was the love of his life. Bianca knew that, so how could she fall for a guy on a slow train to nowhere?

Rudy Bentz always told the parents to "trust the process." In six months, Bianca would turn eighteen. Okay, Alan would trust the process; he'd let Bianca make her own mistakes in romance. Still, that didn't mean he had to play Cupid and track down Darnell at some Friendly's counter where he was serving strawberry Fribbles.

In a windowless office off the great room, Tanya and Julie Haagenson, a supervisor, were talking strategy about Bianca. Tanya's group was entering the third stage of Swift River's four-part curriculum. The kids in the peer group had learned about anger and insecurities in the first and second phases. Now they were starting what many counselors considered the crux: figuring out who they were and what they believed. As Rudy liked to say, they would strip away their emotional baggage and get to their core identities, their beautiful selves. The counselors called this part of the program "shames and blames." Over the years, even students who had held everything together during the first few months at Swift River revealed their darkest secrets during this phase. They admitted to swiping their neighbors' DVD players or pilfering mom's Valium. Sexual secrets came out: guilt over experimenting with friends of the same sex; embarrassment about racking up a thousand dollars on dad's Visa while surfing S&M Web sites.

Julie tied her long black hair in a French twist; her skin seemed to have a perpetual tan. She drove a Jeep and worked as a disc jockey in her free time. Boys stammered and lost their concentration around her; girls unconsciously imitated Julie's habit of sweeping back her hair. Julie had gone through her own reckless adolescence — drugs, guys, everything — before buckling down and studying psychology in college. She worried about a kid like Bianca. In three years of counseling at Swift River, Julie had found that the students who didn't push the boundaries during the fourteen months, didn't slip up and get in trouble, were often the ones who struggled afterward. Julie wanted to push Bianca to lose her cool. Better to make a misstep at Swift River than to wait and do it at home after graduation, with no counselors around.

"The next few weeks are going to be hard on Bianca," Julie told Tanya. "She's busy being Miss Perfect Straight-A Student. We're gonna crack that."

One morning, the sixteen spread across the great room, each sitting at a small table, for a Social Skills Seminar on dating. Bianca looked morose, Mary Alice anxious. Tyrone and D.J. stared out the windows. Julie started by mentioning a few statistics. Nearly one in five kids loses his or her virginity by the age of fifteen. Among high school sophomores, 16 percent have had four or more sexual partners; one in four sexually active teens has contracted a sexually transmitted disease. Things had changed dramatically in a couple of generations, she said. Not long ago, probably when their parents were teenagers, people generally got to know each other before having sex, not the other way around.

Julie and Tanya handed each kid a set of ten index cards printed with words associated with dating and relationships. "If you were to start seeing someone now, how would you like it to happen?" Julie asked. "What would you do first? Don't worry about what you think your parents would want to hear or what we want to hear. Think about your ideal situation if you could start over."

Bianca moved the dating cards around with the tentativeness of a novice poker player laying out a hand. As she changed the order, she realized she'd had only a vague idea of what a real, old-fashioned date was like. Guys she'd been involved with — even Darnell, the best of the bunch — had been interested in getting laid as quickly as possible. It took several minutes to find a sequence that she liked:

> Flirting
> Information seeking
> Group date
> Hold hands in public
> Movie date
> Formal dinner date
> Officially boyfriend and girlfriend
> Going steady
> Engaged
> Married

When she looked at the cards spread out in front of her, she noticed that the order she'd chosen sounded like her father and mother's courtship.

Tanya and Julie handed out a second set of cards, the sex cards. They had terms such as "intercourse" and "hand on thigh." The kids snickered at one of the phrases, "dry-humping." It sounded like something people said in the 1970s.

"Each one of you is the result of someone else's sexual choices," Julie explained. "How many of you have parents who are divorced? Your parents decided to have a child; now they don't want to be married anymore and *you* are the one who has to go back and forth between their houses. How many of you are adopted? Maybe your biological parents had sex once and decided they didn't want to go through with raising a child. You probably don't know who those parents are. Some of you aren't sure if you want to know."

Julie told the kids to put the sex cards in order next to the ten dating cards. "What's the right sequence of things for you? It's not something most of you guys ever consider. You go to a party, you hook up, things happen. We're not naïve; we know most of you are going to have sex soon after you leave here. Many of you have already had sex, but did you talk it over with the other person first? What's the order of events that *you* would prefer?"

Bianca took a couple of minutes to arrange and rearrange the second set of cards by the first.

Flirting
Information seeking
Group date
Hold hands in public          Hand on butt
Movie date                    Hand on thigh
Formal dinner date
Officially boyfriend and girlfriend    Hand on breast
Going steady                  Dry-humping
Engaged                       Oral sex
Married                       Sexual intercourse

There was no correct answer; it was up to each person. Tanya and Julie kept saying that. And yet years of Sunday school had taught Bianca there was a clear right and wrong. The right way was the way her mom had done it — slowly getting to know a guy, dreaming together about the future, having a beautiful wedding. The wrong way was the way she'd gotten involved with Darnell, getting caught half-naked in the back of a movie theater. Bianca had learned in Sunday school that a girl should save her virginity until she got married so that sex was special, even sacred. She hadn't had the chance to find that out because she'd been raped.

At the end of the second hour of the seminar, Tanya and Julie wheeled out a cart stacked with ten-pound sacks of flour and baby clothes. For the next week, they explained, each kid would carry a "baby" to classes, to group therapy, to meals, and to the gym. The flour babies, a Swift River tradition, were meant to show how much work it took to be a parent. More important, carrying an infant around for a week was supposed to churn up emotions from childhood.

"They're not vomiting or pooping, they're not even crying," Julie said. "Think about what a responsibility it is to have a baby. Will you treat it in the same way you were treated? Will you be a different kind of parent than you had?" D.J. rolled his eyes and shrugged. Translation: *a new low — now they're forcing us to play with dolls.*

"You can make something out of this experience; you can give it a lot of integrity and learn something," Julie said, drilling her gaze into D.J. "Or you can treat it as a sack of flour you have to haul around for a week."

Tanya and Julie had decided that Bianca and Mary Alice would get girls; they were given frilly little dresses and Baby Gap clothes in pastel colors. They needed to think about what happened to the happy-go-lucky girls they used to be. Tyrone and D.J. were told they had boys. Tyrone needed to spend time reflecting on the little boy inside of him, the one who kept making excuses for his father. The counselors agreed that D.J. would be tough to reach. Ever since base camp, he'd done poorly on the writing assignments from counselors, perhaps because he had trouble focusing. Carrying a fake baby around might embarrass him, but at least it was a tactile exercise, a break from writing and talking. The counselors hoped D.J. would start thinking about the infant born prematurely to an unmarried girl in New Jersey fifteen years earlier.

The sixteen kids in Tanya's group were soon crisscrossing the campus with their babies. Bianca looked adoringly at hers, whom she named Elena. Tyrone carried the baby in the crook of his elbow and massaged its lumpy back, especially when he thought no one was looking. Mary Alice dressed hers in a crisply pressed striped shirt. It may have been coincidental, but the stripes seemed to make the baby look slimmer.

D.J. carried his baby as far as possible from his body, as if it were about to explode in a puff of hydrochloric acid. He didn't name it and he kept forgetting it in the dining hall, the kitchen, the classroom building. If it had been a real infant, D.J. would've been reported to social services.

*⁊*

On a sunny Wednesday morning in mid-April, the kids gathered for group on a wooden deck behind the great room. It was time to hand back the babies and talk about what they'd gone through for the past week. D.J. found out he'd have to keep his flour baby for several more days, until he could learn to be responsible. "More time with this — this *thing?*" he grumbled. Tyrone, however, looked glum about handing back his baby. He had enjoyed being a father. It felt good to take a baby to classes and the dining hall. The girls in the group smiled, as they had when Tyrone read a letter from his mother in base camp, and they punctuated his comments with a chorus of "*Awww.*"

Bianca locked her arms around Elena, refusing to surrender her. "What's going on?" Tanya said. Bianca said the baby made her think of so many things: her mother and grandfather dying; her grandmother's illness; her life when she was a little girl and everything seemed so blissful.

"Anything else?" Tanya said.

Bianca said she missed Darnell. She still hadn't heard anything from him, but he had promised to wait for her to get out of Swift River.

Tanya interjected. "And . . .?"

And she had almost had a child, a real child. "I wish I had my baby. She'd be a year and a half old."

"That's a lot of responsibility," Tanya said. "You're seventeen, you're not married, you haven't finished high school."

"Part of me wants my baby, but part of me says, 'It's not the right time, you can't handle it.' It's a battle in my head. I think I had a miscarriage because God was telling me I was going down the wrong path."

Tanya let her talk.

"I feel like I have a duty to become a mom soon," she continued. "What if I wait and get cancer? What if I die when *my* daughter is ten? I want to have a baby while I'm young. I don't want my children to go through what I went through."

Tanya told Bianca to hold on to the flour baby for a few more days. She needed to consider what it meant to be a mother. She *was* young. Very young. To be ready to care for an Elena or another child someday, she first had to learn to take care of herself.

# 20

## A Case of the "Fuck-Its"

D.J.'s ROOMMATES COLLAPSED and fell asleep at lights-out time, ten o'clock on weeknights. Maybe it was the hint of warm weather, or maybe it was their meds. Whatever. D.J. stayed awake, tossing back and forth. It was as if he still had stores of energy to burn after seventeen hours of classes and meals, therapy and appointments.

One night in April he was lying in bed when he heard his door creak open.

"Dude, check it out!" A kid named Ezra from the adjoining dorm poked his head in. He motioned for D.J. to follow him. D.J. padded over to Ezra's room, making sure he didn't wake anyone.

Ezra had figured out a way to slice the edge of the window screen with his fingernails; he could lift the screen and then neatly replace it, concealing the damage. It was close to midnight, and the last of the counselors had gone home. The only adults around were the night staff, who didn't create problems for the kids if the kids didn't create problems for them. They made occasional rounds but spent most of their time reading car magazines in the main corridor, about twenty yards from D.J.'s door.

D.J. and Ezra had eyed each other warily for months, but gradually, as they had been put on bans with other friends, they'd come to be confidants. They were from very different families — D.J.'s drove to the Cape for a week of summer vacation and Ezra's flew to Hong Kong — but they had a few things in common. They were young — Ezra arrived at Swift River at age fourteen, D.J. at fifteen. They despised schoolwork. Just as D.J. could while away a day playing Magic, Ezra got so engrossed playing Ping-Pong that he'd forget to do his homework. Although they didn't discuss it, both were adopted. Anyway, the biggest thing, the thing that really mattered, was that they both thought all the therapy and rules and meds sucked. "I'll run away or get kicked out," Ezra had predicted a few weeks earlier. "Either way, I won't be here by the end of summer."

D.J. jumped into his jeans and hiking boots. He stuffed clothes into his bed so that it would appear that a five-foot-eight-inch kid was asleep under the comforter. Ezra put on camouflage gear he had used for Big Mike's wilderness survival course. After slipping out the window and gingerly replacing the screen, they crawled on the ground, under the line of sight of the night staff, then sprinted to a building used for arts and gym. They dashed through the basements of the two dormitories that were being constructed. Then, without a word, they climbed back in the window, high-fiving and shaking off the dirt. Ezra pieced the screen together and they waved goodnight. D.J.'s heart was pounding. Freedom felt great.

During the days that followed, D.J. and Ezra talked casually at meals. When no one else was listening, Ezra shared his plan. They'd steal a walkie-talkie so they could keep track of the night staff. Then they'd run to a store a couple of miles away and break in to steal cigarettes and candy. After that — well, who knew? Maybe they'd drift back to campus and replace the screen before anyone noticed they'd left. Or maybe they'd thumb a ride to I-91, and on to real freedom, to the permanent party Trevor always talked about.

D.J. knew they could pull it off, but something told him not to leave campus. The one time he'd run away from home, the previous spring, he hadn't thought first. He was still paying the consequences — fourteen months' worth.

Jason, the counselor, suspected something because D.J. looked unusually skittish. "There's a kid who has been on meds like Ritalin since age five," he said. "How do we know that, in that early developmental stage, the medication didn't prohibit or enhance the production of other chemicals in his brain, or even alter the biology of the brain? It makes me question whether meds changed his fate."

Three times a week, a white van pulled up outside Swift River's red double doors at the front entrance. It bore the logo of a pharmaceutical distributor. A muscular deliveryman lugged in bags and cartons filled with scores of pills.

CEDU, the grandfather of therapeutic schools, had banned meds, but most programs no longer had such restrictions. When Swift River opened, 60 percent of the students were taking psychiatric medicines. Now, five years later, 80 percent of the students were on meds, from Adderall XR stimulants to Zoloft antidepressants. Kids took 8:00 A.M. meds, noon meds, 4:00 P.M. meds, 6:00 P.M. meds, and 9:00 P.M. meds: tiny Trazodone for insomnia; white bullet-shaped time-released Concerta for ADD; green-and-white Neurontin mood stabilizers. They took oval orange Depakote anticonvulsants for mood stabilization and robin's-egg blue Wellbutrin SR antidepressants cleverly imprinted with words that resembled a smiley face. "Happy pills," students called them.

Kids took lithium and Lithobid, Seroquel and Valium, Risperdal, Effexor, and Prozac. They took 25-milligram dosages, and 100 milligrams and 1,000 milligrams. Some took laxatives to ease constipation caused by medications; others used diarrhea remedies to plug up digestive systems loosened by meds. Some kids took Zyprexa antipsychotics that slowed down their metabolism so much they were in danger of gaining excess weight; they had to take a stimulant like Ritalin to speed it up. "There are pills to take care of the pills that take care of the pills," said Phil the Philosopher, whose bedtime reading included both Kierkegaard and *The Physician's Desk Reference.*

After a few months at most therapeutic schools, chances were a student would be receiving larger doses, or more medications, or both. Swift River, Phil maintained, "throws around Trazodone and Adderall like candy." And Swift River reflected a wider trend. In just a decade, the number of psychiatric medicines prescribed for American children and adolescents had doubled. That spring, a psychologist who came to consult with Swift River supervisors declared that they should think carefully about what all these meds said about the way society views adolescents.

The psychologist was hardly a radical who believed in healing with herbs and tea compresses. Running a clinic out West, he had treated hundreds of people. He'd seen prescription medicines save the lives of schizophrenics and others with rapid mood swings. But he felt that the multinational pharmaceutical companies were looking at America's twenty-nine million teenagers as the next big growth market. He worried about the proliferation of advertisements that showed a young woman walking blissfully through a field, with a teasing message saying something like, *Ask your doc-*

*tor about Tro-zy-nex.* It never stated what the medicine did. It just hinted that problems with relationships, problems with money, maybe bad breath and foul weather — all would vanish with a few milligrams a day. From what the consultant had seen, psychologists, teachers, and, most of all, health insurers were too eager to look for quick-fix prescriptions to address the symptoms (unruly kids) rather than the underlying problems (dysfunctional families). Rudy Bentz was even more dubious about the growth of what he called "pharmacological personalities." He explained, "Kids think, 'If I'm feeling down today, I'll pop in one happy pill and everything's cool.' What we're doing is blocking the emotional world by medicating as opposed to using medications to help with the expression of the emotional world." Ultimately, though, there was little Swift River could do to fight the tide. Most insurance companies paid for meds but balked at paying for anything more than a few counseling sessions.

In Group 23, Bianca and Tyrone were among the four kids who didn't take psychiatric meds. The rest took anywhere from one to six a day, including uppers, downers, mood stabilizers, antipsychotics, and sleeping pills. One day in April, just as group was winding down, the kids got off track. Trevor brought up the issue. He had confounded psychiatrists. A few months earlier, when he'd complained of hearing voices, they'd brought him to a lab and hooked him up to sensors for EKGs. They'd considered a gamut of possible diagnoses, from multiple personalities to posttraumatic stress disorder. (A couple of counselors protested that it wasn't that complicated: Trevor was a confused, frightened boy who had been sexually abused by a neighbor.) "As soon as I get out of here," he said in his mellifluous accent, "I'm going off my meds."

"They're trying to control us," one of the girls said.

"Yeah, the drug companies just want to make money," Willow chipped in — Willow, who had medicated herself with cocaine and heroin.

While Tanya didn't want to shush the kids, she didn't want to encourage an outright rebellion, either. She had mixed feelings about medicines. She worried about the way American kids were plied with pills. But her premed training had convinced her that meds, combined with talk therapy, could help in many cases. Properly prescribed medicines calmed kids, helped them focus, awoke them from depressions, or eased them to sleep, so that counselors could then do emotional work.

D.J., who usually enjoyed trashing Swift River, kept silent during the meds discussion. He had taken prescription pills longer than anyone in the group — three quarters of his life. A few weeks earlier, he had demanded to be taken off meds. "I don't deny that I need meds," he said, "but I just want to feel what it's like to be without them." D.J.'s parents and psychiatrist compromised with him: If he would continue on Ritalin in the morning — to help him focus during classes — he could drop the Wellbutrin. While Wellbutrin was mostly meant to help with depression, it had a secondary benefit of controlling impulsiveness.

One morning, Kate Simmons, the science teacher, cornered Tanya in the mailroom. "What's up with D.J.?" she said. D.J. had started the spring term of science excited about studying radioactivity. At one point, on his own initiative he brought in a book on nuclear submarines. He earned an A-minus for the first half of the term. "Then he went AWOL," Kate reported. He sat in a corner of the classroom reading a paperback. His grades for the second half of the term reflected the decline: homework, F; quiz, F; test, F; outline for final paper, not handed in, which means F. "It's like he's been psychically removed from the classroom. His body is there, but that's all."

Other teachers echoed Kate: D.J. was less attentive in class than usual — and that wasn't saying much. He sat in the back, jiggling his leg and twirling pushpins around in his mouth. He darted out to the bathroom. It was as if his ADD had ADD. In the past few weeks, he'd been caught fondling a girl as they worked in the kitchen, though maybe fondling was too strong a word. They'd clutched each other for a few seconds before someone saw them. He'd been sent to the restriction room to write about what had happened; while he waited on a drizzly afternoon for a counselor to review his assignments, he got bored. So he walked outside, flopped around in a field, and came back with his pants caked in mud.

Tyrone was so frustrated that he, too, spoke to Tanya. "D.J.'s playing attention games all the time. He won't calm down."

"Why don't you talk to him about it?" Tanya said.

Tyrone shrugged. "He doesn't listen."

Things went from lousy to worse for D.J. A supervisor cornered him in the morning, as he walked to breakfast. "I just heard what you've been up to! You better watch out."

Someone had mentioned that D.J. and Ezra had sneaked out and dashed around the construction site a few weeks earlier. In the schoolwide meeting, John Klem, the head counselor, complimented the students for showing respect to one another and the staff. They had come a long way since the nadir of the winter. Well, *most* of them had. He looked over toward Group 23 and locked his gaze on D.J. "This school is in a much better place than it was a couple of months ago. Is it perfect? No. A few kids are bringing it down. Like you, young man."

The counselors ordered D.J. and Ezra to sit on opposite sides of the restriction room and write the truth lists so they couldn't conjure up a common alibi. D.J. came clean right away. He and Ezra had not only sneaked out, but they had also talked about breaking into a store or running away. It was just idle daydreaming. D.J. had already found that he wasn't good at running away.

The counselors put D.J. on a challenge, the second-highest form of restriction. He couldn't go on field trips, see movies, or hang out during free time. Instead, he had to work on assignments for the counselors. John Klem personally ran D.J.'s challenge. Like D.J., John was short and full of energy; he loved rock climbing and disliked writing. Knowing that D.J. froze when he had to write, he devised a series of brief assignments that involved drawing pictures and making lists about feelings.

One assignment was a list of "thirty times in my life I felt I was doing something wrong." D.J. started it:

> when I scratched my great-great-grandma's piano
> when I broke one of my mom's glass animals
> when I ran away
> when I lit a trash can on fire
> when I broke my hockey stick so I could get another

D.J. also had to describe what he was feeling, a standard task for anyone on a challenge. "Right now," he wrote, "I'm feeling hopeless, that I'm going to get dropped. I am feeling angry at myself because I made another stupid decision."

Even during Tanya's time off, her thoughts kept returning to the drama on campus. Some things made her laugh. Phil, for example, had named his flour baby Prometheus. When Tanya asked if he was mocking the exercise, he became indignant. "If you know anything about Greek mythology, you know Prometheus gave man fire. He was punished by being chained to a rock and having his liver being eaten out by a griffon-vulture every day. Since he was immortal, this punishment went on forever. You know, kind of like Tantalus and Sisyphus, except that he was rescued." Tanya had let him keep the name, especially because he seemed so fond of little Prometheus. Then there was D.J. He could be so full of life when he went fishing in a pond or took a trip to the climbing wall at a gym in Northampton. He could be such a troublemaker, too. He was a puzzle. Sitting on her couch, Tanya read a stack of incident reports, keeping tabs of D.J.'s name with a red pen. During his first six months at the school, D.J. had been mentioned only three times. Then his name started to surface regularly. Tanya shook her head as she kept the tally.

In group the next day, Tanya put on reading glasses and thumbed through the incident reports. "Thirty-three in three months," she said, looking up at D.J. "An average of eleven a month. What happened?"

D.J. mumbled something, his dark eyebrows rising and falling.

Bianca asked why D.J. kept sabotaging himself. Several of the others jumped in to the fray.

"You love the outdoors — you want to screw up and see the rest of us go to Costa Rica?"

"You're going to be dropped into some random group. You'll be here till next winter."

D.J. said he had the "fuck-its." He didn't care anymore. Twice the counselors had put him on bans with Tyrone so he couldn't even talk to his best friend. By the time the bans were lifted, Tyrone had other friends. Then he lost the closest thing to a mentor he'd had. Big Mike, the gym teacher, had gotten tired of working at Swift River and quit.

Tyrone tensed up as though he wanted to say something, but he kept quiet. Phil, always the contrarian, spoke up. "You know, I think you're self-destructing on purpose. You didn't want to leave base camp, where you were comfortable. Now subconsciously you feel safe at Swift River and you're afraid of graduating for, like forty-eight days."

Tanya sensed there was more going on with D.J. But who could tell? He was so hard to read. D.J.'s parents called the faculty frequently to ask why he wasn't motivated in classes. One of the counselors suggested that they read a book about adoption, *The Primal Wound*. The book, by a psychologist who had a biological daughter and an adopted daughter, argued that an adoptee never fully gets over the "devastating loss" of the woman who nurtured him in utero for nine months. The book cited a 1985 survey by a California parenting group that found that, while adoptees made up less than 3 percent of America's population, they represented more than 30 percent of the population of special schools, detention centers, and residential treatment programs. "They demonstrated a high incidence of juvenile delinquency, sexual promiscuity and running away from home. They have had more difficulty in school, both academically and socially, than their non-adopted peers." Those adoptees, the author noted, were characterized as "impulsive, provocative, aggressive and antisocial." Another study found that adoptees' problems are strikingly consistent "whether the family is functional or dysfunctional."

During their two decades of work in therapeutic boarding schools, Rudy and Jill Bentz had dealt with scores of adoptees. "Somewhere in their hearts, the kids are convinced they're about to be abandoned again," Rudy said. Jill liked to say that adopted children had trouble bonding with anyone, even well-meaning adoptive mothers. Other Swift River counselors theorized that adoptive parents generally were rescuers. They wanted to overcome infertility or the bad parenting they themselves had suffered, and they were devastated when their plans of saving an unwanted child didn't turn out as they'd envisioned. Adoptive parents and their kids often had starkly different personalities. The parents tended to be older, settled professionals. Therapists had bandied about all kinds of theories about adoptees; one was that by not being breast-fed, they'd been harmed by hormones in cow's milk and additives in infant formula that somehow caused attention deficit disorder. The truth probably was simpler: If the kids had an impetuous streak, it was because their biological mothers and fathers were impulsive people whose temporary relationships had led to accidental pregnancies.

After reading *The Primal Wound*, D.J.'s parents sent e-mails expressing support to the parents of the four other adoptees in Group 23. The book had upset them all; some found it so devastating that they couldn't finish it. D.J.'s parents, who had maintained for years that adoption was not at the root of D.J.'s troubles, no longer knew what to think.

D.J. had always declared that his adoption wasn't a big deal. However, as the infamous 4-20 date approached — along with his sixteenth birthday on April 21 — he started grilling his parents about his birth mother. They didn't know much except that she had been a fifteen-year-old Irish American who wanted D.J. to have a loving family. They tried to dissuade him from his theory that she had gone into premature labor after doing drugs to celebrate 4-20. During several phone conversations with his parents, he demanded that they call the adoption agency and track her down. Just as abruptly he seemed to lose interest in the subject once his birthday had passed.

*⟡*

To help D.J. sort out his feelings, the counselors put him on a challenge. They told him to make lists and draw pictures rather than compose essays, as John Klem had just instructed him to do. D.J. had to come up with "twenty things that are wrong with D.J."

The first came to him immediately: "I belong in a psych hospital." After writing a few lines, he lost interest in the assignment, filling the rest of the page with the lyrics to "Let the Bodies Hit the Floor," by the heavy metal band Drowning Pool.

> Skin against skin blood and bone
> You're all by yourself but you're not alone
> You wanted in, now you're here
> Driven by hate, consumed by fear

In a counselors' meeting, a supervisor raised the possibility of adjusting D.J. to another group. He wasn't a bad kid — not at all — but he appeared to need more time to absorb the lessons on anger and other topics. In the insular world of Swift River, the kids had speculated that D.J. would be booted from Group 23; it had already evolved from flimsy rumor to accepted fact. "Everyone keeps telling me I'm going to be dropped," D.J. said in group. "Why should I bother to try?"

Tanya, too, considered adjusting D.J., but she wasn't convinced it would help. Some kids just needed to get out in the world and grow up. If D.J. insisted on playing games after nearly ten months at Swift Rive — his father would know the exact number, but it had been three hundred-something days — another seven or eight months might just frustrate him.

Tanya had to admit something else: She liked having D.J. in her group. Under the aloof hyper exterior was a tender boy. She'd known that since she first saw him sobbing for his dog, Firecracker, in the woods. In the seven months since then, he'd come to be an important part of the group. Just when Tanya found herself exasperated by his silence, he'd blurt out something insightful. One morning in group, D.J. explained what it was like to be known as the "ADD boy," taking Ritalin and other pills since kindergarten. "My mom was always bringing me to doctors and they kept increasing my dosage or putting me on new meds. I thought she was trying to fix me and since I had to go to the doctor all the time, that must mean there was something so wrong with me that I was unfixable. If I was broken, how could my mom and dad love me? And if my parents didn't love me, there was no way that anyone else could ever care about me."

Tanya squinted at D.J. For months, she'd been trying to find a way to sum up his insecurities. He'd just done it in thirty seconds. Sometimes she wondered if Peanut was absorbing more at Swift River than he let on.

# 21

## REAL FRIENDS

BIANCA WAS BENCH-PRESSING on the Nautilus in the gym one afternoon when a new kid named Jake turned on a radio and started to shoot baskets. He was gangly, with short-cropped dirty blond hair, a baby face, and braces. When the counselors weren't looking, he'd shuffle along in a pimp walk. Back home he probably had been a wanna-be.

A song by Ludacris, a Southern rapper, came on. Bianca knew the Ludacris songs "Southern Hospitality" and "Move Bitch" as well as this one, "Roll Out." Music with explicit lyrics was forbidden at Swift River, but no counselors or teachers were nearby. At the free-throw line, Jake lip-synched a choice phrase: "You take a pick, while I'm rubbin' the hips, touchin' lips to the top of the dick."

"You like Ludacris?" Bianca asked.

"He's chill."

"Where're you from?"

"Atlanta, same as Ludacris. You?"

"From the South, too. Florida."

"It's so damn cold up here," Jake said. "These damn Northerners don't get it. They're cold, too."

They chatted about the nasty weather. It was gray and damp outside, for what seemed like the hundredth day in a row. Jake hated his fucking peer group; he couldn't stand going to friggin' therapy; he wanted to bolt as soon as he could. Bianca thought back to how pissed she used to be. Jake needed to talk, she could see that. She asked if Jake wanted to have an appointment the next night. He did. Definitely.

At first, Jake and Bianca talked about race. Both felt their old friends and families didn't understand the way they'd crossed the chasm of race. Jake, who was white, had gone to a mostly black elementary and middle school, but then, in seventh grade, his parents switched him to a Catholic school favored by rich white kids who wore Abercrombie, listened to 1970s rock, and thought they were hippies. He showed up in his favorite clothes, oversized Sean John shirts draped over low-riding Mecca pants and Nike Air Force One shoes. He wore a long silver chain and listened to rappers like Outkast. The other kids snubbed him as if he were ghetto trash, even though his dad was a rich developer.

Every few nights, Bianca and Jake would sit in a corner of the great room and forget about everyone else. Some of the other girls spread rumors, saying Bianca was going to hook up with the new kid. But Bianca shrugged off the gossip. She was staying loyal to Darnell. Jake's gangster attitude didn't fool her; he was a sensitive sixteen-year-old. And — unusual for a boy — he actually asked questions and listened. Bianca told him about the day her whole life turned upside down, when her mom and dad summoned the three kids into their bedroom. Eight years had passed, but Bianca could still recall every detail. She described the mottled bedspread, the pale light of the lamp on the end table, the vase of yellow gladiolas — her mom's favorite flowers. She would never forget the mournful look on her mother's face as she tried to explain breast cancer to a ten-year-old girl and eight-year-old twins.

Bianca remembered the day her whole family was in her mom's hospital room after the doctor said Teresa would live for one more week. Her mother cried, saying that she didn't want to leave her kids, she wouldn't leave them. Bianca's grandmother reassured her: "You'll always be able to see us through the clouds in heaven." Although Bianca believed that, things kept getting worse after her mom's death. She showed Jake the rap she'd written for Gennarose's class.

> Yes, I've experienced pain, pain so unbearable, talkin' 'bout it'll
> make you cry
> Yes, I've been used, used like some bitch.
> Yes, I've survived through all the shit you hear 'bout on the news.
> That scary shit you shake your head at.

One night, sitting on a couch in the great room, Jake said he'd been thinking about the day his own life changed, his seventh birthday. His father had taken him to Los Angeles for what was supposed to be a special celebration. Jake, too, could recall all sorts of seemingly irrelevant details. He could picture the layout of the hotel room they stayed in and the way the maids puffed up the pillows. He could still hear his father's low voice on the phone. Jake was watching TV in the room when he overheard his father saying, "I love you, honey," and "Yes, sweetie."

"That was your mother," Jake's father said when he hung up.

That was BS, Jake knew. His parents didn't call each other lovey-dovey names. That weekend, Jake and his father dressed up in tuxedos and went to a ball. Jake's father spent a lot of time with a woman who he said was a business colleague. A few months later, Jake's father called in the kids and said he and their mother were getting divorced. With a first-grader's naivety, Jake asked what that meant.

"I'm moving out and your mom and I won't be together anymore."

Jake remembered sitting at the window that day, watching his father walk out and drive away. Jake felt as if his whole world were being turned upside down. His father soon had a new wife — the woman from the Los Angeles ball — and then new children. He missed most of Jake's basketball games, though he seemed to find plenty of time for his new family.

In seventh grade, Jake smoked pot and filched his father and stepmother's vodka. In eighth and ninth grades, he used speed and coke; in tenth, he was caught selling Ecstasy at school. His mother kicked him out of the house, and he didn't want to be with his father. He told Bianca he couldn't get over it: In just a few years he'd gone from a kid who had everything to a sixteen-year-old with two houses and nowhere to live.

The lowest point came when he moved back in with his mom. After an argument with his girlfriend, he went to his bathroom and gulped down 150-milligram Wellbutrin tablets by the handfuls, about forty pills in all. When his mother came home, Jake was lying on the couch in a fog. He told her about his girlfriend, and he admitted that he was no longer a virgin. His mother listened and stroked his hair. It was the best conversation they'd ever had. "Call 911!" Jake blurted, running to the bathroom as he threw up. Dozens of undigested pills spewed onto the floor. That was the last thing he remembered before losing consciousness — all those lavender happy pills smiling up at him.

At the emergency room, Jake had to drink a jello-like solution to soak up the pills. "It's the most disgusting thing," he told Bianca. "I highly un-recommend it."

After being put on bans a couple of times during the winter, Tyrone and D.J. were free to talk again. Even so, Tyrone remained distant. He found D.J. so unpredictable that, in a way, he became predictable. During study hall, D.J. would hunch over his homework briefly, get restless, and thumb through a rock-climbing magazine. Then, with five minutes remaining, he'd resume his homework and get frustrated because he didn't have enough time to finish it. The next day, D.J. would growl about the way teachers picked on him.

Tyrone found another friend, a chubby guy from the Midwest who was also into fantasy stuff. They'd sit around rehashing RPGs, video role-playing games. He was okay, but he wasn't like the guys at home. Once, at lunch, they were talking about how they ended up at Swift River. "You're here because of affirmative action," the boy said. Tyrone let the comment hang in the air. The whole idea was ridiculous. This wasn't MIT trying to open doors for African Americans from New York. It was a school for screwed-up teenagers; if you acted like you wouldn't sneak in opium, they'd admit you. And with two new dorms to fill soon, they probably wouldn't care what you tried to sneak in as long as your parents' checks didn't bounce.

Tyrone kept his distance from the girls on campus. He'd already been burned by two of them — Ashley, who had gotten him entangled in her runaway plot, and Bianca, who had rebuffed him. The rest of the girls in his group were too caught up in dramas of who was whose best friend at lunch and who used to be whose best friend at breakfast. There was one exception: Eva, the newest member of the group. Tyrone and Eva had the same classes every day, starting with algebra, biology, and Gennarose's English class. Eva didn't patronize him, and she didn't lapse into jive talk. She didn't try to impress him with tales of how she'd hung out in the slums of New York and survived to tell about it. She knew when to give him shit, too. Algebra was first period, and Tyrone's brain wasn't in full gear that early. When he shirked the teacher's questions, Eva would raise her eyebrows. "Playing dumb, huh?" she'd taunt. "Come on, Tyrone, we both know that you know the answer."

Tyrone admired Eva's outspoken way in group, too. One day Tanya picked up on Gennarose's observation, asking Tyrone if he held a grudge against girls and women. No, he said, not me. Tanya pressed. Did he feel that his mother tried to dominate him? Or that his sister got more attention from his father? Or that girls had taken over his peer group and constantly shut him down? He folded his arms and didn't answer.

Another counselor, Candice, turned to Eva. Eva had been doing a writing assignment about her sisters and female friends back home, so maybe she could share her thoughts.

"No, I'm good, thanks."

Candice told her not to play games.

"Honestly, I think that girls are back-stabbing bitches," Eva said. "I could name something bad that a girl did to me every year of my life. Girls talked shit about me in eighth grade, saying I was a whore. Even my sisters said it. In ninth grade, my best friend told me to break up with my boyfriend. She said, 'You can do so much better' — then I found out that *she* hooked up with him. Girls here are the same. When I came from base camp, my hair was real long. I loved it. A girl told me I should cut it short; it would look good. After I cut it, she admitted she'd been jealous and just didn't want me to be competition for guys." Eva took a breath. "I hate girls."

The counselors asked Tyrone if he felt he could open up after hearing that. He smiled at Eva. She'd pretty much said it all.

Eva and Tyrone were the only ones in the group whose fathers had never visited. When she felt more comfortable, Eva started talking about her father. One day she mentioned that she used to pray her father would die in a plane crash. When she'd learned on September 11 that he had been in the World Trade Center shortly before the attack but had gotten out safely, the news left her with a mixture of relief and guilt. "I guess I didn't want him dead," she said.

Tyrone couldn't understand Eva's hatred of her dad. He wanted to see more, not less, of his father. Tanya and her co-counselors didn't want to hear about that, though. They said he was protecting his father. Candice gave him an assignment: He had to write a letter to his dad, pretending he was nine years old — the age he'd been when his father was forced to leave the house. Then he had to read the letter aloud to the entire school at closing.

Tyrone screwed up his face in disgust. A week later, though, he walked to the front of the great room at the end of the day. The rest of the kids immediately quieted. Tyrone rarely spoke out; maybe because of that his words carried a lot of weight. Even D.J. froze in place.

"I'm nine. This is the year that everything is horrible," Tyrone explained to the kids. He mentioned several reasons for his predicament: That year, he'd struggled to keep up with the reading and writing in third grade. One of his neighbors, a friend since kindergarten, moved away. Worst of all, his mother got a judge's order to make his father move out of the house.

Tyrone began reading the letter to his father in a quavering voice: "I feel lonely and sad because of the fact that you sleep most of the day. Now you are leaving me. Why? Why did the cops have to come and take you away?" Tyrone peered to the side, as if he could make out his father in the shadows. He was no longer reading the letter.

"Explain it. Is it because of me? Is it because I haven't been good in school? What did I do wrong? It's my fault. I *know* it is."

When Tyrone finished, the room stayed hushed. Several kids, including Eva, had tears in their eyes.

# 22

## RETURN TO INNOCENCE

"WHAT DID IT FEEL LIKE?"

Tanya asked that kind of question all the time. She asked Bianca how it felt to lose the trust of the one adult she needed the most, her father. She asked Mary Alice how it felt to be teased by boys whose acceptance she craved, Tyrone how it felt to be rebuffed by his own father, and D.J. how it felt to be known as the ADD kid.

Tanya liked questions that went right to emotions. She usually avoided the cognitive questions — "what did you think about ___?" — that allowed kids to intellectualize and distance themselves from their feelings. Still, sitting in group therapy in a classroom or library in western Massachusetts, the kids had a hard time connecting with the dangerous games they'd played back home, or the emotional lows they'd experienced.

On a cloudy Tuesday in early May, a day when the damp chill of a New England winter still clung to the air, the time came to bring them back to the moments they'd been trying to forget. The kids were two-thirds of the way through Swift River, starting a workshop that Tanya expected would be one of their most intense days in the whole program. Known as "the return," it was the only one that involved psychodramas, or role playing. "Return to Innocence," a song from the 1990s by Enigma, about the childlike spirit inside everyone, wafted through the library. "Don't be afraid to be weak," Enigma sang.

"Keep pushing them," Julie Haagenson, the supervisor, told Tanya. Over the years, Julie said, even the most reserved students had responded to these psychodramas; something about acting out the past was a release for kids who didn't want to talk. Tanya and Julie had a secret weapon: a six-foot counselor named James. Because of his shock of wavy hair and big blue eyes, some of the kids dubbed him "GQ James." He had grown up in a well-to-do family in Manhattan. He'd rampaged through a hard-drinking, drug-abusing adolescence and gotten kicked out of a prestigious boarding school. At college he was majoring in drinking and on the verge of being expelled when he decided to go sober. He loved acting in Swift River's psychodramas. In previous ones, he'd stepped into the role of a demanding CEO dad, an alcoholic stepfather, and a jocular divorcé. His performances were so convincing that more than one colleague had lamented the absence of Tony Awards for therapeutic school counselors.

When they'd gathered by the fireplace of the library, Julie prepared the kids for the role playing. "This is a chance to look at what your life was like before, to look at the games you played to get attention or manipulate your parents or protect yourselves."

Bianca briefed James quickly: He would play her father, angry about her report card. No one had a script, so he'd have to ad lib. She immediately forgot the world of rural Massachusetts, and she was transported back to a one-story house in Florida.

As Bianca entered the living room, her dad looked up from a stack of papers. His voice was deep. "Bianca, I got your report card. You were skipping classes again."

"So what?"

Her father approached. "Who were you with?"

"None of your business."

"Was it Darnell?"

"Yeah. So what?"

"You drove to see him during school? Without permission?"

"What're you talking about? I have my license. I don't have to ask permission every time I go somewhere!"

"I'm trying to keep this family together. You wouldn't do this if your mom was alive!"

"You don't know what the fuck you're talking about. You don't know how it's been. You don't care." Bianca kicked a chair so hard that it flew up and smashed into a couch. "Fuck this! I give up. You don't understand me!"

She stormed away and picked up the phone. "Darnell? My dad's such an asshole. He doesn't know what it's like. I hate it here. I just want to leave."

Her father stood alone, looking hurt and furious at the same time, still holding the report card.

After her skit, Bianca stood frozen. For eight months at Swift River, she had managed to be the homework-done-early-everything's-in-control overachiever. She hadn't let anyone see the scared, brooding, lonely child she'd been at home.

Julie spoke to her. "There's still a hurt little girl inside of you. When are you going to let that girl be sad?"

"I don't know."

Tanya leaned forward. "How much did you need your dad?"

"A lot."

"How much did you want him just to hold you?"

"A lot," she said, choking up.

"Was all that anger really about your father?"

"My mom wasn't there. She couldn't help me." Bianca covered her face with her hands. "It wasn't fair."

Tanya had a feeling that Bianca was making a breakthrough. She was starting to understand that she'd felt as though she had to be the mother of the house, when she really just needed to be a child. Tanya kneeled next to Bianca and rubbed her back.

⚭

For the next drama, the scene was Dallas, a year earlier. Mary Alice pantomimed her morning routine — putting on makeup and getting dressed. Andy played her fourteen-year-old brother, and Tanner played her brother's best friend.

Mary Alice straggled out of bed after a late night of partying and leaned close to a mirror to brush her hair. She dabbed on blush and eye shadow, then padded into a large closet and ran her fingers over several outfits. She wiggled into a short, hip-hugging skirt, patted it down, then stuck her head and shoulders back to emphasize her bust. She gave a final approving glance. Then she walked down to the living room, where her brother sat with a friend.

"Hey, guys, what's up?"

"Nothin'," her brother said.

"Nothin'," echoed the friend.

"You guys going to the party tonight?"

"Not with you," the friend said.

"What is that thing you're wearing?" the brother said.

Mary Alice walked back to her room, changed her dress, and fluffed

her hair, then returned to the living room. Her voice took on a more Southern flourish: "How's this, y'all?"

"You still look like a slut," her brother said. His friend laughed.

Mary Alice walked upstairs and closed herself in the bathroom. Then
she bent over the toilet. The noise of her retching, and her crying, echoed
across the library.

The psychodrama appeared to be ending and Mary Alice straightened
up, as if preparing to take a bow and walk off stage. Then GQ James, playing Mary Alice's father, strode in from the side. He rapped on the door
lightly, then furiously. "Mary Alice? Mary Alice! Stop that!" He listened,
then rattled the door handle. "Mary Alice, let me in! You're killing yourself."

Mary Alice did a double take, as if seeing her father standing before
her. She collapsed and curled up on the carpet, letting out a moan.

D.J.'s first two attempts at psychodramas flopped. He pretended he couldn't
get the attention of his father and his mother, played by GQ James and
Tanya. He spoke in a flat voice. After a couple of minutes, he shrugged and
gave a look to show he was done with this absurd game.

Tanya, who had been dealing with him five days a week for eight
months, thought that D.J. needed to portray a typical day at home. The
others could think of a dramatic low point, but D.J. was different. He had
been defeated by a series of everyday frustrations. "Come on, D.J.," she
urged. "Show us how it really was." D.J. rolled his eyes and gave out his I'm-
sick-of-this-shit sigh.

"Hey, Dad, wanna do something?" D.J. said to his father, who was engrossed in a football game on TV.

"The Giants are playing, D.J. Why don't you watch?"

"I hate the Giants. Wanna play lacrosse?"

"It's the playoffs. Giants and Eagles. It'll be over in fifteen minutes."

"Then it'll be twenty minutes of overtime, then it'll be dinnertime,
and then nighttime, so you'll say it's too buggy to go outside. Forget it!"

D.J. pretended to go to the basement, where he jumped into a chair.
His mother entered.

"Another video game? I told you no more today."

"But Dad doesn't want to go out. All he wants to do is watch the stupid Giants."

"Why don't you play with a friend?"

"No one lives around here."

"You'll have to find something to do besides videos."

"There's nothing to do. I'm bored."

D.J.'s mother unplugged the imaginary PlayStation.

"Oh, my God! I was in the middle of a game. What are you doing? What the fuck did you do?"

D.J.'s father banged on a door. "What's going on down here?"

"She won't let me —"

"No talking back to your mother!"

"Damien John, calm down," his mom said. "Let's find something to do."

"You know what? Shove it!" D.J. pivoted and ran outside.

As D.J. returned to the semicircle, Tanya nodded. "Well, you got what you wanted — your dad paid attention. That was your game, right?"

"I guess so. Yeah, I did that a lot."

"What do you do around here to get people to pay attention to you?"

"I play games."

"What kind of games?"

"Getting hyper."

"Why?"

"Because I know I'll get attention."

"What are your other games? Refusing to do homework? Running out and rolling in the mud?"

D.J. dropped his head.

"You spent months telling everyone you shouldn't have been sent here. But your games at home got dangerous, D.J. What do you call climbing out a window in the middle of the night and hitchhiking with truck drivers? And looking for someone you met on the Internet?"

Tyrone had planned a skit showing him arguing with his mother, played by Tanya. At the last minute, however, GQ James decided to make things more intense. As Tyrone finished complaining about his mother's rules, the counselor's baritone voice boomed out.

"Son, I was busy today. I couldn't pick you up at school."

Tyrone looked up, surprised. He stammered. "But you forgot me —"

"I had to work late last night."

"You weren't there for me!"

"I have to go now, Son. I'll call you."

"You didn't care about me! You left me all alone!"

Tyrone fell on his side, sobbing. The other fifteen kids watched, transfixed. This was only the second time he'd really allowed them into his life at home.

✍

The kids sat on the floor and ate sandwiches for supper without talking, then formed a semicircle. Tanya explained the next exercise. They had to spread out around the room and write sentences beginning with "I feel shame for . . . ," "I blame myself for . . . ," or "I judge myself for . . ." They had to keep going until they had written everything they could think of.

D.J. stared at the paper. "I blame myself for fucking up," he wrote. "I blame myself for my bed-wetting . . . I blame myself for my adoption . . . I blame myself for no one liking me."

He waited for a few minutes, watching the others write furiously. He went back to the list. "I judge myself as a stupid fucked-up little kid that nobody wants to play with because they have better things to do in their life."

Tyrone sat by a window, his back to the others. He wrote carefully, each block letter gradually taking shape. "I am shameful about yelling at my mom . . . I blame myself for acting stupid . . . I blame myself for not having a good family . . . I blame myself for my dad leaving . . . I feel guilty for not telling my dad how I really feel about him and what he did to me."

Mary Alice plunged in, filling seven pages with her looping handwriting. "I feel shameful for being a slut + letting myself be treated like a little fucking toy, thinking that's all I'm worth," she started. "I feel shameful for my LIFE . . . I feel shameful for sticking my fingers down my throat when I was twelve . . . for having sex with anybody who told me I looked good . . . for being everything that my parents didn't want in their daughter."

Tanya exhaled slowly as she surveyed the room. Off in a corner, Bianca wrote page after page:

I judge myself for being different
I blame myself for Raul's death
I feel guilty about my dad's divorce

I judge myself for being raped
I judge myself for having premarital sex
I feel guilty for my grandma getting sick
I judge myself for having a miscarriage
I feel guilty for pushing my dad away.

The counselors spread out and crouched next to each child. Julie hugged Bianca with one arm as she slowly read Bianca her list: "I judge myself for being raped . . . I feel guilty . . ."

During the workshop, Julie and the other counselors kept small mirrors in their back pockets. Julie pulled hers out and let Bianca gaze into it. "Is all that really who you are? Look deep into your eyes. How did you get so lost? Where did you go? Think about the pain you caused yourself. No, it's not really who you are. So then who are you?"

Julie told Bianca to close her eyes. They were going to do a guided meditation, as the kids did every few months. Julie continued: "Think back to the time when you had your mom and dad, your brother and sister. You were safe. It was a time before you questioned yourself. Do you remember that time, before you knew what death was, before you knew what rape was?"

Bianca nodded.

"There's someone who suffered through this with you, who has been trying to speak to you all along. She wants to come back into your life. Open your eyes and say hello to her."

Bianca opened her eyes. There, on the mirror, was a snapshot of a smiling Bianca at age four, dressed in a pale blue party dress with white trim, her shiny dark hair cascading to her shoulders. Julie continued: "Look how beautiful you are. Would you expect that little girl to be in charge of the whole family when her mom died? Would you expect her to have it all together? Do you blame her for being assaulted in the gym? Do you blame her for being raped?"

On all sides of Bianca, counselors were going through the same exercise with the other kids. Tanya read D.J. his list as he looked in the mirror, then put her arm over his shoulder. "Do you remember the time when you didn't know what ADD was?"

GQ James sat with Mary Alice: ". . . remember a time when you didn't

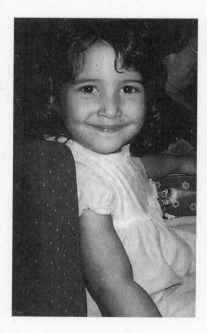

have to look perfect? When you didn't know about bulimia?" Another counselor sat with Tyrone: ". . . a time before your dad left, when your whole family was together? When you didn't know about divorce and court orders . . . ?"

One by one, each kid looked at a snapshot. Mary Alice gazed at a picture of herself wearing jellies and an oversized turquoise T-shirt that matched her eyes, mugging for the camera as if she were posing for a children's fashion line. In his picture, D.J.'s big brown eyes glistened under tousled hair; his lips seemed permanently fixed in a mischievous grin. Tyrone, sitting in a kindergarten classroom, arched his eyebrows. He already had the broad forehead, angular ears, and tightly curled hair that were familiar to everyone at Swift River. There were no hints of the academic struggles to come; his hands were crossed on the open pages of a Dr. Seuss book. He, too, smiled at the photographer.

The stereo played "Everybody Hurts," by REM. Then Enigma came back on, exhorting people to return to a state of innocence.

Sitting by themselves, the kids stared at the photos, crying as they re-

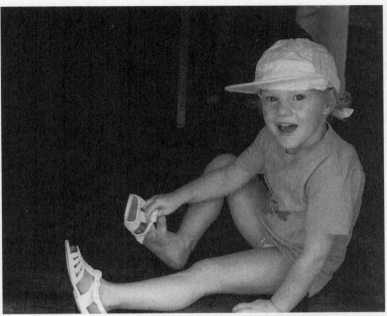

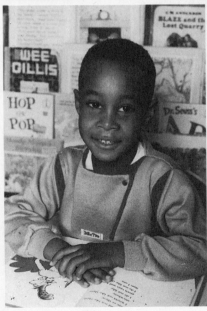

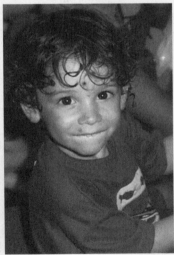

membered a time twelve or thirteen years ago when they were carefree boys and girls. Then, slowly, they came together and sprawled on the carpet in front of the fireplace in a tangle of sixteen bodies and studied one another's pictures. They looked back and forth between the haggard teenage face in front of them and the photo of the giddy kid, as if trying to reconcile the two images.

# PART III

## FORGIVENESS

# 23

## "This Is Not a Test, This Is Your Life"

As the old Toyota whisked south on the Taconic Parkway, past meadows and farmhouses, Tyrone Harriston seemed to transform. He gushed about the sprints he'd been doing in gym, about his work at the school store, the movies they'd seen on weekends. He couldn't contain his glee. For the first time in nine months, he was going home.

Before letting the kids go, the counselors reminded them about the rules for the first home visit. No late-night carousing, no tantrums, and no avoiding their parents. They could see only three friends — friends who had already been approved by parents and counselors. On this visit they had to communicate honestly with their families about the insecurities and fears that were stirred up by being home. "This is not a test," the counselor named Jason had admonished as they left, "this is your life."

During phone conversations over the past few weeks, Natalie noticed that Tyrone had stopped complaining about Swift River. Natalie had a feeling that he secretly liked the place. It was safe and predictable. She had a theory about Tyrone's presence there. "You're a celebrity at that school because you're poor and black. The other kids want to know you because you're an alien." She had worked so hard to get Tyrone away from the pandemonium of his neighborhood, and he ended up surrounded by a bunch of white suburban kids who longed to hang out in his neighborhood. Or at least they wanted the idealized version of it, the music-video version where everybody cruised in limos chugging bottles of Cristal. Natalie wasn't going to gripe about Swift River, though. She had gone and rattled the doors of New York's Board of Education, insisting that Tyrone's high school wasn't interested in actually educating him; it simply wanted to place his name on an enrollment list in order to get the district's money. Natalie prevailed; the

Board of Education had recently agreed to pay 95 percent of Tyrone's tuition at Swift River.

Whenever she left a family resolution at Swift River, Natalie needed to let out steam. She didn't dislike the other parents — she was especially fond of D.J's mother and father. But she wondered why many of them didn't understand the difference between loving and spoiling children. "When their little kids were having tantrums or running out into the street, these mothers would say, 'Mommy doesn't like you doing this, honey.' *No, no, no, no!* When Tyrone ran into the street, he got a spanking. I told him, 'I'll never be able to hit you as hard as one of those cars.'"

In the late afternoon — after getting lost while cutting through White Plains — Natalie pulled up to their two-story house. Surrounded by tall apartment buildings, it looked as tiny and temporary as a piece from a Monopoly set. Across the street was a massive brick public-housing fortress with bars on the ground-floor windows. Tyrone grinned as he gazed through the windshield. "The Projects!" he exulted, as if taking in one of the seven wonders of the world.

Inside the house, Tyrone seemed too big for the dark, low-ceilinged living room and the kitchen, with a metal table for two jammed against the stove. He raced past a cabinet piled high with bills and up the stairs to his old bedroom. It had been taken over by his twenty-two-year-old sister and her toddler. Winnie-the-Pooh posters covered the walls. Tyrone's extra clothes — mostly black, naturally — and his video games had been moved to a bedroom the size of a walk-in closet. Tyrone grabbed his guitar and took it to the front steps, where he practiced chords while watching police cruisers and SUVs with darkened windows pass by.

Soon his old friend Lance came around the corner, and they hugged and talked breathlessly, catching up on neighborhood news. Lance reported on his latest misadventure in the Projects — "like the fortieth time I've been mugged there." He boasted that he'd managed to hand over his wallet while talking the six guys out of pulverizing him. Tyrone sat in the cool May air, transfixed. An hour passed, then another. Tyrone's mother stuck her head out the door. As night fell, she worried that someone with a gun would mistake Tyrone and Lance for gang members. "I don't want you sitting out there in case there's a drive-by," she said. Tyrone and Lance nodded but kept chattering away about friends who had dropped out of school to join the army or stock shelves in the Pathmark.

When Lance asked about the school in Massachusetts, Tyrone said, "It's mad up there. There are some mad girls. There's this guy who is teaching me to play the guitar."

The lights of the Projects flickered on. Tyrone took in the sounds — kids across the street shouting "Yo, bro!" against the backbeat of basketballs on asphalt. Home. He savored the familiar smells, diesel exhaust mingled with spicy Caribbean food cooking somewhere down the block. Not a "dude" resounded anywhere. "You gonna see your dad?" Lance asked.

"Yeah." Tyrone was still deciding what he and his father were going to do, but it would be something mad fun.

The next day, Tyrone played Final Fantasy while his sister braided his hair into long corn rows. Tyrone's two-year-old nephew pranced around in his diapers, knocking a potted cactus off the windowsill in Tyrone's tiny room. At midday, Natalie peeked in to see Tyrone bent over a PlayStation control. "You're doing the same thing you did back in the old days," she complained, but her voice was lighthearted.

"You know that's not true," Tyrone said. "I may be playing games, but I've got people around me. I'm not going back to pattern. Do you see me isolating?" His mother laughed at the way he alternated between the therapeutic jargon of Massachusetts and the street talk of Queens.

Tyrone sang along to hip-hop on the radio. His language changed. "That was some nasty shit," he said of a spring blizzard that had immersed the campus in snow and ice. "You watch out," Natalie teased. "After a few days in New York, you're going to go back to Swift River ghettoized."

Tyrone had hoped he could play laser tag when he saw his father later that day, but his mother nixed the plan. "Your father wants to be part of your life, that's fine. But now he's gonna play games when he wouldn't even read you a book for all these years? No way. Your counselors said you two need to spend time talking. You know that."

Tyrone and his sister talked strategy, then she proposed a compromise to their mother: Tyrone and his father could go see *Spiderman*. People always talked during movies. Natalie vetoed that proposal as well. She stared over at Tyrone, who had been silent while his sister negotiated. She hadn't sent Tyrone to a therapeutic school so he could come home and blow off everything he'd learned. "No. You can go to dinner and look each other in the eyes." If Tyrone had so many questions for his father, he should try to find the answers himself.

✐

Bianca wandered through her house in West Palm Beach. Everything looked the same as it had the morning eleven months before, when the man and woman picked her up and took her away to the wilderness program in North Carolina: the upright piano; her father's books about urban planning lined up like neat skyscrapers; the snapshot of her mother in Portugal. She poked her head into her brother's room. He still had a *Sports Illustrated* swimsuit calendar and a poster quoting Tupac shortly before he was gunned down: *I believe that everything you do bad comes back to you. So everything that I do that's bad, I'm going to suffer for it. But in my heart, I believe what I'm doing is right.* On another wall, Bianca's brother had pinned the newspaper story about Raul's death from the Halloween weekend in 1998. Next to that was another article, a profile of Raul headlined, BOY SHOT IN FIGHT WITH DAD HAD BECOME MODEL STUDENT. A third clipping caught Bianca's eye. It was newer; the paper hadn't yet yellowed. Bianca felt nauseous as she took in the headline: FAMILIES GRIEVE DEATHS OF LOCAL SWEETHEARTS.

The newspaper had reprinted a gauzy, yearbook-style portrait of a black couple. The boy was Bianca's friend Antoine, who was sixteen. His girlfriend had been driving him through town when she lost control of the car and swerved in front of a tractor trailer. Both were Haitian immigrants and "A" students. They were the seventh and eighth teenagers to die in crashes in the county in 2001. The story was dated August 19, which meant that Antoine had died nine months before, just after Bianca started base camp.

"Why didn't you tell me about Antoine?" Bianca asked her brother.

"You didn't know?"

"Why doesn't anyone in this family tell me anything?" Bianca turned her back and went to her room. She was trembling. It was just what she'd told Tanya: Why bother getting close to people when they were going to die?

✐

A couple of days later, on a warm evening, Bianca and her father bought a bouquet of yellow gladiolas. For the first time in nearly a year, they were driving to the Catholic cemetery at the outer reaches of West Palm Beach. Bianca admitted she was nervous — this was the longest she'd gone without visiting her mother's grave — and for the most part they drove in silence.

The spring sun cast long shadows across the cemetery lawn. Bianca and her dad sat and talked by Teresa's headstone, with its carving of the Virgin Mary. Bianca said she'd been furious about being sent to Swift River, but by the time she wrote her flamingo parable in base camp she'd decided to take advantage of the place. Tanya had helped her see that at home she'd kept busy mothering other people and avoided dealing with her sadness and anger. Alan wanted to ask whether she also realized that she had been attracted to aimless boys like Darnell. But Tanya continued insisting he keep his misgivings to himself. He'd spent plenty of time telling Bianca what to do; he still needed to listen.

After a half hour at the cemetery, Alan left to run an errand. He could tell that Bianca wanted to be alone with her mother for a few minutes. To ease her initial feelings of self-consciousness at the cemetery, Bianca usually warmed up with a question. "Hi, how're you doing?" she asked. "Raul's up there, you know. I hope you can show him around."

Touching the gladiolas and looking at the engraved name, TERESA, on the headstone, Bianca spoke evenly. "Mom, I need you so much." The leaves rustled as if responding. She told her mother that she cared about Darnell but she wasn't sure that he was the right guy. She explained the exercise of putting the dating and sex cards in order, then carrying around a flour baby.

When she bid her mother good-bye, she walked a few feet away, to Raul. Crouching at his grave, she wondered aloud, "What's happening up there?" She talked about that Halloween weekend a year and a half earlier, when he had hinted at a bad feeling about going home. She told Raul how much she missed his big grin.

While making sandwiches in the kitchen at 4:00 A.M., Theodor Pandowski told his wife, Janice, that a father-son deep-sea fishing trip would be a great chance for a genuine heart-to-heart. D.J.'s letters from Swift River were so brief and his phone conversations so focused on practical things ("I need a new camera like Mary Alice has") that they didn't have a sense of how D.J. liked school and what lessons he was gleaning from all the therapy.

D.J. opened his eyes long enough to trudge into the minivan, then slept on the ninety-minute drive to the dock as the rising sun bathed the Jersey shore in orange and red hues. D.J. had a way of going from zero to sixty in seconds; in one fluid motion he woke up, bounded out of the car, gathered his lunch, hopped on the boat, and met the other passengers. He was wired. For good measure, he washed down his Ritalin pill with coffee. "It doesn't really make sense to take Ritalin, then drink caffeine, does it?" he asked rhetorically.

As soon as the boat was in open water, D.J. scaled the thirty-foot aluminum ladders up to the flying bridge. In a few moments, he came down, landed a striped bass, then clambered back up. The skyscrapers of New York poked through the fog, and he could see where the World Trade Center had stood.

Watching D.J., Theodor shook his head with a mixture of pride and resignation.

In the minivan on the way home, Theodor tried again. "D.J., we need to talk." He mentioned that the counselors had asked D.J. to deal with the harder truth during this first home visit. What caused his erratic behavior at Swift River? Now that he'd been there for eight months — he was well over halfway through the program — he couldn't get away with simply saying he hated it.

"What's the matter?" Theodor asked.

D.J. pouted. He fiddled with the radio, found an Offspring tune, and pumped up the volume. After a minute he flicked to a different station, then another. "Five more minutes, then we need to talk," his father said sternly. Five minutes passed, then another five. Theodor turned off the radio.

"I don't want to talk right now," D.J. yawned. He reclined in the passenger seat and fell soundly asleep.

The entire four-day visit went like that. Janice and Theodor tried to corner D.J., but he didn't want to go into why he'd rolled around in the mud or why he gave up on classes as the end of each trimester approached. D.J. continued to be, well, pure D.J. When his dad asked him to take out the garbage, he promptly forgot. After the third reminder he did it his way —

by zipping down the driveway on his skateboard, balancing the garbage can in front. Later he sat in the garden beside Janice and tossed pebbles. She asked him to describe the psychodramas.

"It's so dumb. Can I watch TV before we talk?"

Mary Alice's three best friends set the tone for her home visit by stringing balloons and streamers across her bedroom. The next day Lillian drove her to her old high school, on a campus of immaculate brick buildings, to meet with the guidance counselor. Mary Alice thought about her tumultuous sophomore year, when she had gone from making the honor roll and winning a prize for photography to being put on probation for inviting a friend to go "rolling." The school had forced her to take monthly drug tests, though she knew how to time her pot smoking to ensure negative results. All in all, she hadn't made a stellar impression in the guidance office.

In meetings Mary Alice had always been defensive, her arms folded and her jaw taut. But this time she sat back and talked casually, emphasizing her points with her hands. She told the guidance counselor she'd come to realize that she had been insecure at home, too fixated on appearances. She'd been obsessed with impressing the right boys — who turned out to be the wrong boys. "I've thought about it," she said, "and I'm ashamed of the way I used to act." In the peace and quiet of western Massachusetts, she had rediscovered her beautiful self — the little girl inside who loved art and the outdoors. She was determined to stay clean when she left the bubble of Swift River.

After the discussion, the guidance counselor spoke with Lillian. "She's really impressive," he marveled. He would be happy to welcome Mary Alice back after she completed Swift River in October so she could finish her senior year and graduate with her classmates.

Lillian sent an e-mail to several other parents in Group 23. "It's such a pleasure being with Mary Alice," she exulted.

After years of seeing herself as the family's firstborn failure, Mary Alice didn't know how to react to so much praise. It was flattering, sure, but she also felt pressure. Before flying back to Massachusetts, she dawdled in front of the mirror, checking her makeup and trying to suck in her gut. She'd put on more than twenty pounds at Swift River. What if she screwed up and purged again? And what exactly was screwing up? A few cigarettes wouldn't hurt — lots of the popular girls smoked — and a joint now and then wasn't going to kill anybody. She was almost eighteen, and she knew how to handle a drink or two. But could she promise herself that she'd always say no to random sex, or coke, or whatever else came along? What if she went home in October and couldn't live up to everyone's heightened expectations?

✑

Tyrone's father, Lerone, emerged from his white Pontiac at six o'clock on a gray, humid Queens evening. He was rail thin and missing a couple of teeth. Tyrone, waiting on the stoop, was a couple of inches taller than his father. The two hugged quickly, patted each other's backs, then stuck their hands in their pockets. Lerone nodded to Natalie and her second husband, then turned to the Pontiac. Tyrone followed. "Uh-uh," Natalie told her son. "You're coming with us."

"*Aaaagh*, mom . . . ," Tyrone protested weakly, already resigned to losing another argument with his mother.

"It's not a big deal. You ride with us for five minutes, then you have time with your father."

"It *is* a big deal," Tyrone said, but he was already settling into the passenger seat, next to his stepfather.

Tyrone was silent during the short drive. His stepfather dropped them off at a Chinese restaurant on a bustling street. It was the same place that Natalie and Lerone used to go when they were married — with a bar and a lobster tank at the front, full-length mirrors on the walls, and chairs covered in shiny red plastic. Over the years, the restaurant had changed along with the neighborhood. The waiters still talked to the cooks in Mandarin, but now they did their best to speak Spanish to the Puerto Rican and Dominican customers.

Tyrone and his mother waited in front of the restaurant for five minutes, then ten. Rain started to fall, first lazy drops and then a thick curtain. Natalie talked, but Tyrone was busy scanning the sidewalks for his father. Finally, Lerone walked up. He explained that he'd had trouble finding a parking space. Tyrone looked back and forth at his parents, as though he didn't know which one to trust.

Natalie took a table in the middle of the restaurant where she could survey everything. Lerone and Tyrone sat fifteen feet away, in a booth next to the lobster tank. It was early, and there were only a couple of other customers. Tyrone told his father how he had made the honor roll. He talked about running the school store, keeping track of the accounts. Tyrone ordered beef with broccoli and two Sprites. His father sipped a ginger ale.

Tyrone said he wanted to ask about something he'd mentioned in his last letter. "Can you tell me about the divorce?"

"You'll have to ask your mother. She did it. She didn't want me in the house."

"But why did you —"

"She was the one who called the cops. I was trying to make things work out."

Tyrone gave up on the subject after a few attempts and switched back to talking about his life at Swift River. "Our peer group has sixteen kids, it's the only one with more girls than boys. I like some of the kids. Others are a pain." As he continued, phrases like "dyad," "self-study," and "bans" tumbled out. His father regarded him with a blank look. Tyrone stopped himself. When he talked about the school, it came out in a foreign language, like the Chinese waiters talking Spanish.

Tyrone tried focusing less on abstract concepts and told his father about the people he'd gotten to know. He mentioned that a boy in his group, D.J., was having a hard time. "Maybe he needs a friend first," his father said. "Maybe he can't do his work until he has some support. Sounds like he wants you to support him."

Tyrone said that dealing with D.J. was frustrating, but he'd try again.

His father wondered aloud about parents who would choose a school that didn't allow kids to leave for months. "If you're going to be a parent, it means you have to spend time with your kid. You have to spend an hour or two a day with the kid. Otherwise, why bother having the kid?" He didn't look over at Tyrone's mother, but he left no doubt whom he was referring to. "Why be a parent if you're going to send the kid away?"

Tyrone didn't say anything.

"Maybe these parents want the school to do the work for them," Lerone said. "Of course, you are doing good there. It's helping. I like what you told me about the school store."

Outside, a heavy storm inundated the sidewalks. Thunder crashed so loudly that a woman at the bar crossed herself and a waiter dropped a glass.

"Well, I've gotta go get ready for work," Lerone said. "I'll stop by the house with some stuff tomorrow." He paused at Natalie's table and offered a curt good-bye, then turned to the door. On his way out, he handed his son a green slip of paper — the $8.45 bill for Tyrone's dinner. By the time Natalie realized it hadn't been paid, Lerone had disappeared in the gray deluge. She rolled her eyes and sighed as she put the money on the table.

# 24
## MORE THAN LABELS

SHORTLY AFTER RETURNING from their home visits, Mary Alice, Ashley, Trevor, and Andy wandered the deserted streets of an old mill town a few miles from campus. Field trips were sometimes awkward — Mary Alice felt like an inmate on a work-release program, with every stranger gawking at her. Even though they traveled in a plain van without a Swift River logo and wore regular clothes, she felt as if she were stuck in a bright orange jumpsuit emblazoned with FUCKED-UP TEENAGER. Still, this was a special occasion. The kids entered a brick warehouse that had been converted to a café. A counseling supervisor named Tom had arranged for three Group 23 kids to warm up for a sold-out folk concert. Mary Alice had come to support her friends.

Ashley, Trevor, and Andy took the stage. Lest the others forget his nationality, Trevor brought a guitar painted with the Union Jack. He played for a few minutes, his fingers sizzling across the strings. But it was Ashley who brought down the house with a soulful, throaty voice more suggestive of a life filled with whiskey and cigarettes than a pert sixteen-year-old who wore braces. She sang "Yellow," a song made popular by the group Coldplay:

> I swam across, I jumped across for you
> Oh what a thing to do
> And it was all yellow.
> I drew a line, I drew a line for you
> Oh what a thing to do
> Cause it was all yellow.

When Ashley finished, the audience of 150 applauded enthusiastically. Mary Alice, who had been sitting in the front row, jumped up and cheered.

Since the early days on campus, Mary Alice had distanced herself from Ashley, who was a fickle friend, constantly looking for anyone newer and more popular. For a moment, though, all the past slights were forgotten. "You were awesome," Mary Alice said, hugging Ashley. The song "Yellow," which supposedly referred to drugs — specifically heroin — had always given Mary Alice the chills. But she wasn't shaken by the drug allusions now. She was amazed by how cool Group 23 was.

Tom, who had volunteered to shepherd the students on his night off, beamed from the back row. "This is the first time in years that most of these kids have gotten a high without drugs," he whispered to his wife. Tom supervised the final phase of Swift River; soon he would oversee Tanya's group. In the four months that remained, he wanted the students to find a passion for something, to regain the confidence they'd had as little kids. For years, they had been labeled — by their parents, by their teachers, by special education experts. Here in the packed café, Mary Alice wasn't the poor little rich girl with the eating disorder; Ashley wasn't the adopted girl who ached for her birth mother; Andy wasn't the guy who drank and drove to be in with the fast crowd; Trevor wasn't the druggie who had post-traumatic stress disorder, or multiple personalities, or some other condition from the *Diagnostic and Statistical Manual for Mental Disorders*. They were just a bunch of teenagers out for a night on the town.

Not long after the performance, Gennarose noticed Trevor playing the piano in the great room during free time. She listened as he ripped through Mozart and Joplin. He made the old upright sound rich. Gennarose had played the piano for years, but something about Trevor's intensity stopped her short. "Did you play with a band?" she asked.

Trevor looked sheepish. "Well, I played a lot." A couple of years before, he explained, he'd played a solo in front of a large crowd in London. The crowd had applauded, but he could hear only the flaws, the miscounts. He was convinced he wasn't good enough. And that was it — his last time on stage. At Swift River, he'd taken up the piano again and he'd even sent for an application to Berklee College of Music, a top-ranked school in Boston. Gennarose asked to hear a recording of Trevor playing on a grand piano, in a place with good acoustics, instead of the tired upright in a corner of a converted hayloft. As she was leaving, Trevor handed her a cassette. Driving home, she popped it into the stereo. The tape started in the middle of a performance. Someone was playing Rachmaninoff's Third Piano Concerto. As Gennarose listened, she recalled one of her favorite movies, *Shine,* based on a true story of a prodigy who has a nervous breakdown while playing the notoriously difficult Third. Gennarose remembered a line from the movie: "I know life is cruel, but music — music will always be your friend."

Although the concert sounded fantastic, Gennarose wanted to hear Trevor. She fast-forwarded the tape and flipped it over, waiting in vain for the introduction of a young pianist. Then she looked at the program notes on the cover. It was Trevor — Trevor, at age *fifteen* — playing with a famous orchestra in London. "Holy shit!" Gennarose exclaimed. She wondered whether the shrinks who had analyzed and diagnosed Trevor had paused long enough to notice that he was an extremely talented kid.

Tanya wanted to build on the work of the psychodramas, to help the kids rediscover themselves before they had been diagnosed and labeled. She devoted several group sessions to processing what it felt like to reenact scenes from home. How bad had things been? How could these sixteen-, seventeen-, and eighteen-year-olds reconnect with those giggling little boys and girls in the photos? One morning, the group sat on the floor of a second-story meeting room overlooking the campus. A stereo again played "Return to Innocence." Tanya handed back the pictures, then gave everyone a pen and a thick, creamy sheet of stationery. She told the kids to write letters to themselves — to those joyful children who had been betrayed. All the joking and fidgeting stopped.

Sitting quietly with her photo — the wide-eyed, olive-skinned little girl in a light-blue dress — Bianca scribbled away and didn't look up until she'd finished. "Remember what Grandma said," she started. "You're a survivor, you're strong. Turn to her if you feel you can't go on, turn to Dad if you are feeling sad, mad, or happy, tell him what's really going on, he wants to understand, he's always going to be there for you, no matter what."

D.J. wrote slowly and steadily: "Peanut: I'm sorry for everything. The hospital, 2 packs of cigarettes a day, pushing away your family, lying to you and those you care about, pushing you away. Remember when you were 3 and you had the chicken pox? Your parents took you to Sea World and you had the time of your life. You were content with who you were and the love you got from your parents and family, and that was all you needed to be happy. I'm sorry for changing that."

Tyrone addressed himself by his full name: "Tyrone B. Harriston: I need to tell you that your not alone. People don't leave you because of you but because they have problems with them selfs — Dad left because mom and dad had problems, its not your fault. Mom loves you a lot. She tries to help you because she cares and because she loves you."

Mary Alice, who decorated her letter with hearts, was the last to finish:

Dear Precious Angel Mary Alice:
    You don't need to hurt that little girl inside you anymore. It's okay to BE FREE and love yourself and spread your wings and fly . . . You don't have to be scared, you don't have to be someone you're not. You don't have to smoke pot or drink or be the coolest.
    To that little girl inside me, I am *so so* sorry for making you go through so much pain. I starved you and made you throw up and sleep with awful, sleazy guys that didn't deserve you at all and made you get really drunk. Remember all the fun times we have had. Tickle monster with Dad, running around and playing at the lake, doing gymnastics on the beach. You are smart, beautiful, athletic, confidant, artistic, caring, compassionate, loving and lovable. Show the world THE REAL MARY ALICE. Not the fake one that you pretended to be for so long! You don't need her.
    I love you.

The kids put the letters in envelopes, wrote their nicknames on the outside, and gave them to Tanya. No one thought to ask what she would do with them.

Mary Alice took in the tall birch and maple trees, the thick clumps of ferns, the moss-covered stone walls. She breathed in the still, dry air, then grimaced as she smelled the lingering stench of unwashed teenagers — the unforgettable eau de base camp. She had volunteered to return to the woods to help new kids who were struggling.

Watching the kids gather firewood and write with pencil stubs, Mary Alice felt like an anthropologist observing a primitive tribe, a profusely sweating tribe that didn't know much about hygiene. The last time she was in base camp, nine months before, she wheezed from smoking cigarettes and looked skeletal. This time, she was fit from playing soccer and Frisbee. She wore a pink halter and perfectly pressed white shorts. The girls in their dirt-caked base camp clothes glanced warily at Mary Alice while a coun-selor briefed her. The counselor said one girl, Portia, needed guidance be-cause she was scheduled to go to the main campus in a few days but hadn't opened up. Crouching next to Portia, who had tangled hair and a forehead streaked with soot, Mary Alice asked why she had been sent away to Swift River.

"I was really defiant to my parents . . . You?"

Mary Alice avoided tossing out one of her "all of the above" quips. She answered honestly. "Drugs, being really promiscuous, fighting with my parents, eating disorder. I struggled with self-esteem and being superficial, thinking I had to be someone different for everyone."

"That sounds like me. I have an eating disorder, too," Portia said. "I was really sick in seventh grade and I took steroids and gained all this weight and I — were you bulimic or anorexic?"

"Both."

"*Ho!*" Portia said that her parents were doctors and put a lot of pres-sure on her to do well in school and at sports. "I was like, the loser."

Mary Alice nodded. "My mom's a doctor. I used to be a cheerleader and a soccer player. I'm the family fuck-up."

"That's like me. I have a younger sister who is really pretty. She is really skinny. She was actually jealous of me because I was better at cheerleading, art, acting, dancing, and it was kinda weird because I was jealous of *her.*"

Mary Alice leaned against a tree stump. Her youngest sister had just turned thirteen; she was officially a teenager. She lived for horseback riding. Riding gave her a set of true friends; it gave her an escape from the social bullshit of Dallas; it gave her a sense of confidence that Mary Alice had lacked in middle school. It was hard to imagine her out here, wearing the filthy T-shirt and pants of base camp.

A few days passed before Portia made it to the main campus. At appoint-ment time, she prattled on to Mary Alice about her favorite stores. It seemed as if she was aching to say something more. At curfew, Mary Alice hugged her and said, "If you ever need to talk, I'm here for you."

Not long after, Portia stopped by Mary Alice's dorm. Her eyes were red. She sat on Mary Alice's bed and said she'd just made a disclosure to her counselors. The night before she was taken to Swift River, when she thought she was packing for summer drama camp, her boyfriend came over. They were messing around and he pushed her . . .

Mary Alice waited, then said, "I totally understand."

Portia continued: She'd told her boyfriend no, but he kept going until he raped her. Portia said she was in a bind. Her phone call home to New Mexico was scheduled in a couple of hours, and her counselor had suggested she tell her parents about the rape. She was so afraid of their reaction that she didn't want to say anything.

"Do it," Mary Alice said. "They need to understand what's going on with you."

"But they're going to ask me who the guy was. They're gonna want to go to the police. That's how my parents are."

"You don't need to tell them who he is. Just give them the facts. You go, 'I was raped, I want to be honest with you about it, but that's all I'm able to say right now.'" Mary Alice said she'd been opening up to her parents, too, though it wasn't easy. Her mom didn't like it when Mary Alice dwelled on the times she'd felt fat, stupid, or sad. Her dad still made fun of therapy and warm-and-fuzzy discussions about emotions. He liked to remind everyone that the one psychiatrist he'd known had committed suicide. He didn't see any reason for letting it all out with so-called experts if they couldn't even handle their own emotions. Still, Mary Alice said, her family was learning to communicate — one comment at a time.

Portia returned before curfew. "Well?" Mary Alice asked.

"I can't believe it. I told my parents what happened and that I don't want to talk anymore about it, and they were so supportive."

Soon after, Mary Alice found a note on her door. *You actually make me feel like I can succeed,* Portia had written in purple marker. *You tell the truth, not just what I want to hear. You have been a role model for many people here besides me and you should know that.*

Mary Alice had been called lots of things — anorexic, bulimic, spoiled, entitled, druggie, pothead, cokehead, bitch, slut, sleaze, whore, free willy — but she couldn't remember being called a role model.

She liked the sound of it: Role model.

# 25

## "I LOVE THAT KID"

ON A SPARKLING Wednesday morning in the middle of June, a fleet of gleaming black cars — two Cadillac stretch limousines and five Lincoln Town Cars — disgorged forty-two visitors at Swift River's entrance. They were educational consultants from up and down the East Coast — the advisers whom many families hired for guidance on what to do with wayward teenagers. Some had come to see Swift River for the first time; most were returning to find out how it had changed since the early, troubled days.

Students had spent weeks weeding the gardens by the entrance, where marigolds and pansies burst in riots of orange and purple in the sunlight (out back, the work crews had planted impatiens, which they agreed was a good name for a flower in the midst of so many ADD kids). Gardening was an annual ritual at Swift River, but this year it was done with extra attention. The counselors had also overseen a special "deep clean," with every wall, window, and fixture left immaculate. The administrators had ordered the counselors to dismantle a wooden teepee-like structure that was used for sweat lodges by students preparing to go to Costa Rica. In its place, a party-rental company had set up a large white tent.

As the consultants entered, they received leather-bound agendas embossed with their initials in gold. Then they were ushered to the great room for presentations. A sign warned students not to walk up the stairs to the room: SHHHH! CONSULTANTS EXTRAVAGANZA IN PROGRESS.

The first to speak was Elliot Sainer, CEO of Aspen Education Group, Swift River's parent company. Sainer, who had flown in from California for the occasion, reminded his audience that 40 percent of Swift River students came from consultants' referrals. "You are important to us," he said. He traced Aspen's history from a small healthcare group to a fast-growing nationwide company with more than a thousand employees running ten residential programs, four outdoor programs, and more than a dozen special education schools and community outreach projects funded by public schools seeking alternatives for adolescents with behavioral problems. "We're treating kids from some of the wealthiest families in America, very frankly, but also from some of the poorest families in America." Aspen's increasing size, Sainer said, gave it a chance to hire experts to improve the curriculum, train employees, and take on other tasks that would daunt a smaller operation. Referring to the investment of "quite a bit of money" from Warburg Pincus, he made it clear that Aspen would continue to grow. The company planned "a few more acquisitions this year, primarily trying to find programs and locations that broaden our complement of services across the country." Swift River itself would also expand; Sainer pointed out the windows to the carpenters working on two new dorms rising just beyond the great room.

Rudy and Jill Bentz had argued against the expansion, saying that the culture of the program would change. On paper, boosting enrollment to 140 or so didn't seem like a big deal. But throw a few heavy drug users, extreme ODD cases, or vortex kids into the mix and Swift River could end up with the vast underground that had almost destroyed the academy in its first year. Rudy usually made no secret of his fears that venture capitalists — "vulture capitalists," as he called them — would try to wring too much cash from Swift River. He kept thinking of his first boss, Mel Wasserman, grunting, "We need more asses in beds."

Rather than talking about the business end of the school, Rudy told the consultants about the curriculum that he had helped shape. Some in the audience questioned the need to send students to Costa Rica. Couldn't the kids do five weeks of community service in Appalachia, or even in blighted cities of western Massachusetts?

Rudy loved questions like that. He considered Costa Rica the capstone, the experience where all of Swift River's workshops, bonding, and therapeutic exercises came together. "The rain forest just becomes this outrageous, outrageous natural force that the kids need to surrender to," he said. "They come back feeling like they're conquering heroes who have been able to see themselves under fire, to respond with grace and dignity. They come back saying, 'You know, the world is a good place. Yes, we have our pockets of problems and distress and disease but it is a good place if I go and seek it out and bring service to it.'" Several consultants nodded, while others looked on skeptically. Rudy never failed to elicit mixed reactions from consultants and parents.

After three hours of speeches and tours, the consultants sat in the billowing white tent for a lunch of grilled salmon and filet mignon. Then the limos — stocked with fresh-baked pastries and chocolates — whisked the visitors back to Northampton, where the Aspen company had put them up the previous night.

This extravaganza was the brainstorm of a woman who had worked on advertising campaigns for Vidal Sassoon and Bulgari jewelry before being hired by Aspen to oversee marketing in the Northeast. Since applications from distant cities in the West and South had flagged after September 11, the school was anxious to attract more students from places like Long Island's Gold Coast, northern New Jersey's booming suburbs, and the high-pressure towns ringing Boston. All were fertile ground for teenagers struggling with drugs, drinking, and other problems, and all still had plenty of parents who could afford treatment.

Educational consultants were accustomed to being courted by the for-profit therapeutic programs. In the flush days before 9/11, some companies spent tens of thousands of dollars on cocktail parties at consultants' conventions in Tampa, San Diego, and elsewhere. A few schools routinely paid for airfare and bed-and-breakfast stays for touring consultants. At least one group of consultants maintained a Web site that featured favorable comments about what they had seen on their trips — without mentioning that the programs they were touting often picked up the tab.

Still, quite a few of the visitors were turned off by Swift River's hard sell; they wanted information, not pampering. "Glitzy private-sector marketing can make it hard for consultants to learn what a school really does on a day-to-day basis," said Tom Callahan, a former school administrator who skipped the chauffeured cars and drove himself. Although she understood that therapeutic schools needed to woo consultants, Diane Rapp of New York added, "I would rather have had the money that went to limos and filet mignon spent on a scholarship fund."

Aspen executives didn't discuss how much the company had put into the event, but counselors estimated the cost was $40,000 to $70,000, or one student's tuition. (If so, the investment paid off. Within two weeks, the consultants who had visited referred four kids for admission, and three more of their clients were seriously considering Swift River.)

The counselors watched the consultants' tour with conflicting emotions. On the one hand, Swift River's success depended on getting appropriate students, and the best ed consultants knew kids well and screened out those who were dangerous. On the other hand, the staff found something unseemly about a corporate honcho touting the school as if it were an efficient assembly line. Swift River needed to be more than just another business scrambling for customers in a weak economy. Several counselors were furious about the way the sweat lodge they'd built — a structure that had become a symbol of Swift River — had been demolished to make way for a luncheon tent.

Aspen was a privately held company, but curiosity about the financial side of things prodded one staff member to make a back-of-the-envelope calculation comparing approximate annual tuition revenues with salaries, taxes, and other operating expenses. The conclusion: Swift River racked up a 20 percent profit. All the talk about money didn't escape the students' attention. A math teacher and his class figured that if Swift River charged $5,000 a month to 110 students, the school's gross revenues were $183,333 per day, or $763 per hour. (The calculations had educational value because the students learned the difference between "gross" and "net.")

During her first months at Swift River, Tanya hadn't thought too much about being employed by a for-profit company. After all, Swift River offered both a base camp and a Costa Rica service project — something that nonprofits didn't even dream about. But as she watched the two new dormitories take shape, she was starting to question Aspen's priorities. She had begun working at Swift River when it had ninety students; that meant that every student and staff member could know one another quite well. Packing in fifty more students, she felt, would erode the trust and safety. The appearance of the CEO from California could only mean that Swift River would feel pressure to fill those dorms. Tanya also wondered about the way the consultants' visit had been arranged. During six hours on campus, they didn't exchange a word with the primary caregivers, the counselors who dealt with the students day and night.

As summer began, though, Tanya didn't have a lot of time to analyze the state of adolescent mental health care. She was too busy dealing with D.J. After what had seemed to be a breakthrough during the psychodrama, he'd regressed. The "fuck-its" had returned with a vengeance: He was resigned to being dropped from Group 23.

❦

Every Tuesday afternoon, Swift River's top administrators met with a group of specialists to discuss students who were in such emotional distress that they couldn't function in the program. On the last Tuesday in June, the student services team, as it was known, gathered to talk about D.J. There was a feeling of urgency because Group 23 would leave for Costa Rica in two months, and several counselors questioned whether D.J. was responsible enough to go. Rolling in the mud or sneaking out a window was one thing in western Massachusetts, but at the Swift River sites on Costa Rica's remote Osa Peninsula, such missteps could be deadly. (A few months before, a student had taken a walk in sandals — rather than the rubber boots he was supposed to wear — and had to be airlifted to a hospital to treat a bite from a venomous pit viper. He was lucky to have survived.)

Usually the student services team came up with a strategy to help a kid: a change of meds, a community service project, a series of writing assignments. In a few cases, the team decided to expel somebody for dangerous behavior or severe psychiatric problems that Swift River couldn't handle. D.J. hadn't done anything egregious enough to get kicked out. In his case, the team had to decide two subtle questions: Was he understanding the lessons about responsibility, risky behavior, and other subjects? Would he benefit from being dropped and repeating part of the program?

Eleven people sat in the office of the school's executive director, John Powers, including admissions director Anne Favre, supervisor Julie Haagenson, and two consulting psychiatrists. Gennarose was the only teacher. They ran through D.J.'s history — the premature birth, the fire-playing, the bed-wetting till age eleven, the ill-conceived running away. "His very low-key, very sweet parents had no idea how to handle him," Anne Favre explained. One of the supervisors said that D.J.'s parents tried to help him in everything from making friends to boosting his grades — and amid all that help, they ended up doing too much for him. At age sixteen, he needed to create his own successes and stumble through his mistakes. "The parents are very protective and he's very immature."

The group looked over Tanya's tabulations of the incident reports, noting the disturbing rise to eleven per month. Julie said she'd noticed that D.J. had trouble forming bonds with both kids and adults. "That's got to explain his rule-breaking," she said. "It's an attempt to impress others and fit in."

One of the psychiatrists asked how D.J. had dealt with his adoption. The staff members who knew D.J. the best said he'd talked about the subject around the time of his birthday, in April. "He's really been pushing it off," Julie said. "He doesn't really emotionally connect with his adoption and what it means to him."

The special education consultant summarized D.J.'s testing results. There was no doubt that he was smart: Tests showed his IQ was in the "high-average" to "superior" range. But his ability to plan and organize was at the 37th percentile, close to the bottom third. In a test of short-term memory, he could recall three sentences, but when asked to recite a fourth, he flailed. His memory was in the bottom quartile of kids his age. "So if you tell him something, and he has to hold onto it for a minute and consider what to do with it, it's gone," the consultant said. "It's not just organizing, like keeping papers straight and putting them in a notebook that's a struggle for him, but seeing how the world fits together." That helped clarify why D.J. often flubbed instructions from counselors and teachers. He wasn't defiant; he just couldn't retain it all.

John Powers asked about D.J.'s academic performance. Gennarose, who had taught him and kept tabs on his work in other classes, said that he started every marking period smoothly but soon got flustered and gave up. "He'll say, 'I don't understand it, no one's helping me,' even though the teachers and other students are trying their best to help." It was the same with assignments in the restriction room, the counselor said. "We constantly have to be on top of D.J."

One of the psychiatrists observed that D.J.'s insecurities went back to his years of bed-wetting and his frustrations in elementary school: "This is a kid who's been so devalued, he's afraid to open up in group because he's going to say the wrong thing." She said antidepressants had helped. She agreed with Tanya's hunch: D.J. had gotten more impulsive after he'd gone off Wellbutrin and his afternoon dose of Ritalin. While Wellbutrin was an antidepressant, she said, it had attention-enhancing properties that helped calm those with ADHD.

After twenty-five minutes, the discussion wound down. John reminded the others that any action Swift River took would have a significant effect on D.J., his group, and safety in Costa Rica. Everyone needed to weigh the consequences before deciding whether D.J. could stay in Group 23.

As the youngest person, the most recent hire, and the only teacher in a room of counselors, psychiatrists, and administrators, Gennarose hadn't offered too many thoughts. Still, there was much that she wanted to say about D.J. Others saw a restless, reckless kid. They didn't see the D.J. who sat in the hall at night, passionately talking about rock-climbing techniques. They didn't see the D.J. who came up with an original take on Melville's "Bartleby," or the D.J. who sobbed while reading his father's card about fishing for mahimahi.

Although D.J. couldn't sit still for more than a few minutes in a class, Gennarose had watched him in base camp and on field trips. When he was exploring the woods or working with his hands, he was a changed kid — enthusiastic, curious, confident. In November, when the group assembled to build the sweat lodge, D.J. collected sticks and pieced them together for three hours without complaining or losing interest. He'd been completely at peace with himself.

D.J. had an extra burden — the burden of expectations. Gennarose found his parents kind, caring people, but she worried that, as teachers, they put too much emphasis on his academic progress. They called and wrote about his homework; they fretted about his tests; they sent e-mails to the staff to help negotiate extensions for his papers. From what Gennarose could see, many times when the Pandowskis earnestly spoke to D.J. about school projects, he ached to talk about the change of the seasons or about the squirrels and chipmunks he watched longingly from the classroom window. In her short time as a teacher, she'd realized some fundamental things about how kids learn. Some students came across as stupid or lazy, but in fact they just didn't fit into traditional classes taught in fifty-minute blocks.

Maybe it had always been that way. D.J. continued to remind her of Huck Finn, America's most famous adopted kid, who preferred exploring the outdoors to being "cramped up" indoors. At a recent schoolwide meeting, Rudy Bentz had discussed a note he'd received from one of his former students, who was now in his thirties, married with two children, and managing a professional hockey team. He'd cleaned up his life after a stormy adolescence that included a stint at a therapeutic boarding school in California. "I'm living my dream," he'd written. Rudy used that as a way to ask the kids to share their dreams. What would they like to be doing in a decade? They had plenty of ideas, from being an Olympic gymnast to producing rap videos. Mary Alice wanted to travel the world as a photographer. Bianca wanted to appear in a Broadway show. For once, D.J. had raised his hand. He wanted to be in charge of a Fourth of July fireworks display for New York City.

Gennarose, who fantasized about giving up her job in order to sing, liked that about D.J. You could know him for close to a year without truly knowing him. Somewhere under his indifferent facade surged energy and creativity that would let him pursue his dreams.

It was time for the student services team to make a decision. One of the psychiatrists recommended a two-step approach. First, the counselors could demand that D.J. change his behavior, telling him that any more escapades would result in an immediate "adjustment" to another group. Second, they could switch his meds, returning to a combination of stimulants and antidepressants to better keep his impulsivity in check. There was still enough time to titrate, to find the right dosage before the group departed for Costa Rica. John Powers asked the others what they thought. One counselor and specialist after another agreed that for all D.J.'s unpredictability, he had great promise.

The team came to a unanimous decision: D.J. could stay in Group 23, but if he broke window screens or ran around late at night in Costa Rica, he'd be sent back to the United States immediately. Gennarose nodded but didn't say anything. Before wrapping up the meeting, John asked if she agreed with the decision.

"Yeah," she said, grinning. "I love that kid."

# 26

# "LAUGH NOW, CRY LATER"

TANYA CIRCLED UP the kids on a field at the edge of campus, next to the well-worn trail that led through the woods to base camp. At her feet lay a pile of sixteen rocks that she'd collected in a riverbed, some laced with sparkles, some gnarled and lopsided. The sun was setting over the valley; lavender streaks stretched behind the branches of blue spruce and maples. The time for the final workshop had arrived. This one, on forgiveness, lasted twenty-four hours and included a fast and an overnight stay in tents. The kids started with an exercise known as the "boulder hike." Rudy and Jill Bentz had come up with the idea. After a while, the Bentzes had seen diminishing returns in having teenagers sit around and talk abstractly about their troubles. "They need a common experience, symbolically enduring the pain again," Rudy said. "Then they need to learn how to let go."

Tanya handed Bianca a bulky, foot-long hunk of granite, with dark, knobby surfaces. Bianca had so many burdens that she needed the biggest rock. D.J.'s rock had sharp edges. Tyrone's seemed to have a lump in the middle. Mary Alice's was a mutt of a rock, blunt on one side and not very pretty; Tanya didn't want Mary Alice viewing it as a cute keepsake, because it represented all that was odious. When everyone had a rock, Tanya and the other counselors explained the activity. "These are the burdens you've carried for years," said Tom, the supervisor. "Now you're going to carry them; you're really going to feel them."

The kids set off single file down the trail, each ten feet apart, guided by the dim moonlight and occasional beams from the counselors' flashlights. The only noise was the crunch of gravel underfoot and the chirping of crickets. Tanya walked next to Bianca, softly asking questions. "What does the rock make you feel like?" "How is it, thinking about these things?" "When was the time you felt like the burdens were so heavy you couldn't take it anymore?"

Bianca put her arms around the rock. It was getting heavy. Thoughts flooded her mind: She was back home slamming her bedroom door, screaming at her father about how none of this would've happened if mom were alive. She'd known she needed help, but she'd also felt that she had damaged her relationship with him so much that she couldn't reach out to him. She remembered a night when she drove to the beach by herself, sobbing and feeling all alone.

As she hiked, Bianca tried carrying the rock in different positions: under her right arm, balanced by her left hand; in the crook of her left arm, balanced by the right. She remembered the horror of loneliness when she'd had her miscarriage. During the first months at Swift River she had told the story, but not all of it.

It had happened a year and a half earlier, soon after her fifteenth birthday. She'd used birth control pills most of the time, but once in a while she skipped them. Maybe she wasn't thinking; probably she just didn't care anymore. She missed her period but she put off going to her gynecologist, a family friend who had known her mom. When she did go, the gynecologist said Bianca was three months pregnant. He told her to eat well and take better care of herself because she looked worn out. If she wanted, he could talk to her father. Bianca left with an odd sense of assurance. Her high school had a program for pregnant girls. She and Darnell could raise the child.

That night, standing in Darnell's room at his father's house, Bianca broke the news. "You know about my period and everything," she started nervously. This was huge; it was going to change their lives. "I went to the doctor and he gave me a blood test. It was a positive."

"No, this can't happen!" Darnell shouted. "You can't have no baby!"

"Why?"

"You can't!" He pushed her onto the bed.

"What are you doing?"

He slammed his hands into her stomach and pressed so hard that she felt nauseated. He kept pushing.

Bianca left in tears. At home, she went right to her room and fell into a deep sleep. When she woke up she found blood everywhere. She knew that the pregnancy was over. She skipped her morning classes and drove to the doctor, saying she didn't know what had gone wrong. If he was suspicious, he didn't ask. A few months later, she went back to dating Darnell.

The rock felt heavier and heavier. Bianca's arms ached, her fingers tingled. The rock was the miscarriage, the rape. It was the burden of lying and keeping secrets. It was Raul, shot by his own father, and Antoine, crashing into a truck. It was her mother's death. She was sick of death controlling her life. She wanted to dump all of it — the nightmares of the miscarriage, the memories of the girl so starved for affection that she clung to a guy who abused her.

When the boulder hike ended back at the field, Tom and Tanya asked the sixteen students to stand in a circle and hold the rocks out in front of them. Each kid had to come up with a word that the rock represented. A sliver of a moon hung in the sky; the kids could see one another's silhouettes as they struggled to hold up the rocks. Tom pointed at them one by one.

D.J. chose "uncaring."

"Hopelessness," Tyrone said.

"Desperation," said Mary Alice.

"Loneliness," Bianca called out.

Tanya and Tom told the kids to drop the rocks. They thudded to the ground. Then Tom asked everyone to think of a word to express the feeling.

"Liberating," D.J. said.

Tyrone was next. "Confidence."

Mary Alice couldn't settle on a single word, so she came up with three: "Power, strength, freedom."

"Relief," Bianca said.

When the group gathered inside the library, the counselors turned their attention to Tanner. He had a way of giving incisive feedback to other kids that showed he'd been in great pain, yet he rarely talked about that pain. He had won over the guys with his knowledge of Florida gangs; he'd endeared himself to the girls by admitting that, even as a teenager, he slept with his tattered teddy bear from childhood. He was constantly hugging kids and giving them pep talks, yet he retreated to his room to write gloomy rap lyrics. The counselors got to the point: Tanner was hiding so many things. For example, how many of the kids knew about the tattoos on his upper arms? The guys who had seen Tanner bathe at base camp knew he had some kind of marks, but the girls looked dumbfounded. When Tanner played sports or worked out in the gym, he wore a T-shirt, not a sleeveless shirt.

"Do you mind showing us your tattoos?" Tom said.

Tanner rolled up his left sleeve, all the way to the top of his arm. LAUGH NOW was written in crooked block letters. They were a purplish blue and collided with each other so violently that they might have been tattooed on a ship during a storm.

He rolled up his right sleeve: CRY LATER.

Tanner looked at the floor sheepishly as he explained: It happened when he was fifteen. His girlfriend had dumped him, his parents were out, his brother and sister weren't around. A kid at school had told him about "prison tattoos," made with India ink and a needle. Tanner started by dulling his senses with a few shots of Beefeater gin purloined from his parents' liquor cabinet. He was right-handed, so he did his left arm first. That was pretty easy. Then he asked a friend to write two words on his right arm in pen. Tanner traced them with the needle.

Laugh now, cry later. A couple of the other kids recognized the slogan, which supposedly had been tattooed on Tupac's back. "It says everything," Tanner said. "You snort the coke and enjoy it. Then everything gets messed up."

The next day, in group, Tanya told the kids they'd reached the last — and, in many ways, most important — phase of Swift River's curriculum. Now that they'd dealt with their anger and discussed their darkest secrets, they had to get rid of the burdens they'd been carrying for years, just as deftly as they had unloaded the rocks. That meant forgiving all sorts of people whom they'd blamed for their drug use, anorexia, adoption, depression, anxieties.

Mary Alice was willing to start on the road to forgiveness. She forgave the boys at school for teasing her and calling her "free willy." She forgave her father for belittling her eating disorder, and her mother for making too much of it. D.J. forgave his birth mother for deciding on adoption, and his parents for treating him like a sick kid who needed to be cured. Tyrone forgave his mother for kicking out his father.

Bianca said she was willing to forgive her mother for dying, even willing to forgive God for letting her mother die. But she could not go further; she couldn't forgive Kenneth for raping her. How could she ever do that? She explained it: "For so long, I've been thinking it was my fault for saying hi to him, for talking to him, for going over to his house. I've been telling myself that I could have stopped it by shouting louder." As she talked about it, Bianca realized she was missing the point. She didn't need to forgive Kenneth — she might never reach that point. She needed to forgive herself.

At a school meeting on a Monday evening, Bianca looked up from her spot on the Group 23 couch to see Cody, a blond Californian from her chemistry class. Cody knelt down before her as everyone watched. "Bianca," he said in his booming voice, loud enough for the whole school to hear, "would you like to go to dinner with me?"

Bianca blushed. Tomorrow, as everyone knew, was date night. The kids who had just returned from Costa Rica were allowed to take someone to dinner in downtown Northampton. Bianca hadn't expected to go — unlike Mary Alice, who practically strutted around with a sandwich board that advertised AVAILABLE FOR DATE NIGHT — JUST ASK! Cody, who would graduate at the end of the week, was unlike any guy Bianca had hung out with at home. His family had a lot of money, and he'd done all sorts of drugs. If he'd gone to Upper Creek High School in West Palm Beach, Bianca figured, they would have been with completely different cliques. But in chemistry he'd charmed her with his humor.

"Sure, I'll go with you," Bianca said. A couple dozen kids clapped and cheered.

On date night, the counselors paired each of the students who was about to graduate with someone he or she didn't know well. This was a time for getting to know a person, not for gossiping with an old friend. Date night had several purposes. First, it was a reward for students who were doing well. Second, it was a lesson about having fun without having sex or doing drugs. Jill Bentz, who came up with the idea of date night, had been struck by the number of teenagers who'd had sex without ever going on a date. "Dating is outdated," Jill lamented when she trained counselors. "Kids have no idea how to get to know someone from the opposite sex, what to look for in a partner, or how to build a long-term relationship."

When she returned from classes the next day, Bianca put on her favorite red dress and a heart necklace from her mom. It had rained all morning, but the skies cleared in the late afternoon. With two vans waiting, eleven couples gathered in a circle outside Swift River's front door. They draped their arms around one another's shoulders with Tom, the supervisor who oversaw kids as they went through the final phase of Swift River. Tom, who had spent a couple of years in the Peace Corps, was one of the most popular counselors. Looking around the circle, he recited the rules: "This is a social date, not a sexual date. We want you to enjoy yourselves, to have fun without going overboard." He nodded at another counselor and added, "We're going to trust you, but we'll also be nearby."

As Bianca's van approached Northampton, which a magazine had dubbed a "lesbian mecca," the kids cheered at the sign for a small road called Fruit Street. "Stop, I need that for my collection!" one of the boys called out. The others laughed. He had been a kleptomaniac at home; his bedroom was reportedly stuffed with street signs, traffic lights, store mannequins — anything that hadn't been nailed down, and many things that had.

As the kids set off, Tom handed each couple twenty-five dollars to spend as they wished. Well, almost as they wished: no cigarettes, no joints from street dealers, no hip-hop posters with guns and half-naked vixens. Nobody at Swift River had cash, so to Bianca the crisp bills felt like the MegaBucks grand prize. The first stop was a pizza parlor with tall stools. Cody told Bianca about the Costa Rica trip. They'd hiked in the rain forest, they'd taken horseback trips, they'd gone on a kayak trip with tents lashed to their boats. It was brutal, he said, and at the same time it was amazing.

After dinner, they sat on outdoor benches watching people cruise the sidewalks: college students, homeless men, women in pairs kissing each other. Bianca couldn't concentrate on the parade of characters. She was wondering about life after Swift River. "What happens next?" she said. "What happens when you leave?"

Cody said he didn't know. He figured he'd face the same temptations — mostly drugs — that had gotten him in trouble before. He couldn't promise that he'd stay off everything, but he thought he'd be more moderate.

Bianca had done her best to look as if she had things under control, but she didn't feel that way. Mary Alice's incessant talk about eating disorders made her feel fat. And constantly reliving the past made her wonder about Darnell. He had finally sent her a letter, addressing it to "my one true love." Although he had promised to work in an urban job corps program, then go to college, the letter said that hadn't panned out after all. Instead, he'd worked briefly in an ice cream store, then at a record shop, but he'd lost that job after getting into a fight ("Don't worry, I won"). He'd abandoned his plans to study and was thinking of joining the army. "You know, college was not for me," he wrote. Bianca missed Darnell, but she was afraid that things wouldn't be the same between them after graduation. And she worried that she'd get in trouble again.

"I know about the kids who graduate and do well, but others . . . ," Bianca said to Cody, her voice trailing off. They'd both seen alumni return for graduations every two months. Some wanted to prove that they'd made it; they were in college and staying clean. Others, quite a few, came back with snarky smiles, boasting about the drugs they'd scored. At the last graduation, one girl brought something — pot or coke — to share with friends. Rudy Bentz practically dragged her to the parking lot. Then, his face red with anger, he'd announced a ban on alumni returning to campus.

Bianca and Cody walked to a store that sold funky clothes and furniture. In the basement, they crouched on an oversized chessboard, pushing around three-foot-tall knights and bishops. They spent their remaining money on ice cream cones. Back in the van, Bianca let the evening's reports wash over her as the kleptomaniac and others drifted in.

"Yo, I had a vanilla Coke."

"Hey, wasn't Ariel supposed to be here tonight?"

"That's the new Coke? How was it?"

"It was chill."

"How come Ariel didn't come?"

"Yo, check out my sunglasses. They cost six bucks."

"Ariel was on restriction again."

"You sure you didn't steal those glasses?"

"She was crying. She wanted to go on date night."

"We went to a store with lesbian sex stuff. They had these, like, leather whips. *Shee-it!* I wanted to steal one so bad."

When the kids were quiet, one of the counselors, a short woman, haltingly backed the van out of its parking space. "Anything behind me?" she asked nervously.

"Just a bunch of people in wheelchairs," quipped the kleptomaniac.

Bianca shook her head and settled back. The van cruised up the dark road to Swift River. Bianca looked at Cody, who was working the other passengers like a city councilman. She realized it was strange: She was nearly eighteen and she'd been seeing guys since she was fourteen, yet she'd never gone on a dinner date before. It was as if she had skipped the middle steps, had gone from saying hello to — bam! — sleeping with a guy. When Bianca and Cody returned to campus, he'd go to the boys' dorm and she'd go to the girls' dorm to tell her roommates about her first date.

# 27

## LIFE'S A PERMANENT PARTY

IN MID-JULY, Trevor emerged at the front of the great room, wearing a tuxedo with long tails. His fingers rippled across the piano keys, and he sang a song he'd written. A large banner, trimmed with sparkles, fluttered over the makeshift stage and a hundred students applauded thunderously. The parents of Group 23 sat expectantly in the two front rows. This was their last visit to campus before graduation. ("Seventy-one days left till they come home," as D.J.'s father happily noted.) The next morning they'd have a family therapy session and then they'd take the kids home for their second and final home visit. But right now it was show time.

The group was putting on the "personal challenge," an off-off-off-Broadway production. The point was not to produce a professional performance; it was to push each student to deal with an uncomfortable situation on stage for a few minutes, in front of everyone. If a boy loved to play guitar in front of an audience, then he would not be asked to play. If a girl relished speech making, she wouldn't get to open her mouth. Mary Alice, who had taken dance lessons since kindergarten, wouldn't dance; she'd sing "Yellow Brick Road." And because she obsessed so much about her appearance — because she'd already persuaded her parents to buy a new evening dress and shoes with stiletto heels for this occasion — she was instructed to dress casually and go barefoot.

Tyrone, who kept quiet and blended in with the walls, had to recite an original poem, then prance around in front of the crowd. And out with the black pants, black shirt, and black boots; he'd have to wear bright colors. The most unusual assignment went to Bianca. Because she was a perfectionist who agonized over every detail, she wouldn't even learn what she was to do until an hour before curtain time. That way, Tanya argued,

Bianca could let loose and enjoy herself while others prepared. She would be freed of her perfectionism.

Once the students found out what they had to do on stage, they were in charge. They had figured out the order of the show, written introductions of one another, and decorated the stage. In essence, the performance was to be a test for Costa Rica, where the kids would have to organize their days and work together as a group.

Just before the show started, Bianca learned of her challenge: She had to read a poem about friendship that her mother had written twenty years earlier. She walked on the stage and read it with vigor, her words ringing out. Tyrone wore a shirt with red and blue boxes on a white background as he performed. Mary Alice, barefoot, sang in near-perfect pitch. But the show stealers were Trevor and Tanner. Although Trevor had regularly played the piano in the great room, he had refused to sing, so Tanya gave him a special challenge. He had to write a song with an uplifting message — no hip-hop-style war-storying — then set it to his own music and sing it while playing the piano.

The crowd went wild as Trevor finished his song, which included a refrain that said, "I'm ready to just be me." He crossed the stage and walked to the front row. "Hey, Mum," he sang as he stepped forward. "In this song my story's been told, but one last thing if I'm not too bold. I love you." He got on one knee, removed the boutonniere from his jacket, and presented it to his mother.

Tanner's assignment was similar. When Tanner was sad, he'd sit alone and write melancholy raps — raps that he'd practice alone in a soft voice because he was too shy to get on stage. For the personal challenge he had to write one that didn't celebrate drugs and violence or use foul language. Then he'd have to perform it without musical background. He worked on the assignment fervently during dorm time and on weekends. Now, with his friends, parents, and brother and sister watching, he started in a slow, halting voice.

> I am an eternal soul warrior
> Born eighteen years ago on a beautiful day in South Florida
> Eighteen years later, I know what I am, and that's greater than what
>     I was before, and it's glorious
> So here's what tha story is

I'm not this mean rapper guy that you probably might think and
    judge me for
That last line was just to prepare you for all the beautiful things that
    I am about to lay on the floor
That's right, you heard it, "beautiful things"
Say it a million times and I will not get jinxed
And you see no gold links
I don't need the material blings
For you to see the golden heart that's pumping inside of me

As the kids cheered, Tanner picked up the tempo. Walking toward his family, he let loose in the rhythmic, sing-song style of a participant in a poetry slam.

Dear dad and mom
My love for you is why I quit with the wrong
Chose a new path for my life to be on
My love for myself is why I'm here right now singing this song
Mom and dad, your support helped me find all the positive
    qualities that I always have had

Tanner's mother was weeping. His father, a giant of a man with forearms like wooden clubs, was teary-eyed.

I'm hoping that none of the fire inside of me burns out
And I stay open
To the things that I've learned
In this beautiful bubble.

*⌘*

On the last Thursday in July, the day after the personal challenge, Tanya split the students and parents into groups for family therapy. Tanya ran a group with the New Yorkers: Tyrone and his mother and Ashley and her parents. Tanya started with Ashley, who had alternated between showing affection for and ambivalence toward her parents. She was still sorting out what it meant to be adopted. "I feel worthless," Ashley said, explaining that she couldn't get over the sense of being abandoned by her biological mother.

"We give you our love, we give you our support," her mom said. "But you're like a sieve — it goes right through you."

Tyrone's mother, who was sitting next to Ashley, joined the conversation. She looked across the circle at Ashley's parents. "When they're young, every child assumes, 'Mommy and daddy are mine.' When that assumption is shattered by reality, it's like a sea of negative stuff just comes washing over them."

She turned to Ashley. "The definition of mother is someone loving and caring and nurturing, and your mother couldn't do that. She gave you away. She discarded you, right?" Tanya wasn't sure what Natalie was getting at, but she trusted Natalie's insights. That's what made multifamily therapy more spontaneous than regular family therapy — the facilitator never knew how things would unfold.

Natalie looked Ashley in the eye. "Every time you look at yourself in the mirror, you feel there's a flaw somewhere. You think, 'How can anyone love me when my own mother didn't want me?' Am I right?"

Ashley nodded in recognition.

"You're afraid to accept other people's love because you're afraid that they'll discover the flaw, the thing that made your mother give you away. Is that what it's like?"

Ashley kept nodding. Tanya let things take their course, though she still had no idea what Natalie was trying to say. Natalie was supposed to be sitting two seats away from Ashley, but she was on a roll and it was best not to interrupt.

"The fact is, you don't know the truth," Natalie said. "And when you don't know the truth, you can make it whatever you want. I'm going to tell you something, Ashley. When I was about your age — I was fifteen — a man pushed me into the back of a store and raped me. I got pregnant. I couldn't offer anything to a child. I shared a bedroom with two brothers, I insulated my shoes with cardboard, and I lived with a stepmother who hated me. It was 1969, and abortion wasn't legal in New York until 1970. It wasn't that I didn't want my baby, but I couldn't even provide milk. I put her up for adoption. Like your real mother, I wanted that girl to have a better life than I could offer. I think of my child and I wonder if she's wrestling with doubts about whether she was loved, and if she knows that I had to do something drastic to save her life. That's how much I loved my daughter — so much that I gave her up."

Ashley started to speak, but Natalie hadn't finished. "Don't assume that you did something so horrible that your birth mother abandoned you. Maybe she just wanted you to be able to eat. Look, you have two parents that give you all the love and all the material things you want. You, Ashley, *you* have what I wanted for my daughter."

Ashley lowered her head as tears ran down her cheeks. Across the way, her parents were crying, too.

Natalie and Ashley went to the middle of the circle and hugged. Ashley's parents joined them. The four stood together, embracing. Tanya looked over at Tyrone. Still in the bright red and white shirt he'd worn on stage the previous evening, he was beaming.

✍

Five days later, while the group was away on the second home visit, Trevor's mother called, her voice quavering. Trevor had overdosed while snowballing, injecting a mixture of cocaine and heroin, in the bathroom of a Burger King in London. He had almost died. Tanya couldn't speak when she heard the news. Trevor had been sober for nearly a year. When he'd said his seventeenth birthday had been his best ever, no one doubted his sincerity. He'd become a mentor to Swift River's newer kids, telling them to relinquish their secrets, just as he had done. Tanya had been holding something that had arrived for Trevor — a thick packet with an application to Berklee College of Music. She had wanted to believe that his dark days were over.

Trevor returned with a hangdog look to a campus abuzz about his overdose. The gossip wasn't malicious; it was fueled by concern and curiosity because Trevor, with his easygoing personality, was one of the best-liked kids on campus. More than one student, losing a soccer game or tripping during a crucial moment of Ultimate Frisbee, had taken to shrugging it off with "Life's a permanent party."

In group, Tanya asked Trevor to explain what had happened. Rather than starting with his customary "Whatever, Tanya," he hung his head. He had been planning for months to drink and smoke pot during the second home visit, nothing more, so one night he told his parents he was going shopping. Instead, something prompted him to pawn his beloved turntables for a fraction of their value. He went to the house of an old mate and drank vodka. Another of his mates, he'd learned, was dead — stabbed in a seedy neighborhood during a drug buy. It was scary to be back in London, Trevor said. With the money from his turntables, he bought heroin and cocaine and ended up at a Burger King bathroom with a girl he'd known before. Holding a hypodermic needle, she dared him to try a snowball. The needle contained far more of the mixture than he'd ever tried.

"That American school got you scared?" the girl taunted.

Trevor injected the mix. A few minutes later, he blacked out. While riding in an ambulance to the hospital, he "coded" — his heart stopped.

Trevor assured the group he was grateful to be alive. On his last day in London, he'd gone out with his parents to buy hiking gear for Costa Rica. He wanted Swift River to give him a second chance.

The group looked stunned. Everyone remembered him in base camp defiantly announcing he would go back to drugs, back to clubbing and raves. But they also had more recent, more vivid memories of Trevor playing guitar and piano late at night, and handing the boutonniere to his mother. "We love you, Trevor," someone said. The others echoed it. After group, Mary Alice summed up the fears of many of the kids: If Trevor could fall so far, what about everyone else? If Trevor nearly killed himself when he ventured away from Swift River, what about *me*?

Trevor wasn't the only one who had struggled during the second home visit. Tanner, the baseball player's son, sheepishly admitted that he'd drunk most of a bottle of whiskey he'd found in his parents' liquor cabinet. Eva, the everything kid, had smoked cigarettes. Andy, in what seemed to be a sentimental touch, came back from Long Island with a children's picture book in his suitcase. Tanya opened the book and found a snapshot of his girlfriend in skimpy clothes. A couple of weeks later, Andy's parents noticed that someone had gotten into his E-trade account and sold stocks that he'd gotten for his bar mitzvah. Andy admitted that he'd done it from Swift River's computer room.

Tyrone didn't volunteer much about his second visit home, so Tanya pressed him in group. He'd hoped to spend time with his father, and his mother had given her okay. But when he arrived in Queens, his father said he had to head out of town. Certain that pent-up anger was making Tyrone depressed, Tanya tried to provoke him to let out all the bile. That would be better than storing it up inside. "But, Tyrone, you *wanted* to see your father," she said, almost taunting. "He wasn't there for you again."

"I was busy with my friends. I didn't have time to see him, anyway."

One visit ended on a positive note. Sitting in the kitchen in West Palm Beach, Bianca had told her father she'd been thinking about Darnell. She watched her father's reaction as Darnell's name came up. Alan didn't lose his cool, didn't fulminate, didn't bring up the time he'd found them sleeping together. He listened to Bianca declare her eternal love for Darnell, then waver ten minutes later. Bianca said she was frustrated because Darnell hadn't followed through on his plans to sign up for the job corps or enroll in college.

Bianca didn't say anything about her most profound doubts. In the letter with his digital picture at the top, Darnell had proudly proclaimed, "I ain't cheating, baby." Bianca wondered if she could take him at his word.

"Please, Bianca, think about couples who are completely different from each other, who have different ambitions," her father admonished. "Those are typically the couples who end up having a lot of trouble." But he quickly added, "It's your decision," just as Tanya had told him to.

Alone in her small bedroom, looking at the deflated metallic balloons Darnell had given her for her sixteenth birthday, Bianca reviewed the jumbles of impressions from a year at Swift River. She thought about arranging the dating cards during the seminar a few months earlier: flirting; information seeking; holding hands in public; formal dinner date . . . She and Darnell had skipped right from flirting to sex. Bianca remembered the silly, but completely enjoyable, Northampton date night with Cody. She remembered her discussions with Gennarose, who had pointedly asked her if Darnell was truly special or if he just seemed like a prince compared with the guys who had abused her. She thought of questions Tanya had asked her as they sat in the dorm hall night after night: *Could you spend the rest of your life with him? If you did, what would your life be like?*

Bianca steeled herself, then picked up the phone. "I need some time alone," she said in a steady voice that didn't leave room for contradiction. "I hope you understand. I still want to be friends."

"It's okay, babe," Darnell purred. "I thought you'd feel that way. No worries." For a guy who had just been dumped, he didn't sound heartbroken. In fact, he sounded like someone who'd already lined up another girl.

When Bianca told her father about the breakup, he praised her for being mature. A year before, he probably would have at least got in an "I told you so." This time he restrained himself. When he made his weekly call to Tanya, though, he said he felt like dancing on the ceiling.

A couple of days after his return from London, Trevor was summoned to the headmaster's office. Rudy and Tanya gave him the news: He wouldn't go to Costa Rica with Group 23 or graduate with them. He was being "adjusted" to another group and he'd have to spend an extra six months at Swift River. They'd discussed it with Trevor's parents, who agreed that he needed more time in a structured place to address the causes of his drug use.

Tanya felt torn. Trevor was so talented that he'd shown the administrators how to thwart hackers into Swift River's Web site. And he had come so far, talking about being molested by the boy next door, and by doing so he'd made it easier for others in the group to be frank. She couldn't imagine Group 23 without his incandescent grin. On the other hand, if he walked out of the doors in three months, he might overdose again.

Tanya was curious about something. Trevor was a smart kid. Why would he go from a year of abstinence to the highest dosage of heroine and cocaine he'd ever tried?

"I didn't care if I died," he said.

That night, with every student watching at closing, Trevor was supposed to announce that he would be changing peer groups. Tanya had figured that he would be humble; maybe he'd help others by admitting that he was dealing with a serious drug problem. Instead, he let loose a tirade. "This place has fucked me up the ass," he growled as students listened in hushed disbelief. "I did all that work, and this is what I get. I never should have come here."

Tanya drove home in tears.

The next morning, the gentle Trevor reemerged. He stood up during a meeting in the great room and apologized for his outburst. He promised he'd make the best of the extra months at Swift River. "Tanya, I don't know what I would have done without you," he said. The room erupted in applause.

After the meeting, Tanya's sixteen kids remained in the great room. It was time for group, so they arranged their chairs in a circle. Tanya told everyone to take a deep breath. She was going to share a poem her father had written years before. She'd recently read it to her dad in his sickbed. It reminded her of Trevor.

My erudition
In words
At length
Of wisdom
Love
Compassion
Matter little
If my behavior
Sucks

A counselor came to take Trevor downstairs to his new peer group. All the kids got up and hugged him, just as they had four months before, when he'd made the disclosure about being molested. On his way out, he dragged his heavy wooden chair to the side. The fifteen remaining kids pushed in their chairs and closed the circle.

# 28

## PURA VIDA

WEARING KNEE-HIGH BOOTS for protection against deadly pit vipers, D.J. crept along a trail in the rain forest. The heat felt like a slap in the face, the humidity soaked through his clothes. Clouds skidded overhead, occasionally covering the full moon, and lightning flashed in the distance, over a tangle of mangroves. It was a Friday night in late August, and they had finally reached Costa Rica. Everyone walked in single file on a narrow path. Several of the kids ahead of D.J. grumbled about the muck and the mosquitoes. But D.J. was engrossed, peering into crevices and tidal pools. "Tyrone, check it out!" he called, pointing to an owl perched on a branch.

The group followed Luis, a short, spry guide with a pencil mustache. D.J. had sized him up in a few seconds: a cool guy with no pretensions who loved the outdoors. Luis toted a foot-long machete in a leather holster. With one quick slash, he whacked the top off a coconut and with a couple of chops he made spoons from the husks, so the kids could drink the cool milk and chew on the white meat. Luis's gaze sweeping across the horizon could spot two-toed sloths reclining in branches thirty feet above the ground, the way Mary Alice scanned a crowd of teenagers and picked out the bulimics. "*Mira!*" Luis said, pointing up at a gnarled tree. The chattering stopped. One by one, everyone followed the beam of his flashlight, trying to see what Luis had found. D.J. crouched and looked straight up to see a bluish boa constrictor with a white belly slipping through the branches. The boa was at least five feet long.

"*Mira!*" Luis repeated a few minutes later, and the kids looked at two tree frogs mating, their eyes glowing scarlet in the light as if they were mortified at being caught in the act. The amorous amphibians brought a nervous snicker from everyone. "Hey," Phil scolded, "you're breaking the sex agreement."

The trip to one of the most inaccessible areas of Central America was the chance for the staff to reinforce all the lessons the kids had learned about anger and forgiveness, trust and teamwork. The experience began with an eight-hour bus ride from Costa Rica's capital, San José, through a misty mountain pass and along rutted roads to the largely unspoiled Osa Peninsula, which jutted out on Costa Rica's Pacific coast near the border with Panama. The bus arrived at night and the kids walked blindfolded one by one to a rustic lodge that used to house tourists who traveled on motor-cycles. That walk was meant to echo the hike to base camp thirteen months earlier, when the kids were scared, lonely, and essentially blindfolded — they had no idea what to expect.

The Costa Rican trip, like other phases of Swift River, was meant to "artificially ignite fear and anxiety" a few final times. Students were put through one physical, mental, or social challenge after another while cop-ing with a foreign language, unfamiliar food, and a climate of extremes, from overpowering heat to torrential rain storms. They inevitably went back to pattern, becoming cranky, clingy, or alienated. At this point in the program, though, they were expected to figure out how to deal with set-backs. By finding an appropriate word in a Spanish-English dictionary, by tying the right knot while lashing their belongings on a kayak, by persuad-ing several friends to help build a campfire in a windstorm — by using their own skills or the help of their peers — they would taste success.

Swift River based the Costa Rican program at several sites on the Osa Peninsula, one of the most biodiverse regions in the Western Hemisphere. At eight degrees north of the equator, the peninsula had 3,100 species of plants, 375 species of birds, and 124 of mammals. The commercial hub, and the starting point for the Swift River program, was Puerto Jiménez, a honky-tonk town of five thousand people surrounded by rain forest on one side and the Golfo Dulce, or Sweet Gulf, on the other. Puerto Jiménez had the peninsula's only health clinic and high school, and a couple of rusted stop signs that were usually ignored by a stream of bikes, scooters, horses, and taxi-trucks — pickups with makeshift roofs of plastic sheets to shield passengers from a sudden downpour. The average yearly income, mostly from seasonal construction work and bean farming, was $3,000. Down-town Puerto Jiménez consisted of one barely paved street lined by a clutch of discos, storefront churches, and an Internet café where eco-tourists and down-and-out gold miners jostled for sex, salvation, and painfully slow on-line connections.

In Costa Rica, each Swift River student carried a journal and a workbook that opened with a quote from Margaret Mead: "Never doubt that a small group of thoughtful, committed citizens can change the world. Indeed, it's the only thing that ever has." To many of the kids, that sounded like typical adult hyperbole. But the Costa Rican staff explained that one person could make a difference. The staff told the story of a determined American who had worked with teenagers at a wilderness program in the United States and volunteered in the Peace Corps on the Osa in the 1990s. He had a dream of combining his interests in counseling, environmental education, and sustainable development by bringing American teenagers to Costa Rica. Then, in 1998, he heard that a faltering school, Swift River, was redesigning its curriculum. He pitched the idea to Rudy and other administrators. By coincidence, they had recently sent kids to the Appalachian Trail, and they were intrigued by the possibilities of the rain forest.

The Costa Rican program was born. The founders dubbed it *pura vida,* an expression that loosely translated to "the good life." Each week was increasingly difficult, starting with a stay in the rustic lodge by the gulf. During the second week, the kids moved to a farm that could be reached only by a one-hour horseback ride along muddy trails. In the third week, they paddled ocean kayaks and camped. The fourth week, students scattered around town to stay with families. For the fifth and final week, the parents visited for family therapy and planning sessions for life after Swift River.

Along the way, a team of instructors and wilderness counselors taught the kids Spanish, anthropology, and biology. They emphasized experiential education, so that a mangrove estuary became a makeshift classroom. The American students also spent time building their confidence while constructing schools and giving English lessons to children. As their command of Spanish improved, the kids had to work on a research project about an issue that was close to them, from abuse to alcoholism: They had to interview Costa Ricans, then write up and present their findings. The staff constantly tried to draw therapeutic lessons from the kids' daily ups and downs.

Throughout the five weeks, Swift River tried to expose the kids to American and Costa Rican role models, starting with the staff, which included several former Peace Corps volunteers. The newly appointed director of the Costa Rican program, a tireless woman named Anita, had grown up in several countries and worked in the Peace Corps in Africa. She spoke six languages and didn't mince words in any of them. Then there was the kids' perennial favorite: Luis, the guide who rode horseback, fished for lunch, hunted for dinner, and wound down from a day of work by riding a bike with his young son. Rounding up the Americans, he'd call out, "*Vamos, chicos.*" The kids saw him as a savant with a machete. "Americans move too fast," he'd say as he jounced around on horseback. "The parents hand over their kids to nannies, and they never really bond."

Although the Costa Rican program had the back-to-basics feel of base camp, there was a significant difference: This was for real. Even the most distant point of base camp was no more than fifteen minutes by all-terrain vehicle from the infirmary and the comforts of the main campus. At base camp, the counselors cajoled and goaded the kids, dispensing spices and brown sugar like gold coins; anyone who behaved well could spend fewer days in the woods. This time, the students were in charge. They divvied up the cooking, cleaning, and other chores. They ran a nightly check-in to settle conflicts and hold each other accountable for following the rules. Costa Rica didn't offer reduced time for good behavior; the only reward was a sense of inner satisfaction.

Halfway through the five weeks, a peer group's head counselor and teacher — Tanya and Gennarose, in this case — flew in. They both knew that Costa Rica could make or break a group. Some groups reacted to the stressful situation by unifying. Others fell apart, breaking the no-sex-no-drugs-no-violence agreements they'd tolerated for so long in Massachusetts. Kids who had been cooped up on campus sometimes couldn't control their libidos in the *pura vida* land of sultry climate and scanty clothes. Group 22, which had gone to Costa Rica a month earlier, had imploded in scandal. A boy and girl had been groping in the dark like a pair of lustful tree frogs. Another girl had witnessed the tryst but kept it a secret. They were a couple of weeks shy of graduation. Despite their parents' pleas, Rudy Bentz kicked out all three students. (Because kids inevitably mistook the phrase "pura vida" for an excuse to go wild, the counselors had changed the name of the program to *Rio Rapido*, Spanish for Swift River.)

In every program where he'd worked, Rudy had noticed the same phenomenon: One or two students inevitably got in big trouble just as the end neared. Rudy had a theory about that. First, a surprising number of kids didn't know how to embrace success; they feared it. Second, after all those months of storming, norming, and forming, the students became anxious about the next dramatic step — leaving. "Some kids are scared shitless of separation," he said. "They figure, 'If I leave first, I won't have to say good-bye.'" The counselors knew about that mentality, but they could do only so much to prevent it.

✍

Far from classrooms, D.J. was liberated. The transformation started on the ride from San José. As the bus crawled through industrial neighborhoods on the city's outskirts, D.J. sat in the back. He stared out at storefronts shielded by steel gates and used-car lots fortified by concrete walls and con-certina wire.

"Paterson," he said, as if in a trance.

"Who?" Tyrone asked from across the aisle.

"This looks like Paterson, New Jersey. That's where I ran away to."

Still peering out the window, he told the story. "I could've gotten killed three times. One, when I hitched with the first truck driver. Two, when I got a ride in the next truck. And three, when I walked around the city."

The adventure had started at an intersection when D.J. flagged down an eighteen-wheeler at an intersection. "Are you running away?" the driver asked. "If you are, I'll have to report you." It was 1:00 A.M. on a Friday, a school day. "No, I'm supposed to go see someone," D.J. replied. The driver let him in. D.J. got off at an exit ramp so he could take another highway to Paterson. That's where the girl lived — the girl he'd been messaging on AOL. He thumbed a ride from a second trucker, a sketchy guy who mut-tered a few words.

There, sitting in a bus in Central America, nearly four thousand miles from home and almost a year and a half after the runaway, D.J. revealed details that he'd never shared with anyone. He had brought along a three-dollar pocketknife for protection. That seemed absurd to him now: a 116-pound, fourteen-year-old fending off a truck driver with a flimsy pocket-knife. And that wasn't the worst of it. When his parents came to pick him up after he'd run away, a therapist suggested they take him to an emergency room so he wouldn't hurt himself. It was a weekend and the ER didn't have a shrink on call, so D.J. sat around doing nothing for forty-eight hours.

Then he went to the psychiatric hospital, a dingy gray place encircled by a tall iron fence. The wards were locked and some of the teenage patients mumbled to themselves. D.J. explained to a psychiatrist that he'd run away after playing with a lighter. The psychiatrist said D.J. needed to promise, in writing, never to play with fire again. Once he signed the agreement he could leave. D.J. took things literally, though. He said he couldn't promise that he'd never, ever do something. He held out for five days before signing.

D.J.'s focus shifted in a split second. "Cool!" he said, seeing a familiar sight outside the bus. "McDonald's *auto-servicio.*"

In the wilds of the Osa Peninsula, D.J. and Tyrone resumed their friend-ship. A typical adventure started soon after daybreak with D.J. summoning Tyrone from breakfast so the two could follow a procession of leaf-cutter ants marching determinedly down trees, through lawns, over roads, and finally down a two-inch-wide hole. D.J. diverted the ants by building road-blocks of mud, carving trenches in the soil, and dumping water in their way. He stood back and watched in amazement as they scurried around waving antennae and passing urgent messages. After five minutes, they'd collect themselves and resume their inexorable march.

D.J. and Tyrone seemed to draw energy from each other. They could be silly one instant — hooting and snorting as they quoted lines from *The Simpsons, South Park, and Futurama* — but then they'd shake off the goofi-ness and take charge. They built campfires and cooked meals without being asked. At nightly logistics meetings, they solemnly determined who would haul provisions the next morning. One day the kids awoke at four to help a conservation group that protected baby sea turtles as they hatched from eggs on the beach and waddled to the sea. D.J. and Tyrone were the first ones dressed. They gingerly carried the inch-long hatchlings as the sun rose, and they probably would have stayed for a week if a counselor hadn't insisted it was time to leave.

During a three-hour hike through the forest, D.J. carried a backpack that appeared almost as large as he was. He made a walking stick, he ex-plored caves at the foot of a waterfall, he dashed ahead on a rocky river-bank. The other kids flagged, but D.J. dashed back to giddily report that he had seen howler monkeys skittering through the forest canopy. "Today was the best day I've had in a long time," he wrote in his journal. "It was so amazing in the forest. Saw different types of cool trees, a snake, a poison dart frog, four Jesus Christ lizards, spider monkeys, white-faced and squir-rel monkeys. It's like I'm in a dream that is very realistic."

The Costa Rican staff used the rain forest as a metaphor to reinforce the concepts the kids had been learning in Massachusetts. The staff stressed that species in the forest were interdependent, just like members of a family or a community. In biology class, students sat on the floor of an open-air room with a tin roof as an instructor talked about parasitic, opportunistic, and symbiotic relationships. Not everyone grasped the concepts. D.J.'s hand shot up to explain. To illustrate a parasitic relationship, he pointed outside to an enormous strangler fig that straddled a larger, older tree. D.J. explained: The strangler sends down roots and gradually takes over, finally choking its host. But, he added, even parasitic relationships have benefits in nature: Unlike the original trees, the fig trees bear fruit, which attract monkeys and bats. The animals eat the fruit without helping or harming the trees — the definition of an opportunistic relationship . . .

That led to a discussion about the kids' own opportunistic and parasitic relationships. A half-dozen kids spoke at once, reminiscing about opportunistic friends who used each other for drugs and sex, or parasitic kids who constantly mooched from someone's stash. The instructor asked about symbiotic relationships, and again D.J. raised his hand. "That means that everyone depends on everyone else," he said. Again he gestured outside, to the heliconia, orange-and-yellow lobster-claw flowers. He observed that particular species of hummingbirds had adapted to fit into particular species of heliconia. The hummingbirds drank the nectar, but at the same time they pollinated the flowers. Without the hummingbirds, the flowers would die; without the flowers, the birds would die. "Tell 'em, D.J.!" somebody cheered. He looked a bit embarrassed, but mostly he looked proud.

A couple of hours after class, D.J. was still thinking about symbiotic relationships. He remembered that one species of hammerhead sharks swim to the Bahamas every year, where they are met by fish that pick off their barnacles. The instructor asked D.J. how he knew so much about the topic. "Every summer I watch *Shark Week* on the Discovery Channel." The instructor shook his head. This couldn't be the D.J. he'd been warned about — the immature, reckless boy who'd almost gotten kicked out of the group. "That kid," he marveled, "is *pura vida.*"

Ever since Tanya had accepted the Swift River job, she had been looking forward to the Costa Rican trip. She often thought about how much she had matured during her service project in rural Thailand; she wanted to work with the kids and their parents in the rain forest so she could share the lessons she'd learned about community and Americans' culture of entitlement. On a more personal level, Tanya had to admit that she missed seeing her kids. There were more than a hundred students on campus, with new ones walking in from base camp every few days, but the place seemed empty. Sure, Trevor was still around, but Trevor, too, was adrift without the group. His smile looked forced, and it was obvious that he was still livid about being dropped. The campus was edgier without the guru group. At one point, Tanya ordered a particularly snooty boy to clean up a mess of scraps he'd left in the dining hall. "Yeah, right," he snapped. "You're taking out your shit on me because your dad's dying."

Tanya had reluctantly told the Swift River supervisors that she might not be able to go to Costa Rica. Her father's cancer was much worse. He hadn't eaten for the past month and he couldn't even swallow water. Hooked up to an IV tube, unable to paint, write poetry, walk, or talk, her swarthy father had shrunk to an eighty-five-pound skeleton. A week before she was supposed to fly out, her mother called from upstate New York. It was midnight and Tanya had just returned from her parents' house. Her father had suffered two seizures in less than two hours. The hospice nurse said he might not make it through the night. They'd been dealing with his illnesses for so long that Tanya knew how to read her mother's tone. "I'm coming," she said.

She reached the house shortly before dawn. Her father's eyes were open, but she didn't know if he saw her. His skin was yellow. He had a seizure. Two minutes went by and he didn't breathe. He started breathing, slowly and laboriously. "Don't be afraid," Tanya said soothingly. "We'll be okay." Half an hour later he had another seizure and he didn't breathe again. He died at age seventy-one, ten years after he was first treated for cancer.

When Tanya returned to work three days later, she was surprised to find a message from Bianca's father. Some Swift River parents called and sent e-mails constantly, demanding instant advice about their kid's college application essays or midterm grades. But Bianca's dad rarely made unscheduled calls. This one sounded ominous. He needed to talk with her about "something important."

# 29

## "I CAN'T GO
## THROUGH THIS AGAIN"

I had a dream last night. My dad told me I was going to some type of camp. I was kind of angry. I had to walk up tons of stairs to get to this camp and when I got to the top my dad was there and the people had tricked him so he had to stay. I raised hell then, kicking, punching and screaming and told my dad, "We're going to get out of here."

It was the weirdest dream that I've remembered in a long time. Anyway, today we're going to do some community service.

— Bianca's Costa Rican journal, September 5, 2002

THE STAFF of the Costa Rican program liked to say that all of a group's dirty laundry, the final bits of dreck, the remaining shames and secrets, came tumbling out in the tropics. The staff's reverent tone suggested there was something magical in the air, some truth pollen spread by hummingbirds, but the real reason was more prosaic. In the rain forest, the kids were stuck together day and night in tents and primitive cabins, sharing outhouses or ditches when bathrooms weren't available, colliding with each other at every turn. They had no one else; this wasn't the campus, where they could find solace among newly arrived Swift River kids who were too awed to call them on their phoniness and game playing. "You could hide on campus," Anita, the director, told them, "but you can't hide here."

Bianca had always had a reliable bullshit detector — maybe because by tenth grade she herself had mastered the art of lying to her dad about her late-night forays with Darnell. After going through the months of base camp, group therapy, workshops, and family seminars with the rest of the kids, her detector was finely calibrated. She could tell when someone in the group was full of it. And from the start of the Costa Rican trip, she had no doubt that two girls, Ashley and Mary Alice, were positively steeped in BS. Ashley was a terrible liar; her exaggerated emotions, from sobbing to giggling, gave away everything. By the second week, she was too bubbly.

Mary Alice was a bit more subtle. When she was concealing something, she became defensive. And when she wasn't protesting, she blabbered anxiously about her favorite topic: herself. Over a breakfast of fried bananas, Bianca could hear Mary Alice chattering about her plans for life after Swift River: "I'm going on a semester-at-sea program in New Zealand . . . I'll visit with the aborigines in Australia, which I've always wanted to do . . . I'm going to volunteer for a group that works with kids with eating disorders . . ." Ten minutes later, Bianca clenched her teeth as Mary Alice prattled on: ". . . I'm going to get back into snowboarding . . . go to Africa . . . definitely take photography courses, and do some painting . . . yoga . . . dancing every weekend . . ." Although these sounded like enough projects to last through her twenties, Mary Alice still hadn't finished talking about what she would do in the ten months remaining until she went to college.

Bianca and Ashley were doing community service, painting a classroom in a two-room schoolhouse, when Ashley went into full giggle mode. She told Bianca she was having a *wonderful* time in Costa Rica. "I think there's something you need to get off your chest," Bianca admonished. "You can put on that facade for everybody else, but I know you. Come out with it. You'll feel better. I'll probably get mad but it doesn't mean I'm not gonna be your friend." Ashley just laughed.

Bianca briefly thought about reaching out to Mary Alice, asking her to share what was prompting her nervous jabbering. She decided not to bother; Mary Alice would only snap at her. Anyway, Bianca had a feeling that Eva the Everything Girl would eventually say something. Because she was a recent arrival to Group 23, Eva didn't sugarcoat her criticisms. She made it no secret that she thought half the girls in the group were full of crap; she was especially brutal with Mary Alice. More than one kid had surmised that they were rivals because they were alike in many ways: They came from fancy suburbs, they were pretty blondes, they were obsessed with appearances.

During the second week, the kids were staying in narrow bunk beds in a farmhouse where two-inch-long cockroaches scuttled along the walls at night. All the kids' nerves were on edge — except D.J.'s and Tyrone's; they were so content with the long hikes and the heaping meals of fried chicken and plantains that they seemed oblivious to the roaches. The counselors predicted that it was just a matter of days before tempers would flare. Sure enough, during a morning check-in, Eva spoke up harshly.

"Do you have something you want to say, Mary Alice? Like about your bulimia coming back?"

Mary Alice bristled. "Why are you always asking about my eating disorder? I can't even look at a fucking pancake without you asking if I'm purging."

Bianca gave a knowing nod to Eva: *accusation confirmed.* They held their tongues. The next night, Mary Alice said she needed to clear up something: Six weeks earlier, on her second home visit, she had sort of purged.

Eva challenged her. "Sort of? How do you *sort of* purge?"

Ignoring the question, Mary Alice explained that being back in Dallas was difficult because her family and friends had such high expectations. Her mother, especially, acted like everything was fine. She trotted Mary Alice around as if to impress friends with the new, improved model that had been shipped back from the fucked-up-teen-fixit school in Massachusetts. One morning Mary Alice skipped breakfast and gobbled down chocolate bars. Feeling bloated and disgusting, she went to her bathroom, locked the door, and forced herself to throw up.

"That's not 'sort of purging,'" Eva corrected, but she softened her voice when she saw Mary Alice sobbing.

Once the dirty laundry started emerging, it didn't stop. The Ohio girl spoke up during group at the farmhouse. On her second home visit, she admitted, she had gone for a ride with four kids. She wanted to impress them so badly that when they broke out Bacardi Silver rum and Marlboro Red cigarettes, she joined in. They drank a bottle, then two . . . then five. And since she was being honest, she thought *everybody* in the group should be. She looked across the circle at Ashley, who was intently studying the floor. Maybe, she said, Ashley should tell everyone that she'd kissed Andy.

The heads of thirteen other kids and three counselors swiveled to look at Ashley. She lowered her gaze and admitted that it was true; she had kissed Andy. She wanted to clear up two other things, things that had happened when she was home, several weeks before. She'd called an old boyfriend — the one who had raped her and shoved her down a flight of stairs — because she wanted to hook up again. Ashley paused. The only sound was the incessant chirping of crickets.

She continued: While playing around with her old cell phone, she found her dealer's number in the speed dial. Her parents had cut off the cell service. She called him on another phone and told him to have a bag of coke ready as soon as she graduated from Swift River.

The kids sat for a couple of moments in stunned silence before unleashing their fury on Ashley.

"Do you know how much it's going to suck when we turn on the news in a few years and see that you're dead of an overdose?"

"Look what happened to Trevor. He was dead for four and a half minutes. He was lucky to get a second chance."

"Yeah, what if *you* don't get a second chance?"

When she had time to write in her journal, Bianca let out her frustrations about Mary Alice and Ashley. *Why are they doing this to themselves? What's going to happen after Swift River? They're probably going to go back and do the same old shit.*

The next afternoon, when the kids had a quiet hour to work on Spanish assignments, Ashley lay on the top bunk in the girls' room of the farmhouse. Suddenly, her voice echoed through the building: "I just want to get out of here!" Another girl screamed. Ashley was holding a disposable razor in one hand; blood dripped from the other. The counselors dashed in. They found that Ashley had given herself a half-inch cut on the wrist — an attention-getting nick, not one meant to be deadly. Just in case, though, the counselors put her on suicide watch; she had to be within view of an adult at all times.

After dinner, the group was scheduled to put on a performance for farmhands who lived nearby. None of the kids was in a festive mood, but there wasn't a way to cancel the performance and spread the word because the farmers didn't have phones. At 8:00 P.M., Andy strummed the guitar and Mary Alice, substituting for her onetime friend Ashley, sang the Coldplay song, "Yellow," in Spanish. The Costa Ricans took turns singing ranchers' tunes, trying for a festive air to dispel the Americans' gloomy mood.

Bianca performed her rendition of the MTV "La-La Awards," which was sprinkled with Spanish phrases that drew laughter from the Costa Ricans. Tanner the teddy bear was usually timid about performing, but this time he paced back and forth, and belted out his rap from the personal challenge.

> I'm proud of myself
> Where do you think I'm gonna take me?
> To the streets? No

I'm gonna change things
I'm gonna shine on this world like I'm doing right now, can you
    blame me?

Tanner had started the trip by admitting he had a fear of swimming in the ocean (a friend of his had once been nicked by a shark). But after a few days he'd plunged into the surf. Costa Rica had emboldened him. Now he was letting loose, rapping like a pro. None of the visitors understood English well enough to follow the lyrics, but it hardly mattered. They could read his story in his body, in the jailhouse tattoos that peeped out from his T-shirt. The thirty people stomped their feet and clapped to Tanner's beat.

I long for love, so love's what I create
I could be fake
But I'm not
Let me just reiterate
The statement
I'm making
Number one on my agenda is to never be faking
And I claim it a great thing
You're watching a masterpiece, just short of a miracle in creation
Not the challenge I was faced with tonight
But the bad things I'm replacing with good in my life.

After an hour, rain pelted the tin roof. A couple of kids pulled Ashley out of the chair where she was slumped. She sang "The Rose" in a tremulous voice:

Some say love, it is a river
That drowns the tender seed.
Some say love, it is a razor
That leaves your soul to bleed.

In the morning, Ashley complained of pains in her legs. Although the staff was dubious, a counselor rode with her on horseback to the airport in Puerto Jiménez, then flew to a hospital. For several days, doctors tested Ashley. They agreed that physically she was fine. When she returned, she alternated between moping inconsolably and laughing as if nothing had happened. During check-in, she explained her mood swings by saying that she kept fantasizing about the mother who had abandoned her. The three other adopted girls jumped in. "Why can't you let it go?" said the gullible girl, who had spent her first month of life in an orphanage before being adopted. "My mother and father are my parents. They raised me."

Willow, the small-town girl, was the only one who had met her biological mother. "I'm nothing like my birth mom," she said. "She came over to my house and looked at all these photos I have in my room. She was like, 'Who are these girls, your friends?' I'm like, 'Friends? The photos are of me, starting when I was in nursery school.' She's supposed to have all this stuff in common with me — she's supposed to be my *mother* — but she can't even recognize a picture of me."

D.J. had sat through check-in without comment, as usual. When he cleared his throat and started speaking in an even voice, everyone looked startled. He told Ashley that he had two theories about adoption. "Number one, adopted kids have a pain inside. That won't ever go away. But number two, adopted kids are optimists. Their mothers could have aborted them but they made the harder choice to go ahead and be pregnant and give birth and find out about adoption. They did it so the baby would have parents who really wanted a child."

It was the first time in months that he had mentioned adoption. The group looked from D.J. to Ashley. Tears slid down her cheeks.

No one in the group embraced Costa Rica with as much gusto as Bianca. She enjoyed the wet-towel feel of the steamy climate, the smell of coffee beans roasting, the constant screech of howler monkeys in the treetops. She doused her meals with hot sauce and danced to salsa music. She liked the assortment of blacks, mulattoes, and whites, the mixture of leather-skinned gold miners and children riding bikes with freshly caught red snappers dangling from the handlebars. She plunged into Spanish conversations, summoning phrases she had learned and forgotten in middle school. When the peer group stayed on the farm, Bianca awoke at five each morning to help milk cows. Then she wrote in her journal, sitting on a veranda with a sweeping view of the Golfo Dulce and the mountains that formed the Costa Rica–Panama border. Bending over the journal, she listened to the scarlet macaws excitedly gossiping about the day ahead.

After breakfast, Bianca volunteered to cook with the farm's matriarch, Doña Sabina, a stout woman who parted her hair down the middle and gathered it in a tight bun. Doña Sabina rarely spoke, but Bianca was a fear-

less communicator, miming and using her hands when she couldn't remember a Spanish word. Doña Sabina opened up enough to tell her life
story matter-of-factly: She was born in an area with no electricity; her
mother died when she was two; she was sent from one relative to another;
she was beaten by a brother-in-law; and then she was left as an orphan at
age twelve when her father died.

Doña Sabina stopped talking and looked at Bianca. "I love your hair,"
Doña Sabina said. "It reminds me of the one thing I remember about my
mother: her thick, straight hair." Not long after, a counselor noticed that
Bianca had started parting her hair in the middle and wearing it straight, in
the traditional Costa Rican style.

For Bianca, Costa Rica was a time of joy mixed with melancholy. The
other girls were talking about forging new relationships with their mothers
after graduation — getting their nails done together, going for espresso, activities they'd scoffed at before. One minute Mary Alice would deride her
mother as a superficial Dallas socialite; the next she'd mention their plans
to attend a retreat on women and assertiveness. These girls had spent so
much time hating their mothers. Didn't they ever stop to think how lucky
they were to have mothers to confide in — even to argue with? "I think
about my mom in the past tense and everyone else thinks in the future,"
Bianca observed in group.

Her thoughts swirled. She'd focused on her mom's absence so much
that she'd failed to see that her father had tried his best to be both father
and mother. As the farm stay ended, she spent a restless night interrupted
by the dream of her dad being taken away.

The next morning, the first Friday in September, Tanya and Gennarose
were scheduled to arrive to help with the final three weeks. The Costa Rican
staff took Bianca in a taxi-truck to the Osa Peninsula's airport, which consisted of a landing strip and a soda stand. Bianca kept asking why she'd
been singled out to make this trip, but no one gave her a direct answer.
When Tanya and Gennarose stepped out of a twin prop plane, Bianca ran
up to them. "What's going on?" she shouted over the engine's roar. "What's
wrong?"

"It's better for your father to tell you," Tanya said. Her long blond hair
blew sideways in the wind from the propeller.

"How's *your* father, Tanya?"

Tanya said he'd died seven days before. They stood on the tarmac and hugged.

The counselors took Bianca to the staff house a few blocks away. She sat on a patio surrounded by women staff members she'd gotten to know, including Tanya, Gennarose, and Anita. They made small talk for a minute. Tanya faced Bianca and clutched her hands. "We arranged a special call with your dad. He needs to tell you something. It is very difficult news —"

Bianca started to cry, although she didn't know what the news was.

Tanya handed Bianca an unfamiliar phone number. Her dad answered and said he was in the hospital in Tampa. He'd been feeling exhausted; blood tests showed that he had leukemia. They'd caught it in the early stages.

"Dad, tell me what this means," Bianca pleaded. "Don't sugarcoat it, please."

He said he was taking hemoglobin to strengthen his immune system. He'd gone to the same hospital where Bianca's mother went — the one a few blocks from their college campus — to start chemotherapy. There were good omens everywhere: The doctor was someone they all liked; he had treated Bianca's mother. The doctor was pleased with his progress and said he had a great chance of recovering fully.

When Bianca hung up, her face was pale. "I don't believe this is happening, I don't fucking believe it!" she yelled. "I can't go through this again!"

The counselors wanted Bianca to have support, especially from women who had dealt with tragedies. Bianca knew that the director of the Costa Rican program, Anita, had been eleven when her only brother was hit by a car and died. At age twenty-nine, Tanya had just lost her father. Gennarose had two friends who had successfully fought leukemia, and she told Bianca about their recovery. Another woman, the Spanish instructor, sat quietly. Her best friend from childhood had been diagnosed with leukemia. After a remission that lasted several years, she had died.

The women consoled her for a few minutes. After she finished crying, she said, "It's weird, he's just down the hall from my mother's room . . ."

It took her a moment to complete the thought. "The room my mother died in."

Tanya said that they'd already reserved seats for Bianca and one of the

Costa Rican staff members on a flight to San José and then on a connecting flight to Florida if she wanted to leave right away. Bianca asked to think for a while. Her father, surrounded by relatives, had told her to take care of herself rather than rushing back.

She rested in the shade of the porch for a minute, then announced her decision: She'd stay for the kayak and camping trip. Group 23 had become like her family. She needed them more than ever.

That night, the gullible girl suggested an activity. She wanted each kid to sit for a while with someone who had been a close friend a year before, at base camp. She pointed to Bianca, then Tyrone, and told them to catch up on what they'd been going through since their friendship fell apart. They sat in a hammock and chatted away as if they'd been waiting to reunite. Bianca talked about her trepidation about the kayak trip, about life without Darnell, about her father's health. Tyrone talked about how he'd finally lost his fear of going to classes. He planned to find a different high school when he returned to Queens — a smaller school — and finish his junior and senior years. Listening to Tyrone, Bianca thought about how much he'd grown up. He looked comfortable with himself and with others. She'd even watched him playfully tossing Mary Alice — *Mary Alice,* his opposite — into the ocean.

During the next five days, the group kayaked from point to point, sometimes through mangroves and open water. Shoulders straining and backs aching, they paddled through foot-high waves for six hours a day, stopping to eat lunch or camp out at pristine beaches edged by coconut palms. Deadly yellow-and-black sea snakes slithered past the kayaks. Several times the kids saw dolphins swimming by. At one point, Tanya said she wished her father would send a sign. "Holy shit!" Gennarose yelled, pointing to a dolphin dancing and shimmying. "Dad!" Tanya called out. Bianca laughed.

Bianca seemed to draw on a secret reserve of stamina. Stabbing her paddle in the water, her kayak skimming over waves and surf spraying her face, she led the others day after day. At night, she plunged into cooking, cleaning, and hauling kayaks, even when others offered to give her a break. She kept to herself, though, and didn't say much.

When the kayak trip ended, she sat alone with a Spanish-English dictionary and a copy of her mother's poem — the one she'd read aloud during the personal challenge. "Hold me in your arms, God," it said. Bianca translated the poem into Spanish, then wrote it in delicate calligraphy as a present for her favorite teacher, Gennarose.

Early the next morning, as the other kids got ready to spend a week with Costa Rican families, a taxi-truck pulled up to take Bianca to the little airport. As Bianca promised she'd make it to campus for graduation, Tanya did her best to keep her composure. Throughout the spring and the summer, Tanya had felt that Bianca was strong enough to put the past behind her. The counselors and teachers had done about as good a job as they could. But now she didn't know if any program could prepare a seventeen-year-old for what Bianca faced.

# 30

# "YOUR CHILD
# IS NOT FIXED"

THE COSTA RICAN STAFF had a surprise for the girl who had bellyached about how much she needed tinted moisturizer, designer clothes, and a top-of-the-line SUV. They had chosen the poorest host family for Mary Alice. When a taxi-truck dropped her off, she faced a one-story house made of wooden slats punctured with holes as big as a fist. The roof was a rusty patchwork of corrugated metal. The front door creaked open to a living room so small it could hold just two chairs and a card table. There wasn't a light switch; the occupants had to reach up and turn a bare bulb in its socket. Three tiny bedrooms flanked the living room. The entire 900-square-foot structure could have fit in the nanny's wing at Mary Alice's house back in Dallas.

This was the home of sixty-five-year-old Virginia Guerrero, known to everyone as Doña Virginia. She lived with a fifteen-year-old granddaughter, an eight-year-old grandson, a six-year-old granddaughter, and a constantly changing cast of cousins, nieces, and nephews who stopped by and stayed over. As Mary Alice set her backpack down at the entrance and took off her boots before entering, a counselor watched her face for signs of revulsion. Far from it. She smiled and cooed at the tiny chicks scuttling in and out of the front door. She admired the mango and coconut trees towering over the house. Doña Virginia explained that there was no running water and no bathroom, just an outhouse under the broad leaves of a banana tree. Taking a shower involved hoisting a plastic jug from a well, then carrying it to a makeshift wooden shelter. Mary Alice found the whole place incredible. That's what people didn't understand about her. She liked the good life, yes, but she also enjoyed people and things that were *real*. You couldn't get much more real than this.

Doña Virginia kept bustling around. While making coffee on a stove heated by scrap wood, she told Mary Alice about herself. A widow, she had ten grown children, thirty-six grandchildren, and thirteen great-grandchildren. She had never flown in a plane and never driven a car. When Mary Alice's turn came, she offered her story in a blend of English and Spanish: She was the oldest of four children. "*Mi familia* is *caos* in *la casa*," she said. It's chaotic at my house, she meant. "*Mi familia* is *diferente* from *Costa Rica familias. Muchas presiones* from *los padres*." There is a lot of pressure from my parents. "*Quiero aprender* from *ustedes*." I want to learn from you.

Doña Virginia, her grandchildren, and two visiting nieces nodded thoughtfully. They had hosted twenty Swift River students in four years, so they knew much more than they let on about high-pressured American families.

✒

Before dropping off the kids, the staff gathered the group for a discussion. Anita asked why they thought they were being sent to live with host families.

D.J. had just learned that he was going to be assigned to a couple who, like his parents, had one boy. "You want to put us with a family that's the same as ours," he suggested, "so we can see it with an outsider's perspective." Mary Alice guessed that Swift River wanted to continue the lessons of simplicity that had started in base camp. Tyrone had another theory: "We're supposed to be giving something to the family, bringing them lessons about our culture."

Anita said everyone was correct. Yes, the staff wanted American teens to appreciate how much they took for granted — but in many ways that was the least important part of the home stay. And yes, they were supposed to give something to the families — by teaching English phrases to children, for example. Of course they needed to learn how to use their wits in all kinds of uncomfortable situations. Soon they'd be back at high school or away at college, going to parties where they'd feel pressure to do drugs, have sex with strangers, or prove themselves to cool kids who liked to drink and drive.

More than anything, Anita said, Swift River wanted them to rethink their notion of home and family. A home didn't need to have broadband access, wide-screen televisions, and a Cherokee or Explorer with a topped-off tank waiting to be borrowed. Being part of a family didn't mean breezing in and demanding money or retreating to a bedroom to communicate with Instant Messenger buddies. It meant being interdependent, like the species of the rain forest. The counselors wanted the kids to watch several generations cooperating as they cut firewood, prepared meals, and dealt with the joys and the hardships of getting through each day together.

Anita pulled Mary Alice aside and told her that she'd have a writing assignment during her home stay. Anita started to explain it. "You spend so much time telling us about all the things you're going to do, trying to impress us —"

"My parents always tell me how I've had the perfect life, and how lucky I am."

"We're not talking about your parents, Mary Alice. You're almost eighteen. What about *you?* Who *are* you?"

Mary Alice soon filled up a page, then two, then ten of her journal. She made lists on two facing pages:

| *What's Real about Me* | *What's Fake about Me* |
| --- | --- |
| doing yoga | talking in a Southern accent |
| helping others | makeup |
| dancing | tight clothes |
| photography | trying to be someone I'm not |
| singing | feeling insecure and paranoid |
| running | shopping every week |
| snowboarding | obsessing in front of the mirror |
| being outside | trying to fit in |
| respecting myself | thinking I'm okay and everything's fine |
| reading at a café | |
| going to church | |
| not changing who I am and what I stand for | |

Mary Alice quickly took to life at Doña Virginia's place. She read to the eight-year-old grandson and tickled his cousins. She biked to the beach with a flock of little kids, then spent hours swimming and building sand castles. The children didn't have a soccer ball, so she took them to the yard and kicked around a deflated basketball. In a sweltering house with a tin

roof and no running water, it was hard to look good. But Mary Alice noticed that Doña Virginia's family liked her fine, even when she was soaked
in sweat. "It doesn't matter to them that I don't have any makeup on," Mary
Alice told the counselors who checked in on her. The Costa Ricans certainly
didn't care about her eating disorder. In a family that barely had enough
food, no one had the luxury of bingeing and purging.

On a Wednesday morning in early September, Tanya picked up the kids
from their home stays so they could work on community service projects,
ranging from building a sidewalk at a high school to assembling a topo-
graphical map at an environmental agency. Shouting over the noise of
the taxi-truck, Mary Alice said she realized she had spent her life trying to
fit her mother's vision of the perfect daughter. "She's always saying I'm
spoiled, but she has four closets full of clothes. She says I always want more
things, but *she's* the one who has to drive around in a Lexus. She says I'm
obsessed with my appearance, but *she's* the one who got a nose job." Tanya
told Mary Alice to slow down, but she couldn't. "My mother wanted me to
play sports so she could say I made the teams. She wanted me to have certain friends so she would look good. She wanted me to say my eating disorder was fine so she could tell her Bible study class that I was cured. It's like I
was her success story." When Tyrone hopped into the taxi-truck and sat
next to her, Mary Alice barely paused to greet him before continuing. "I'm
not going to let her control me anymore." She said she understood things
she had never grasped before. She wasn't a broken girl who had to be put
back together like Humpty-Dumpty. She was just someone who needed
compassion from her parents.

For the rest of the day, as Group 23 built a concrete sidewalk for a final
community service project, Mary Alice buttonholed one kid after another
to share her epiphany. "I figured it out: It's not the kid who is screwed up,
it's the parent."

A day before the parents were to arrive in Costa Rica, Tanya got an alarming call from Rudy Bentz in Massachusetts. The campus was in an uproar.
Kids had admitted to sneaking in drugs after home visits, plotting to run
away, and behavior that stopped just short of having sex. Seven students

had been expelled. Thirty — a record for Swift River — were on self-study, sitting at a mirror and writing about their transgressions. A handsome boy named Dylan had boasted about fooling around with several girls, including two in Tanya's group.

Tanya rushed to the community service site. She pulled aside Eva and Willow, who were shoveling wet concrete into a wheelbarrow. She sat them at tables so far apart that they couldn't see each other. "Truth list," she commanded each one. "I want everything." Her harsh tone left no doubt that if they failed to divulge their secrets, they wouldn't graduate in two and a half weeks. This wasn't about a couple of girls who had been duped by a smooth-talking Lothario named Dylan; it was about cleaning up the school.

Eva and Willow spent four hours in the shade with nothing more than water and slices of papaya. In group that afternoon, Willow said she had something to disclose. She had broken the sex rule right before leaving campus — by giving someone oral sex in the woods behind Swift River's main building. "It was Dylan. He said he loves me."

A few seats away, Eva gasped. She was about to tell the group that *she* had messed around with Dylan just before leaving campus. They had sneaked outside and he'd felt her up while saying he loved her.

Everyone looked at Tanya to see if she was angry. Instead, her expression was surprisingly serene. She hadn't put much stock in the constant praise, or the criticisms, of the "guru group." She didn't expect perfection, just honesty. And now, at least, the kids were being far more honest than they'd ever been at home.

Still, Tanya had a nagging sense that there was even more going on. Although Ashley and Andy were on bans, guilt was etched all over their faces. Tanya kept trying to see what they were up to. While talking to someone else, she'd crane her neck and look for Ashley and Andy. She couldn't catch them at anything. Whenever she so much as hinted at her suspicions, they indignantly asked why she kept picking on them.

The Costa Rica staff called the final week of Swift River the "personal challenge for parents." Most of the mothers and fathers had never been to a developing country, and often they became nauseated as the prop plane bounced over the clouds and landed in Puerto Jiménez. By then the students knew their way around. They could order food and make small talk in Spanish. That upended family relationships: Parents had to depend on sons and daughters who had been undependable for a long time.

When the Group 23 parents arrived — looking dazed from the puddle-jumper flight, the heat, the potholed roads — Anita, Tanya, and Gennarose met with them on the deck of a hotel surrounded by palm trees. "Swift River is the start of a long process," Anita cautioned. "Your child is not fixed." Over the years, more than one mother and father had assumed that they could drop off a struggling teenager for fourteen months, then retrieve a happy, well-mannered son or daughter, as if they were picking up a car from the mechanic. Anita stressed that the kids weren't the only ones who still had work to do; a parent might have to continue treatment for depression or alcoholism.

Tanya noticed that the parents had changed during the year she'd been working with them. Although D.J.'s mother and father were still eager to offer him tips for succeeding in the remaining year and a half of high school, they first listened to his tales of the Osa Peninsula. Mary Alice's parents, Burns and Lillian, remarked that they had cut back on their golf outings, trips to Europe, and other "pleasurizing" to spend more time with their children. Lillian had given a lot of thought to her own upbringing and how it had influenced her parenting style. She remembered the pain of growing up as an only child feeling isolated in a divorced family, embarrassed because she lived in a small house in the wrong part of Dallas. "So many parents are living through their kids. That's what I ended up doing."

Then there was Tyrone's mom. She was just the same as she had been when she dropped him off at base camp. She chattered away with Costa Ricans in a rapid-fire mix of Spanish and New Yorkese. She shared pointers for buying cheap plane tickets. And she couldn't stop putting her arm around her son, even though her head no longer reached his shoulders; he had shot up at least an inch since base camp.

Most of the parents praised Swift River. A couple of them appreciated it more when they stumbled into a pack of kids from a new school for wayward American teenagers that had opened in Costa Rica. Standing in a hotel lobby, several of the kids puffed on cigarettes; one growled at a counselor to "fuck off." At nightfall the boys and girls held hands and sauntered off to the beach, and it was safe to assume they weren't searching for a turtle hatchery.

Every day the Swift River parents and kids gathered in the classroom with the metal roof for seminars about communication or discussions about life after graduation. One morning they received an e-mail from Bianca in Florida. Anita read it aloud.

> The plane ride was fine and I didn't get hit on by any guys (you can stop worrying, Tanya).
>
> My dad has already lost weight and is a lot paler. It hit me hard when I looked at him holding the newspaper and his hand was shaking and his voice was weak. I told him about our adventures in Costa Rica and that he and I will go there some day.
>
> Over the weekend my best friend asked me to her eighteenth birthday party at a hotel two hours away and my dad said to go and have some fun. So I went. It was kind of pathetic, all the people were just sitting around getting drunk and smoking and acting like dumb asses (excuse my language, I can't think of a better word). I stayed for at the most 10 minutes and went home.
>
> Anyways, my grandma and grandpa came and I sat with my grandma and she held me like I was a little girl. My grandpa helped out with taking my dad to the hospital every day for a shot that helps you regain your immune system and he got dad a shower chair, because the other day my dad fell in the shower. He didn't get hurt, but when my brother went in to check on him, he was in a towel; kneeling by the bathtub and said that he was fine. My uncle sat us down and told my dad that even though he doesn't want us to know about all this and worry, we're going to anyways, so he is going to have to ask for help.

Anita choked up. She took a few moments to regain her composure before finishing.

> Since then my dad has been asking, and I'm not the only one helping. My brother is, and my Nana, and grandma and grandpa and uncle and my sister. When my mom was sick, I was just so much more oblivious and my parents hid a lot from me. This time, I'm seeing the full effects of chemo and I'm scared as hell. I think the hardest part for me is not being able to touch my dad. He has no white blood cell count and no immune system, so he is susceptible to every germ.
>
> Every night I go to bed praying that this isn't happening, but every morning I cry because it is.

I can't express the love I have for all of you guys. Say hi to all of
your parents from me and my dad.

Love always, Bianca

*ↂ*

"*Uno, dos, tres* . . . cheese!" Mary Alice's father shot pictures of Doña Virginia and her grandchildren, then the Texans and the Costa Ricans admired
the images on the back of his digital camera. Mary Alice had returned to
Doña Virginia's tiny house with her parents. As the children tugged at her
arms and legs, Mary Alice led a tour, showing the well were she had collected water as part of her daily chores and the room where she had slept —
a nook smaller than their laundry room back home. "*Mi casa es pobrecita*
. . . ," Doña Virginia explained as Mary Alice translated: "My house is very
poor but it has a lot of love." The old woman complimented Mary Alice's
parents on their daughter's manners and set out a homemade cake with
bright pink frosting.

Burns and Lillian presented Doña Virginia with a suitcase full of pots,
pans, and clothes. Then they gave her a photo of Mary Alice and her three
siblings. Doña Virginia removed a snapshot of her own family from a
frame that sat by her bed and slipped in the Chamblisses' photo. She in-
spected the picture. "Your cheeks were fuller then," she said, looking disapprovingly at Mary Alice's trim face and body.

The Chamblisses produced a gift for the children: a soccer ball. Soon
Mary Alice and the four children were kicking it around the muddy yard
while laughing and bantering. The Chamblisses shook their heads in
amazement as they tried to decipher their daughter. Was this the same
Mary Alice who had started a diary two years before by referring to "my
fucked-up life"? The same Mary Alice who was having sex with strangers
on a church trip the previous summer?

During the week, parents and kids had to work on contracts about life
after Swift River. The contracts listed thirty questions: What would the curfew be for a kid who moved back home? What kind of rules would there be
about bringing boyfriends or girlfriends over? If a kid got a car, who would
pay for gas and insurance? If parents banned cigarettes at home, did that
apply to smoking somewhere else? Mary Alice was willing to discuss drugs
(she wouldn't do them) and cigarettes (she couldn't make any promises).
She reflected on what she'd learned about her own neighborhood by living

at Doña Virginia's. "Kids have way more money than they need, that's the problem. Because there's so much pressure, kids who aren't secure get into bad relationships and drugs." But when Lillian happened to make an off-hand comment about the last semester of senior year, Mary Alice exploded. "I don't want to go back to Dallas!" she screamed. "I can't survive there. Do you fucking understand?"

D.J. vacillated too. He eagerly showed his parents around on a hike, pointing out a trail of leaf-cutter ants, but he pouted and whined when they asked about the homework he still owed his chemistry teacher.

Only Tyrone sailed through the parents' visit. Sitting at a picnic table, he and his mother pored over the contract and saw eye to eye on every point: He would finish his final year of high school; he would follow his mother's rules as long as he lived in the house; he would talk to her instead of isolating in his room. On one subject — his father — he and his mother agreed to disagree. Tyrone didn't want to hear any more criticisms about his father. Not from his mother, not from Tanya, and not from his peers. He planned to get together with his dad from time to time; he'd see what happened from there. That was nobody else's business.

"Tyrone, you're seventeen — you're almost a man," his mother sighed. "At your age, I was living on my own because I'd moved out to get away from my stepmother. You know how I feel about your father and you know that won't change, but I'm never going to tell you how to feel."

On the eight-hour return bus trip to San José, Andy wore a bead necklace and a T-shirt with the sleeves cut off. He had the cool, detached aura of the guy who drank and drove through Long Island at ninety miles an hour. Ashley, who was still banned from talking with him, had connived to sit a few feet away. She giggled and flirted. "Why is it that they call it underwear for boys," she asked no one in particular, "and panties for girls?"

In San José, the group threaded through crowded streets on the way to a souvenir-shopping trip at an outdoor market. The Ohio girl sidled up to Tanya and said she needed to confess a secret: She and Ashley had been planning on stealing something from the market. Tanya did what her training told her. She pulled Ashley aside, dropped to the end of the line, and made an open-ended statement: "There are things that you need to tell me." Ashley seemed nervous. She looked away. Her response surprised

Tanya. "I can't tell you because other people will get in trouble and they won't be able to graduate."

"Ashley, you don't know that," Tanya answered, but even as she did she wondered what Ashley was concealing. Not graduating? For *planning* to shoplift? Tanya tried to fish for more information, but Ashley stonewalled. Uncertain about what was going on, Tanya bluffed. "I already know the truth," she said. "Ashley, what is it going to feel like to get on the stage for graduation and know that you're being dishonest?"

While the others went out to dinner with Gennarose that night, Tanya sat on a bench and talked with Ashley. Ashley said she was tired of holding on to secrets. She admitted that since arriving in Costa Rica, she and Andy had had sex three times in bathrooms and outhouses — once when their parents were just a few yards away. Tanya had resolved not to take the kids' actions personally, but this time she felt insulted. She had practically left her father's deathbed to fly to Costa Rica, and this was the way the group was behaving?

While she finished with Ashley, Tanya told two of the Costa Rican counselors to try to get Andy to own up to what he'd done. After a half hour they were flummoxed. The kid hadn't done anything wrong, they said. Tanya took over. She sat with Andy and waited. He was calm and casual. "You guys are ridiculous," he objected. "What you are doing is ridiculous."

Tanya ordered Andy to come clean about everything that had happened. An hour passed. It was eleven o'clock and Tanya was hungry and tired. She'd had enough of his me-first attitude. Trucks rumbled by outside. She told him he could stay up all night, but he wasn't leaving till he came clean. Besides, she said, she'd already learned everything — *everything* — by talking to Ashley. "The least you could do is say it yourself and not make me say it for you."

That worked. In a matter-of-fact voice, Andy recounted the bathroom sex. His account matched Ashley's. Tanya was so disgusted that she had to turn away. Andy had one request: He wanted to call his parents at home on Long Island and tell them what he'd done. "I don't want it coming from anyone else."

Tanya summoned everyone to a meeting room for an impromptu group. Ashley spoke first, crying as she admitted to having had sex with Andy. "*What?*" Mary Alice gasped. The others sat dumbfounded.

Andy echoed her story without showing any emotion. He said he might as well put it all on the table. Visiting back home two months earlier, he'd drunk beer and smoked pot. He'd also kissed his old girlfriend, breaking the rules for a home visit. He'd lied about that to everyone, including Ashley.

The kids had suspected Ashley and Andy were fooling around a bit, but sex in bathrooms? Three times? It was Tyrone who voiced their collective shock. "How could you do this to yourself?" he asked Ashley. Then he turned to Andy. "You were doing so well. Why did you mess it up?"

Andy hung his head. "I've been asking myself that. I don't know."

"I think you do," Tyrone countered.

The others chimed in heatedly. Eva was the most vocal. Andy might think it was his business and no one else's if he broke Swift River's rules. But it wasn't so simple when you'd spent more than a year with other kids and they'd trusted you and told you things that no one else had ever heard. No, Eva said, Andy was a brat who didn't think about anyone but himself.

Group 23 had gone from sixteen members to fifteen after Trevor's overdose. Tanya assumed it would soon shed two more. To let Ashley and Andy graduate after having sex in the final weeks would send a message to other students that they could pick and choose which of Swift River's agreements to follow. That cafeteria-style approach had landed many of them at a therapeutic boarding school to begin with.

The group arrived at an airport outside of Boston after midnight the next day. As the groggy, grouchy kids spilled into the terminal, they noticed a short, tan teenage girl with long wavy hair parted in the middle. "Bianca!" several of the kids cried, running to embrace her. Bianca got in a few words, explaining that her father was still going through chemo so he would be too drained to attend graduation in a week. The others babbled about the Costa Rican families and the parents' visit. One of the girls blurted out details of the scandal involving Ashley and Andy, who hung back from the rest, heads drooping. Bianca shook her head in disgust, but she could top that news.

"Guys, things are crazy on campus." She detailed the spate of expulsions and restrictions. She prepared them for the most devastating part. "You don't know about Trevor? You'll never believe what he did."

# 31

## CONQUERING HEROES

IN THE HIERARCHY of Swift River students, none were as exalted as the kids returning from Costa Rica. Their skin was bronzed, their muscles sculpted from kayaking and hiking; they wore seashell bracelets and shared private jokes about sex-maniac tree frogs hooking up; they peppered their conversations with mysterious references to dancing dolphins and a machete-toting guide named Luis. The kids were, as Rudy liked to say, "conquering heroes." They strummed guitars and bided their time. "*Vamos, chicos*" — one week till graduation. The heroes no longer went to classes, no longer did work projects, no longer lived in the dorms. Instead, they left campus in a van every night to sleep in a faded old skiers' lodge consisting of one large room for boys and another for girls, each with lumpy bunk beds surrounded by tattered posters of snowy scenes. The others at Swift River didn't know what it looked like. The very name of the place — Remington Lodge — packed so much mystique among younger students that it might as well have been the Four Seasons.

Of all the rituals at Swift River — sweats, dress-up Sunday dinners, personal challenges — nothing came close to the rituals for the kids in their final week. The school honored them at one event after another, starting with their first day back, when they sat in front of the great room and each kid talked about a favorite moment in Costa Rica. At another meeting, Rudy handed them "Rio Rapido" T-shirts with a map of the Osa Peninsula and a list of the peer group's names on the sleeves. Then there was date night — when they, the oldest peer group, got to ask kids out for an evening in Northampton. The final week sent a message to other kids on campus: You, too, can be heroes if you stick it out.

With the acclaim and the freedom, though, came new duties. On the first morning, as the fifteen kids in Group 23 straggled to breakfast at the lodge, Rudy stopped by for a meeting. He hugged everyone, including Andy and Ashley, and congratulated the group for succeeding in Costa Rica. He singled out Tyrone for emerging as a trustworthy leader and D.J. for thriving in the outdoor classroom. "I've come to cheer your success, but also to ask a favor," he said. "The campus is in an uproar, as you've heard. The school needs you more than ever to be role models, to be positive. If you see someone struggling, let them know that not long ago, you, too, were there struggling. We don't want you to be fake, but we do want you to tell them the good things about Costa Rica so they have something to look forward to." He paraphrased Thoreau: "We need now to walk among the higher order of being."

The kids wanted a full account — no sugarcoating — of what had gone wrong while they were away. Rudy gave it. During August, a perfect storm had welled up, a perfect emotional storm much like the one that had roiled campus half a year earlier, in the winter from hell. The counselors had pieced together the story through truth lists. It began with a boy who had managed to hide three hundred dollars in the lining of his pants before being sent to Swift River. He'd retrieved the money on moving to main campus and had slipped it to a friend who promised to buy heroin during a home visit. The friend lost his nerve and instead bought a case of cough syrup for "Robotripping." He'd smuggled it to Swift River in a backpack. And that's when Trevor came in. After hearing about the plot, he stole the leftover cash and the cough syrup and tried to get a buzz.

That wasn't all. Trevor had learned that the infirmary had a drawer stuffed with Adderall pills — the extras from kids who had left the school or changed their prescriptions. Knowing that there was a time on Sundays when one nurse worked alone, he'd set up a scam to top all scams. A buddy faked an asthma attack in the nurse's office, falling off a stool and wheezing, "I can't breathe!" As the nurse helped the boy use an inhaler, Trevor pretended to trip and rammed his shoulder into a wall at the infirmary entrance, making a foot-wide hole. He stuck his head in the wall and acted as if he'd lost consciousness. As the nurse rushed from one crisis to the other, Trevor's friend grabbed the Adderall — enough to provide a prolonged high for their friends. They divvied up the booty, sixty-one pills. Trevor spent a day crushing and snorting Adderall. Finally another kid, worried that someone was going to overdose, told a counselor. While searching Trevor's room, the staff found a stash of cough medicine under his mattress. All kinds of secrets soon surfaced on truth lists — including what Tanya had confirmed: Willow and Eva had fooled around with the same guy before flying to Costa Rica.

Several of the kids cried as they listened to the saga. Rudy said he had no choice but to expel Trevor. "On a personal level, I love the kid. He's a precious guy. But on a clinical level, we cannot let him back. We can't provide him the care he needs."

After the meeting with Rudy, two vans deposited the kids on campus for the first time in five weeks. They walked in to find the foyer plastered with handmade posters welcoming them back. They also saw a restriction room packed with kids who had broken the sex and drug agreements. They spread out to help. Mary Alice spoke to girls she'd gotten to know, encouraging them to tough it out till Costa Rica. Tyrone and D.J. didn't proselytize, but while playing hacky-sack with other kids they described the hikes and horseback rides in Costa Rica with just enough detail to tantalize skeptics.

Bianca caught up with her friend Jake, the boy who had told her about overdosing on Wellbutrin. She was still worried about life after "the bubble." How could she find a boyfriend who treated her well? How could she stay strong when her father was sick? Jake didn't have easy answers, but he assured Bianca that if she kept asking those questions she would be on her way to doing well.

Bianca had been through so much that she no longer held back her thoughts. Counselors asked her to join group therapy because other kids needed the "harder truth." One afternoon she sat in a group of students who had been chosen to discuss loss and grieving. Two counselors were trying to get a boy to talk about how he had been affected by his father's death. The boy spoke slowly, mechanically: "My father had a heart attack when I was nine. I didn't really know him."

Bianca took over the questioning. "But how did you feel about it? What did it mean to you?"

"It was a long time ago and it didn't affect me."

Exasperated, Bianca stopped the conversation. "This is bullshit! You have no emotion! You sound like you're talking about someone else's dog dying."

The boy seemed to wither in his chair. Bianca spoke evenly. "You can't fool me. I was like you, trying to act like I didn't give a shit, like I didn't spend every day thinking about my mom. It was a lie. I don't care what you tell everyone in this room, but you're lying to yourself. Your dad died and now you're here. Stop pretending you could deal with it."

Looking away from Bianca, out the window, the boy started to sniffle. At the end of the group, he admitted that he hadn't been honest. He had tried to act as if he was too macho to be affected by his father's death. He thought he'd fooled everyone.

The final week passed in a blur of campus celebrations and field trips to restaurants and parks. In a school meeting, the students from the group sat on the floor in a circle and talked about what they'd learned during Costa Rica. During "legacy night," as the group's final Tuesday closing was known, each kid gave away a favorite memento to a newer student while offering words of encouragement. But Group 23 had an unsettled feeling while the other thirteen kids waited for Swift River to decide what to do about Ashley and Andy.

Two days before graduation, Rudy ordered Andy to pack his bags and go home. He was eighteen and he'd finished his academic requirements for high school, but he didn't deserve to stand up on the stage at graduation.

Ashley, though, was to be given a last chance. On the day before graduation, she went to the headmaster's office for a meeting with her parents. Rudy and Tanya said she could stay at Swift River if she agreed to be dropped to another group that would graduate in eight months. The staff wasn't punishing Ashley, Rudy emphasized, but everyone agreed that some important messages hadn't reached her the first time around. She needed to understand more about who she was and why she kept taking risks.

Without reacting, Ashley went to wait in a hallway. A few minutes later, someone noticed that she was gone. The staff checked the bathrooms and the dorms. A counselor who was friendly with Ashley had a bad feeling, so she dashed out of the front door. Tanya followed, grabbing a supervisor's car keys and jumping into his pickup truck. She didn't realize until too late that it wasn't automatic. She had driven a stick shift just once — thirteen years earlier. The gears screeched as she lurched and bucked along country roads.

They found Ashley, still in her beach sandals from Costa Rica, hiking across a pasture. Swift River counselors could restrain students only in an emergency, so for half an hour they took turns walking next to her, talking to her gently and reporting her location on a walkie-talkie. "What about that little girl in the picture?" Tanya asked as she kept pace with Ashley. "What would she want for you now? Are you really making good decisions for her?" Ashley strode forward in silence, looking straight ahead. A third counselor drove up in a van with kids from the peer group. They shouted at Ashley to come back. Ignoring them, she veered into the woods and waded through a stream. Even when a sandal fell off, she kept going.

As Ashley approached a road, a counselor warned that she'd be restrained if she got near the traffic. Ashley reached the pavement and lunged toward an approaching car. Running to help, Tanya watched Ashley turn toward her and freeze for a moment with an almost beatific smile. Just as the car stopped, she threw herself on the hood. Tanya and one of the other counselors grabbed Ashley and held her for five minutes while waiting for the police. Ashley kept thrashing around as a policewoman handcuffed her.

A year after confiding her runaway plan to Tyrone in base camp, Ashley had made good on it. She would spend graduation day about twenty miles from campus, under psychiatric observation in a hospital.

That afternoon, Tanya gathered everyone at the Remington Lodge for the last group. By tradition, this was the time when kids talked about what they liked the most about each other; it was a way of dealing with separation anxiety. It took a few minutes for everyone to calm down and focus. The group agreed they liked D.J.'s sense of adventure, his boyish smile, and his joy at learning about animals; they liked Tyrone's integrity and unfaltering confidence, Mary Alice's empathy with younger students, and Bianca's piercing honesty. "We're never going to sit in group together after this," Eva said as her sometime archrival, Mary Alice, started to sob.

"When I think of the future, I think about going back to the same shit, and it scares me," Mary Alice said. She steadied herself and looked at Tanya, that big lovable goose of a counselor. "I'm gonna miss you, Tanya. I wish I could put you in my pocket and take you home."

After group, Mary Alice surprised Bianca by asking to talk. "We've had some crap get in our way," Mary Alice said, sniffling.

"Both of us made everything get in the way," Bianca said. "We're so much alike."

"I'm sorry," Mary Alice said as they hugged. "I love you, Bianca."

The staff decorated the main building for graduation. In the middle of the foyer, a table was set up with photos of thirteen of the kids cavorting on a beach. They didn't include any hint of Ashley or Andy, as if the two of them had been airbrushed out of Group 23, just like Trevor.

On the foyer wall was a framed front page of the 1917 *Daily Hampshire Gazette*, which marveled at the $50,000 farm that had opened on the site, complete with a dairy, stables, barn, and other buildings. Sending the members of Group 23 to Swift River had cost the parents, as well as school districts in New York, New Jersey, and Vermont, close to a million dollars. (In the case of Phil the Philosopher, the tuition was paid by his parents' employer, the federal government. The family was posted overseas, and a psychologist found that Phil needed special services). It was still too early to predict what the families and the taxpayers would get for that money. Swift River had devoted two years to devising an "outcomes project" that would measure kids' communications skills, self-control, and self-esteem throughout the program and years later. The administration said it would be the most thorough and accurate evaluation of student progress at any therapeutic school. But the project was still mired in the design stage. (A University of Idaho study of nearly 900 teenagers who had been sent to wilderness intervention programs found "significant reductions" in behavioral and emotional problems. But the study was simply a comparison of questionnaires given to parents and kids at admission and at discharge from the program. And the research was funded in part by the very programs that were being evaluated, raising questions of objectivity.) Rudy and Jill Bentz maintained that the school had given the kids the tools to go out and live happy, productive lives. In the family resolution in July, Rudy had told parents about his 10-80-10 theory: 10 percent of graduates soared, 80 percent did quite well, and 10 relapsed. "I don't want to scare you, but the children may falter after graduation, they may regress a bit," he had warned. "But they can never ever plummet back to the bottom where they were. It's impossible."

The tumultuous summer had left some staff members cynical, however. "It's not like a new kid walks out the door after fourteen months," a gym teacher grumbled. After working in base camp and on campus for three years, he had come to believe that when Swift River succeeded, it was simply because kids matured. "But the school can't tell parents it's just a matter of maturation. Otherwise, who is going to pay eighty grand? The parents would feel like they're being ripped off."

Even the staff members who knew the kids the best couldn't agree about how well Swift River had worked. Supervisor Julie Haagenson rolled her eyes as she thought back on her quarrels with Mary Alice over mirrors and makeup. She was well aware that eating disorders persist for years. "You hear story after story about how these girls do fantastic in a program, then they go home and stick their fingers in their throats." Even worse, she said, Mary Alice was returning to "artificial-land," her wealthy neighborhood where everyone appeared perennially cheerful and impossibly thin. Gennarose lowered her voice when she thought of Mary Alice back in Dallas: "Honestly, I think she's gonna fuck up. She's too caught up in the Southern society woman bullshit. It'll be too much pressure for her. She might either have a relapse of her eating disorder or go back into drugs." Still, she believed Mary Alice would be able to pull out of it eventually. "With the skills she's learned, the relapse will be shorter."

When Mary Alice's parents had filled out the application for Swift River, they listed their goals: "To improve self-esteem, get in touch with her issues, respect herself and others, property, and life, find direction and a sense of purpose, gain healthy skills for dealing with anxiety and stress, to make better decisions." While Tanya had seen Mary Alice make great progress, she figured it would take a while for the lessons to kick in.

Those who had worked with D.J. were divided. Julie couldn't hide her frustration with D.J., who struck her as too impulsive. "I don't have a whole lot of hope for him," she said. Gennarose wavered. She thought of D.J. careening around the rain forest, reciting facts about leaf-cutter ants. She'd seen the charming boy in him, the Huckleberry spirit who couldn't abide being "cramped up." But D.J. was going back to a competitive private school, a difficult place for a kid who couldn't sit still. "He needs a mentor and he needs to find a passion for something that's not a video game. He needs to meet the right friends. If he doesn't, if he finds himself isolated again, then he's going to fuck up."

Even Bianca stirred disagreement. Tanya had no doubt that she was going on to great things. Gennarose concurred: "She's a star." Julie, though, was dubious of anyone who appeared to be a Swift River poster child. "I wish we could have cracked her," she said. "Some kids like Bianca are so smart and so charming that you don't know when they're being sneaky and dishonest. Those kids are more self-destructive than the kids who go around punching walls." Julie had reason to worry. She had been proud of her work with a boy, a heavy drug user, who had graduated a couple of years before. He'd done wonderfully at Swift River, where he had support around the clock. A few months after returning home, though, he smashed his car into a truck so hard that he flipped over. The cops found heroin stashed in his glove compartment.

Tyrone was the enigma. While Tanya thought that he had learned a lot about himself, he seemed to plow through Swift River more out of loyalty to his mother. By frequently pointing out that the rest of the students were different, Tyrone had given himself an excuse not to look past those differences. "He missed out on the experience of truly connecting to people from other backgrounds," Tanya said. She wasn't surprised; she knew that kids who felt abandoned by a parent had trouble trusting others. Julie insisted that if Tyrone didn't get enough out of Swift River, it wasn't the staff's fault. "He didn't fully embrace what we were teaching here. He was just doing his time."

Gennarose didn't want to hear any of their nay-saying. Tyrone's mother, in her comments to the staff in Costa Rica, had gotten it right: Tyrone was no longer isolated. Without giving up on his father, he had found a way to get along with his mother. Even more, in the middle of the rain forest, he had taken charge. He was a leader — no small feat for a boy who had all but hibernated in his bedroom through the first two years of high school. "That kid," Gennarose said, "is gonna rock."

# 32

## "You Have Your Little Girl Back"

GROUP 23, WHAT WAS LEFT of it, circled up for the final time. It was the first Friday in October 2002, graduation day. Bianca, Mary Alice, Tyrone, D.J., and the rest of the kids — thirteen in all — stood in the foyer with Tanya and Gennarose, arms draped on each other's shoulders. "Take a couple of deep breaths, get into the here and now. Nothing else is going on, no place is as important as this circle," Rudy said, starting the group's final guided meditation. "We're going to take a little journey. Come back to base camp and smell that campfire. When did you know? When you were sitting on shadow in the woods? When did you know? When you went to your first group at base camp and started telling your life story truthfully?"

On one side of the foyer, mullioned windows looked out to the classroom building, the soccer field, and the path to base camp. On the other side, windows in the double doors of the main entrance looked out to the curving driveway and, beyond that, the road home. Everywhere, maple leaves were tinged with crimson and gold. Rudy continued. "When did you know? When you were on solo? Did you have some hope about the future when you walked in from base camp? Or when you took your first shower on campus? When you sat in your first class here did you think, 'Hey, I'm not the dummy I'm supposed to be. I *do* have a brain'? Did you think it when you were in the sweat lodge, jammed among your friends? When was it? The first time your parents visited? The night before you went on the first home visit, or when you got to Costa Rica? When did you forgive yourself? Was it just this morning when you got dressed to come to campus for the last time? When did you know you were perfectly okay? Did it take until right now?"

Rudy's traditional graduation-day pep talk was supposed to help the kids concentrate before giving their speeches. As with everything about guru group in the final weeks, though, graduation day wasn't following the script. Just as the kids got settled, Bianca let out a shriek. *"Dad!"* She had expected just two guests, her grandmother and her twin, Bruno, but her father's doctor had okayed a surprise trip. Bianca ran to embrace Alan, who wore a baseball cap to conceal the baldness caused by chemo.

In the great room, the peer groups sat on white folding chairs, one group after another all the way to Group 30, newly arrived from base camp, in the back. As rousing, brassy processional music played over the loudspeakers, Group 23 filed past the cheering, hooting crowd. Bianca's father kept his cap on. "We have colds, we need to sit away from him," the mother from California told an elderly relative in a stage whisper that could be heard two rows away. "He has leu-*kee*-mi-a."

From the side of the stage, Tanya watched the kids wistfully. She knew it would be strange not to see them around the school — and perhaps never to see or talk to them again. Graduates didn't buy Swift River sweatshirts or come back for reunions; they didn't dream of sending their children to their beloved old therapeutic alma mater. At best, they turned their backs on the place and remembered the lessons they'd learned. Terminating with a client in one-on-one therapy was difficult enough, but now Tanya was terminating with thirteen on a single day.

Mary Alice, still tanned and glowing from Costa Rica, wore a full-length strapless blue gown, pearl earrings, and a pearl necklace. Bianca wore a knee-length red dress with sparkles, topped by the silver heart necklace that her mother had given her. Tyrone had on black trousers and a shiny black button-down shirt and a black tie. D.J., too, wore black slacks, black shirt, and tie. He no longer had a baby face; the acne that once blotched his cheeks had cleared.

The parents and grandparents settled on chairs in the front three rows. Mary Alice's parents sat at front row center. Mary Alice had remained unpredictable during the final days in Costa Rica. She'd lash out at her parents, then embrace them. She'd talk about joining her mother at meetings of an eating-disorder group in Dallas, then insist that she would *never* live in Dallas. Mary Alice's eighteenth birthday was just six days away. Legally, at least, she would be an adult in most ways. Burns said she was getting to the point in her life when she would have to work things out for herself.

Bianca stepped up to the lectern to receive an award for her academic work, then returned to speak. She surveyed the two dozen parents and grandparents sitting in the front rows and the hundred students behind them. "Picture this," she said in a lilting voice. "You're in a hospital room looking through a glass wall at your mother. She's sleeping. For once, she's not hallucinating from the meds or throwing up from the chemo. She looks so weak. You can't go into the room and hug her or lie with her; you're too young. A barrier is holding you back, but it's not holding you back from the horror of your mother's suffering.

"That was me eight years ago. I didn't know what to do. I turned away from my family. I built up false hopes with fake friends. I yelled, I screamed, and tried so hard not to show the tears. I knew I needed help but I couldn't ask."

Bianca said that she had learned to talk about her struggles and ask for help. She turned around and glanced at the twelve kids seated behind her. "I care so much for each and every one of you; all of you have always been there for me and are my true friends." Then she nodded to her brother. "Bruno, we have been together for nine months longer than anyone in this world. You're my twin brother and I can't even express all the love I have for you. Dad, I'm really happy that you came too, it means a lot to me and I don't know how to express my thanks to you and my love for you. I cherish our relationship so much."

She looked up at the soaring ceiling — up beyond the ceiling, it seemed — and swallowed hard. "Mom, I know you're watching over me and you're proud of me." Even in the back row, kids who didn't know Bianca were dabbing their cheeks with tissues. "You're my inspiration and hero. I love you so much and I miss you so much."

Mary Alice stood at the lectern and took a breath. "Fourteen months ago I came here still high from all the drugs, still tired from all the sex and throwing up I'd done the night before. I had nearly died inside." She spoke about breaking all the rules at home. Then she looked at the newer students in the back. "Some people think that this place isn't reality, that we live in a bubble. I can tell you that this is the realest place you will ever be, and that if you do not take advantage of what is around you then it will come back to haunt you down the road."

She glanced to the side. "Tanya, you are the first person who has truly understood me and my struggles. I don't know how to comprehend all that you have given me and the rest of the peer group, even in the midst of your own struggle. You are the strongest, most amazing person I have ever met. I'll carry you with me wherever I go."

She turned and looked at the front row: "To my parents: You have your little girl back."

Tyrone hadn't said much to anyone about his speech. When he walked to the lectern, the rustling in the room stopped and the kids sat upright, just as they had when he'd stood in the same spot five months earlier to read aloud the letter to his dad from his nine-year-old self. Tyrone's mother clasped her hands and his stepfather smiled. Although Tyrone's dad had talked about visiting, the last day had arrived and he hadn't made the four-hour trip from New York.

Tyrone started in a voice so low that the audience leaned forward to hear. "Loneliness, fear, pain, anger, isolation, sadness. These are the feelings I brought here with me. I brought them because that's all I knew." As always, he was a man of few words, but his poise said much more. He raised his voice. "I thank my family for being there for me, especially my mom. You took time and did work to help me when I was struggling. I love you."

For days, D.J.'s parents had fretted. Would he finish his history paper in time to stand on the stage at graduation? Would he forget to write his graduation speech, then get up there and ad lib and mumble? They didn't have to worry. Not only did he turn in his history paper, he wrote out his speech a couple of days early.

In his black outfit, D.J. looked somber. He started his speech by talking about his time at Swift River. "It's been hard and I didn't make it any easier on myself," he said. Tyrone and several others grinned at that, remembering his antics. "Not until the end of the program when I started taking risks and standing up for myself did I truly feel happy. In Costa Rica I dealt with my impulsivity and stayed calm. Never thought I'd say this, but I'm gonna miss it here." He looked to the audience. "Mom and Dad, I love you and I can't wait to get home."

D.J.'s mother wiped her eyes. D.J.'s father grinned; the exile was over, all 403 days of it.

❧

While the graduates bustled out the front door — first Mary Alice, dashing for a plane to Dallas, then Tyrone, lugging duffel bags of black clothes and ducking to fit into the dented Corolla — other students clutched them or offered high-fives, as if trying to squeeze in a few more precious seconds of inspiration. D.J. bounded into his minivan, scooping up his dog, Firecracker, without a look back. Bianca walked slowly through the foyer and held her father's elbow to help him keep his balance. Fourteen months before, she'd angrily turned her back on him as she started at Swift River. Now, lingering at the front door, she looked like someone who was afraid to leave.

❧

Bianca stared out at the landscape she loved — perfectly flat lawns spreading in all directions, with occasional stands of wild lantana bushes and royal palm trees. It was the day after graduation, a Saturday, and she was driving home from the West Palm Beach airport with her brother, their father, and grandmother. New England had been its usually morbid, gray self when they flew out a little after dawn, but the temperature in south Florida was in the seventies. The sky was light blue, with cumulous clouds jouncing above the Everglades like massive SUVs.

As they headed inland to the newer suburbs, Bianca noticed the construction that had started since her last visit. Every few miles, bulldozers scraped the earth to prepare the way for strip malls and housing developments. Her grandmother pointed out a large Eckard's drugstore, bedecked with balloons, that was celebrating its grand opening. A Wal-Mart was going up nearby, and at every other intersection new fast-food restaurants, nail salons, and drive-through banks were taking shape.

Sitting in the backseat, Bianca was silent. She was taking in different landmarks, ones significant only to her. They passed a sheriff's substation tucked behind some trees. She'd gone there in ninth grade to file a report after being assaulted in the gym — but she'd changed her story and refused to press charges. A few minutes later, the car passed the Friendly's where she and Darnell had worked. Across a vast expanse of parking lot stood the cinema where they had been caught nearly naked.

A few minutes later they swept by her old high school, a peach-colored building rising from a black ocean of parking spaces, with islands of portable classrooms in front. Her father was saying that the school had 1,200 students when Bianca started; now it had 3,000, with more squeezing in every month. Many were escaping the sprawl of Miami; as they arrived, they brought the sprawl with them. Bianca wasn't listening. She was remembering how she used to dash to the car she and her brother shared, then sneak out for a rendezvous with Darnell. Her brother always parked the car at the outer edge of the student lot. She'd try to return it to the same space, then run back for world history class.

They swung into her neighborhood. Not long ago it had been filled with idyllic memories: the schoolyard where she and her mom had played hopscotch; the park where she and Bruno had passed hours squirming through play structures; the lawns where they'd spread blankets for picnics. Over the years, though, it had taken on darker overtones. Near the park was the house where Kenneth had raped her at fifteen. As a sixteen-year-old, she'd gone to the park and cried about her life.

As the car pulled up the driveway, Bianca listened to familiar sounds: the whine of someone across the street power-washing his house, the roar of another neighbor assailing the curbs with a weed trimmer. It was the music of Saturday-morning chores in Florida, grating but immensely comforting.

Bianca stepped into the air-conditioned stillness of the living room and walked past her mom's piano, past the kitchen table where her father had sat that morning when she was taken away, screaming that she hated him. Now clusters of pill bottles and stacks of leukemia pamphlets covered the table, and computer printouts of white and red blood cell counts hid the kitchen counter.

In her brother's room, mounds of dirty clothes covered the floor; the place never would have passed a Swift River dorm inspection. The old Tupac poster still hung on one wall, facing the newspaper clippings about Raul and Antoine. Bianca crossed a hallway to her small bedroom. On the top shelf, a dozen dolls gazed out keenly, like students waiting for a teacher to step back into the classroom. The lower shelves brimmed with soccer trophies and certificates and ribbons from debate tournaments. Summer clothes drooped from hangers in the closet. They all were exposed; the sliding door, which she had kicked down two years ago, was still missing from the frame.

Familiar pictures were taped to the edges of the mirror above her bureau: Bianca and Bruno at age two in matching green overalls by a Christmas tree; Bianca the toddler cuddling with her mom; Bianca prancing in her flower costume in kindergarten; Bianca and her sister twirling batons in middle school.

Bianca glanced over to see her father in the doorway, the same spot where he had stood on that morning at the start of summer vacation, with the large man and woman looming behind. Now his clothes hung loosely on his body. His green eyes were lighter, his skin pale and wrinkled around his eyes. With his oversized baseball cap askew on his nearly bald head, he resembled a kid playing dress-up. There was something different about Bianca, too. She looked her father in the eyes when she talked. She stood straighter, more assured. Yet she was more like the girl she had been ten years ago, the girl who smiled out from the old snapshots.

When her father spoke, his voice had its usual deep tone, but it was not much louder than a whisper.

"Everything look the same?"

Bianca nodded. They could hear the thrum of lawn mowers, power-washers, and weed whackers. Just outside, the hedge bore the gap Bianca had made by sneaking out late at night. She leaned over and tried to raise the window but it wouldn't budge.

"Hey, Dad, maybe we could take the screws out so I can open my window?"

Alan studied her. "Yeah," he said. "I guess I trust you." He smiled and turned back to the hall.

# "So Many Fake People in the Real World"

Well look up from the ground and see who's laughing last
I do what it takes to pull me through.

— Drowning Pool, "Told You So"

THE HANDWRITTEN ENVELOPE that arrived in Dallas in the winter of 2003 had a Massachusetts postmark and no return address. *Dear Precious Angel Mary Alice,* the letter began. *You don't need to hurt that little girl inside you anymore. You don't have to be scared, you don't have to be someone you're not. You don't have to smoke pot or drink or be the coolest.*

It was the letter Mary Alice had written to herself after going through the psychodramas and staring at her childhood photo. Ten months had passed since that day, and four months had passed since she'd graduated from Swift River. She had forgotten about the letter. "Remember everything that you learned at Swift River," it urged.

Mary Alice sat alone in her cavernous bedroom, running her fingers over the thick stationery. She *had* tried to remember the lessons, but it was difficult. At her parents' urging, she'd returned home and enrolled in a small alternative school. For a while, she had seemed to hold it all together. "I'm doing great!" she had insisted in an interview while cruising in her SUV. She spoke enthusiastically — probably too enthusiastically — about her new life at home. She was spending time with her family, volunteering at a children's shelter, helping girls with eating disorders, setting up a darkroom, looking for a dance company to join. In a note to a friend who was still at Swift River, she talked about how many kids back home were drinking and doing drugs. "God, there really are so many fake people in the 'real' world," she added. Later, in a letter to Portia, the New Mexico student who had called her a role model, Mary Alice offered a hint of her struggles.

"It is definitely really hard being at home and not falling back into old patterns."

By then she had fallen back into some of her patterns. She lost about fifteen pounds; her clothes hung loosely on her body. "I think it's because she's become a vegetarian," her father observed. Her mother, though, knew what was going on. Ultimately, Mary Alice admitted that her eating disorder had resurfaced. Later, when she went on a study-at-sea program for teenagers, her temperament fluctuated wildly. Neither Mary Alice nor her parents had informed the program's director that she was bipolar and had decided to stop using her mood stabilizers. Mary Alice's family enrolled her in Swift River's alumni program, which allowed her to have weekly phone conversations with a counselor on campus for a year (the program cost parents $2,000). The counselor told Mary Alice that she should expect setbacks, but she needed to talk honestly with her parents and drop the everything-is-fine facade.

A year after finishing Swift River, Mary Alice moved a thousand miles away from home to attend a liberal arts college. Feeling besieged by term papers and social pressures, she dropped out and spent the winter of 2004 working as a ski instructor. Then that spring, a year and a half after Swift River's graduation, something seemed to jell. She returned to college with new resolve. She found that she could focus on her classes. She stuck with a boyfriend who, her family and friends agreed, was responsible and loving. Mary Alice now plans to work with children.

*Peanut,* read the slapdash handwriting, *I'm sorry for everything . . . You better never forget when your grandparents rented the pontoon boat in Florida and you went on a mini-safari and they let you drive the boat with your feet. Remember to be true to yourself and never forget about little Peanut. I will always be with you.*

When D.J.'s letter arrived in New Jersey, he was struggling through junior year at his old school — the school where his dad taught. His mother was tempted to intervene with teachers, to ask for extensions and take charge of D.J.'s homework. Instead, she let D.J. seek help from his school's learning disabilities specialist. It wasn't easy, but by the spring of senior year D.J. caught up. He has been accepted at a college noted for its hands-on classes and outdoor education programs. He hopes to become a wilderness guide.

Although D.J. fell out of touch with most members of Group 23, he and Tyrone spoke by phone every couple of weeks. One Saturday morning, D.J. took a train from the suburbs and then a subway to visit Tyrone in Queens. It was his first solo trip to New York. The two played video games, goofed off at a guitar store, and hung out with Tyrone's old friends. D.J. didn't ask about Tyrone's father, Tyrone didn't ask about D.J.'s classes, and both had a great time. D.J. repeated the visit every few months.

Tyrone enrolled in an alternative school in the Hudson Valley that offered small classes. The New York City Board of Education paid for his tuition and the daily two-hour round-trip bus ride. Most of the other kids were "hard cases" who had been kicked out of their regular schools, said Tyrone's mother, Natalie. She had to smile when Tyrone griped that he was different. He'd said the same thing while surrounded by rich white students at Swift River. "At the new school he's just another poor black kid," she observed, "so he's not a celebrity anymore."

Tyrone's family noticed improvements in his attitude, even his body language. One day, for example, a great-uncle stopped by. He saw Tyrone smiling for the first time since elementary school. "The boy's got teeth!" he bellowed. Natalie noticed other changes. For one, she could finally have real conversations with Tyrone. One evening he admitted that he'd smoked pot for the first time while at his best friend's house. Natalie thanked him for experimenting in a safe place and for being honest. She had smoked more than her share of joints and cigarettes as a teenager, so she felt it was hypocritical to scold her eighteen-year-old son. "Swift River saved him," Natalie said recently. She thought back on the days when Tyrone seemed to be living in a cave, isolated from everyone and sustained only by junk food and computer games. "He had so much anger. If he stayed home, he would've been one of those guys who keeps a knife by his mattress and decides one day to stab his mother."

Tyrone has applied to colleges and hopes for a scholarship to study computer programming. Although he had planned on seeing his father regularly, they rarely get together. Tyrone says they are both busy.

*Hey Sweetie-Pie!* the letter to West Palm Beach started. *How have you been doing? . . . Turn to dad if you are feeling sad, mad, or happy, tell him what's really going on, he wants to understand, he's always going to be there for you, no matter what.*

The letter came at a time when Bianca needed all the encouragement her Swift River self could offer. Chemotherapy had wasted her father's body. He had started preparing for a bone marrow transplant, the same operation that Bianca's mother had undergone before dying. Though Bianca liked living with her twin brother again, she felt smothered in her childhood home. "This house smells like death," she complained. "I need to go to a place where there's some life." Going back to Darnell was out of the question; he had admitted cheating on her. She started dating a guy who was almost ten years older, didn't have a steady job, and already had two children from previous relationships.

A year after finishing Swift River, Bianca fulfilled one of her dad's dreams: She enrolled in college — the same college where her mother and father had met as undergraduates. She joined the drama club and maintained a 3.8 average. Her father was thrilled.

Alan's euphoria didn't last. In the winter of 2004, halfway through freshman year, Bianca called to say she was pregnant. Alan could barely respond. Bianca was a nineteen-year-old college freshman with no income, no savings, and a dismal record of choosing boyfriends. (Gennarose, hearing the news, managed to blurt, "Holy shit!") Several relatives urged Bianca to consider abortion or adoption. Bianca hadn't intended to become pregnant at such a young age, but she quickly decided it was her destiny. She remembered the aching feeling she'd had while carrying around the flour baby, thinking about the deaths of her mother and her friends Raul and Antoine. Bianca is now looking for an apartment with her boyfriend and preparing for motherhood. She hopes to finish her degree in drama.

While at Swift River, the kids in Group 23 often mused about meeting in a warm, sunny place for a reunion. They did have a reunion in Florida sixteen months after graduation, but for a reason no one had expected: the funeral of Tanner, known as the "teddy bear."

This story of what happened was pieced together from relatives and friends. Tanner proudly told others in Group 23 that he had stayed clean most of the time after Swift River. He enrolled in music school, which he loved. He planned to have a doctor remove his "Laugh now, cry later" tattoos. In January 2004, an old friend who had used and sold drugs asked if he could stay in Tanner's apartment, saying he needed Tanner's help as he started a new life. Tanner and his parents reluctantly agreed. A few weeks later, Tanner started vomiting after drinking cognac. His new roommate did nothing. Two other friends phoned the apartment but ignored Tanner's request for help. The next day one of Tanner's buddies stopped by and insisted on being let into the apartment. He found Tanner dead on a couch and his roommate busy weighing pot and separating it into baggies.

"The whole story is appalling," Tanner's mother wrote in an e-mail. "His death is directly attributed to human negligence. My son, who would have called 911 for a hurt dog . . . Tanner did not always make good decisions, but probably the worst decision was his choice of 'friends.' He always saw the ultimate good in people. He liked to walk on the edge, but he trusted the wrong people to see that he did not fall." Tanner was twenty years old. After catching the roommate hiding drugs and cash, the police charged him with five felony drug counts.

Among the scores of well-wishers at the funeral were five members of Group 23, including Bianca, Trevor, and Willow. Bianca, in her first trimester of pregnancy, had trouble approaching the casket for most of the service. She couldn't deal with yet another death. When she finally did glance in, she saw that Tanner was going to be buried in the electric-blue suit he'd worn at graduation. Somehow that comforted her.

The others at the funeral said they'd gone through emotional rollercoaster rides since graduation. After being expelled from Swift River, Trevor had gone to a detox program, then moved back to London. He had enrolled at the same music school as Tanner. Willow, the adopted girl from a small town in New England, had gone back to using drugs and living with her abusive boyfriend for a while. But she'd recently told her parents that she wanted to go to college and start anew.

Tanner's death prompted the remaining fifteen kids of Group 23 to reconnect in a flurry of e-mails and visits. The tragedy seemed to jolt several of them out of the self-absorption of adolescence and into adulthood. Eva, the "everything kid," is completing her senior year at a public high school, where she has found a guidance counselor she trusts. Several colleges accepted her, and she wants to study psychology and law. Phil the Philosopher is finishing high school at a private academy, where he has dazzled teachers with his intellectual prowess. He is enrolling in a prestigious college. He continues to proselytize for his Chillisism movement, though it now emphasizes spirituality, not pot smoking. He remains its only member.

Perhaps the biggest surprise is Andy, who was kicked out of Swift River two days before graduation. He returned home to Long Island, then went to a college in another state. He partied excessively at first, but low grades and a summer of grueling classes moderated his habits. Now half-way through college, he hopes to go into business. Andy briefly saw his old flame Ashley and reports that she is finishing high school and working.

After Tanner's death, the mothers and fathers of Group 23 reached out to each other by phone and e-mail. They continue to hone their parenting styles. With Mary Alice away at college but three teenage siblings still in the house, Burns and Lillian Chambliss look for early signs of drinking and other recklessness; they do their best to express love through activities and words, rather than credit card purchases. Lillian helps raise money for an eating disorder awareness group. Burns has reduced his hunting and golfing trips and other "pleasurizing." In New York, Tyrone's mother kept a promise she'd made to herself long ago: At the age of forty-nine, as her son finished high school and her grandson entered kindergarten, she completed her bachelor's degree.

D.J.'s parents are getting ready for the prospect of an empty nest. D.J.'s father plans to visit the town in Connecticut where he lived as a six-year-old refugee from Eastern Europe in the summer of 1954. He is curious to learn what happened to a couple who offered to adopt him.

In Florida, Bianca's father received good news from his doctors before scheduling his bone marrow transplant: He had beaten his leukemia and would recover. Eleven years had passed since his first wife died. He decided to move on, literally and figuratively. He fell in love and got engaged. In the spring of 2004, he sold his house. While packing, he found a box of letters Bianca had sent from Swift River. She had written one of them for Father's Day 2002, a few weeks before Alan found out he had leukemia. "Dear Dad," she wrote, "it was really nice to realize that our relationship has grown because both of us have been so open with each other about so much. If I'm crying or laughing, I don't really think it makes much difference. Just talking about mom brings me closer to you."

The Academy at Swift River constantly reinvents itself. After Group 23's graduation, two new dorms opened, the school lengthened its program from fourteen to fifteen months, and it increased its fees to $85,000. All that happened just as an economic recession and fears about air travel cut down the number of applicants. The school struggled to "make the numbers" and keep 135 students enrolled at a time. Many counselors complained that the admissions office accepted kids who wouldn't have been given a second look during flush times.

The pressures took a toll on everyone. During a snowstorm in the winter of 2003, Rudy Bentz stepped out of his Ford Explorer to wipe the back windshield. "I would've used the rear wiper," he quipped, "but one of our loving-kind-oppositionally-defiant kids broke it off." Soon after, Tanya Beecher sat in a café in a town near Swift River. There were dark lines under her eyes and her face was pale. She had just mailed out Group 23's "letters to myself," but her mind was on Swift River's current students. Several girls had cut themselves. A group of boys had broken toilets; others had sneaked into a crawl space in an ill-conceived plot to escape. "The place was awesome with ninety students when I started," Tanya said, "but it's overwhelming now."

A few months later, Tanya quit Swift River to work at a pilot project for at-risk high school students. And in November 2003, about a year after Group 23 graduated, Rudy and Jill Bentz left the school amid what a press release cryptically called "organizational changes." The Bentzes refused to talk publicly about their departure. Some staff members said Rudy had been too controlling and reluctant to allow colleagues to suggest new therapeutic approaches. Others said that he had clashed with management over the push to keep up profits.

On a fall day a year after graduation, three girls from the guru group sat gossiping over coffee in midtown Manhattan. Glancing across Broadway into a deli's window, they spotted a thin woman with shiny hair down almost to her waist bustling behind the counter. The girls ran across the street yelling, "Gennarose!"

Gennarose Pope greeted them with hugs and a hearty "Holy shit!" She had burned out on Swift River, where she taught, ran the humanities department, and trained new staff members — for $29,000 and three weeks' vacation a year. She had quit to take odd jobs in New York while pursuing her dream of writing music and singing. "The best thing about Swift River — the only good thing — was the kids."

During my first visit to the Academy at Swift River in June 2000, several students amazed me with tales of their miraculous turnarounds: the gun-toting gang-banger who selflessly built a playground in Costa Rica; the Ecstasy-dealing gamine who became a devoted daughter. And so on. They told me the tidy stories of conversion and redemption that a journalist on deadline pines for. As a writer — as a parent — I sorely wanted to believe in miracles.

But the more time I spent on the campus, the more I realized that the truth is often untidy. Swift River isn't capable of magic. It takes kids in trouble and tries to give them the tools they'll need to face life's many uncertainties.

When I visited Mary Alice in Dallas not long ago, I could tell she was still torn, still deciding who she was. Before venturing out to a restaurant, she spent a half hour putting on makeup. She talked a hundred miles an hour about her future while driving almost as fast. And yet she had changed in important ways. Rather than screaming or cursing at her parents, she spoke to them about her struggles. I kept thinking back to my first glimpse of her more than two years before — slumped in the back of her parents' rental car, bleary-eyed and reeking of cigarette smoke, her sallow face taut as a snare drum. "This is Mr. Marcus, who will be writing a book about your group," her mother offered, trying to elicit some kind of reaction. Mary Alice glanced at me in a daze.

D.J. and Tyrone are still far more comfortable discussing the family dynamics of *The Simpsons* than their relationships with their own parents. These days, though, they walk with confidence and laugh easily. I remember the D.J. I met in the Swift River admissions office three summers ago: a confused, lonely, angry fifteen-year-old who had recently run away from home, hitchhiked with two truck drivers, and ended up in a psychiatric hospital. Soon after, I watched Tyrone walking out to base camp. He was a scared boy who couldn't own up to his own difficulties. "I'm just here for the academics," he insisted. He saw nothing wrong in staying up till 4:00 A.M. every day playing Final Fantasy. Tyrone didn't deny that he had skipped school for two years — but it took him a long time to understand that he'd also skipped life.

I'll never forget Bianca's blend of naivety and callousness that first summer. She had been taken from her bedroom at dawn and put through a six-week wilderness program; she believed she had nothing more to learn. She was irked at her mean father, the ogre who had banished her from the house. Never mind that she had sneaked out of a window repeatedly, or that she was cutting classes and lying to her teachers. Or that she'd been arrested, half-naked, in a movie theater.

Because the father and the journalist in me desperately wanted the students in Group 23 to succeed, Bianca's pregnancy, followed by Tanner's death, made me cynical about Swift River and other therapeutic programs. Had the kids changed, or had I been deceived? Maybe the school really was little more than a fancy holding pen for messed-up teenagers, as a gym teacher had remarked.

Now that I've had a chance to reflect, I see that despite the glowing testimonials, despite the late-night workshops and family therapy and hundreds of pages of emotional-growth curriculum, Swift River can only do so much. Sometimes it's simply a safe place for boys and girls to grow up for fourteen or fifteen months. Skeptics will say that makes it a very expensive babysitting service, but I have no doubt that if the kids had remained at home, at least a couple would have overdosed on drugs. Perhaps they would have killed themselves, or someone else, in drunk-driving crashes.

Tanner's parents don't blame Swift River for his death; they watched Tanner blossom during his time in Group 23. They remember the words from the rap he performed in July 2002. With the crowd cheering, he chanted, "I chose to come to this strange place / It's probably the best choice in my life that I will ever make." He'd felt comfortable with all sorts of people at Swift River; while other students asked popular counselors or teachers to introduce them at graduation, Tanner was so unpretentious that he had been introduced by one of the women from the kitchen staff. And Bianca credits the school with making her face all the traumas she had lived through. She has her own reasoning to explain her pregnancy at age nineteen. She has long felt certain that God will cut her life short with cancer. She wants to spend as many years as she can with her child. Bianca is finding her own way to cope with tragedy. A few weeks ago, she drove to the cemetery to visit her mother's grave. First she informed Teresa that she was going to become a grandma. Then she spoke about her friend Tanner, who could reminisce about his gun-toting gang acquaintances one minute and his ragged old teddy bear the next. Looking at Teresa's headstone, Bianca asked a favor: "Mom, can you show him around Heaven? You're really gonna like him."

The shocking twist in Bianca's life made me see that Swift River isn't — *can't be* — about removing all the obstacles from a kid's path. It is meant to help her deal better with those obstacles. While a person, especially a teenager, can gain maturity and sensitivity during a therapeutic program, there are often deep needs and scars that no counselors can heal.

Swift River could teach Bianca to respect herself and communicate with her father, but it couldn't replace the mother she'd lost or the baby she'd miscarried. It could help her talk honestly about the past, but it couldn't undo a rape. The Bianca who recently met me for lunch in Florida was confident and caring. I am certain that she will be a better woman, and a better mother, thanks to the fourteen months she spent in a converted dairy barn in the hills of western Massachusetts.

*For updates, see* www.DaveMarcus.com.

# Memo to Parents

AT THE START of this project, I assumed I knew most of what I needed to know about adolescence. After all, I'd spent years as an education reporter, swooping into schools to spot trends. I'd written my college thesis on Americans' yearning for community. And of course I'd had the best training of all: I'd been a teenager. My friends and I had done some stupid things — including shoplifting a *Penthouse* magazine at a drugstore with surveillance cameras — but like most teens, we'd survived. So I arrived at the Academy at Swift River with a couple of preconceptions. One, kids who had been sent away to a private school for wayward teens must be spoiled. Two, they had self-involved, absentee parents. As a guidance counselor told me, "Behind every fucked-up kid is a fucked-up parent."

Researching this book consumed me for four years. I hiked and biked with the students, camped and played Ping-Pong with them, visited their homes and prowled malls with them. When tragedy struck someone we'd all loved, I grieved with them. Along the way, I abandoned my simpleminded stereotypes about the kids and their parents. It's easy to write off "troubled teens" and their incompetent, indifferent parents. It's difficult, even harrowing, to recognize that often they are normal teenagers and normal parents dealing with normal problems.

My journalistic project became a personal quest. I'm the father of two young children who are sweet, obstinate, smart, and uncontrollable — all during a typical ten-minute car trip. I constantly agonize about my parenting skills. (It gives me little comfort to know that fifty years ago an American historian wrote, "In no other country has there been so pervasive a cultural anxiety about the rearing of children.") As I plunged into the research, I felt a sense of urgency. Well before my son and daughter reached middle school, I needed to learn about adolescence from the true experts — the kids who were struggling.

I set out to answer key questions:

1. Why had these kids gotten into so much trouble at home and at school even as their friends and siblings thrived?
2. How could their parents have helped earlier?
3. What lessons can the rest of us — teachers, religious leaders, lawmakers — draw from a fourteen-month program that most people can't afford?

Whenever I mention the first question to my friends, they want someone, or something, to blame; they inevitably ask *who* is at fault, *who* screwed up. Was it bad parenting, bad genes, or bad luck? Many assume, as I used to, that these kids are a product of baby boomers who indulge their children. Phyllis Steinbrecher, an education consultant who has worked with families for nearly thirty years, traces her increasing number of troubled adolescent clients to narcissistic mothers and fathers who were raised after the upheavals of the Kennedy assassinations, Vietnam, and Watergate. "These parents don't know how to set rules because they've broken so many themselves since their childhoods." Others have a dramatically different theory: that overprotective parents don't let their children make, and learn from, mistakes.

I've come to see that it's not a simple matter of parents who are too lax or too strict. The overwhelming majority of the Swift River parents I met were neither narcissistic nor uncaring. Several suffered from what psychologists call "emotional unavailability" — they couldn't empathize with their children. Some were reeling from their own upbringings, financial predicaments, or bad marriages. Quite a few were wrestling with addictions, depression, or anxiety disorders themselves.

What's especially frightening is that children can go awry even when their parents seem to do everything right. Some kids have biochemical or genetic problems — significant learning disabilities, attention deficit–hyperactivity disorder, bipolar disorders, schizophrenia — that can't be cured by milk-and-cookies moms and stay-at-home dads. While many teenagers learn to work around such setbacks, other kids become defined by their disorders. They see themselves as broken. This is especially true with adopted kids, who often suffer from attachment disorders and problems with impulse control. "Not everything that affects a child's mental health is within a parent's control," psychologist Daniel Kindlon of Harvard University's School of Public Health observes. "Good parents can raise bad kids and bad parents can raise good kids."

Then there are outside factors, from peers to beer commercials, from violent video games to cable TV shows with unbridled sex. Children are growing up in a society where adults have higher expectations of them but provide less support; where many communities offer little sense of community; where the media glorify violence, sex, and alcohol, then tell kids to abstain.

Again and again, parents' influence is marginalized. Teenagers have always pushed the limits, but in recent years the limits have expanded. In my time, in the 1970s, the temptations were so much milder. The *Penthouse* we shoplifted at age sixteen, or attempted to, was Disneyesque compared to what a twelve-year-old can find in seconds today on the Internet by Googling "sex" and a smattering of choice words. Now any girl can surf "pro-ana" sites, which advocate anorexia and bulimia, for tips on avoiding food or inducing vomiting. I'm not a prude, but I was astounded to see drunk, barely clothed college kids groping each other on MTV's *Spring Break* one recent afternoon, when my first-grader could have been watching. Swift River parents who had once let their imaginations run wild while listening to

Tommy James and the Shondels croon "I think we're alone now" were stunned when their preteen children belted out Prince's lyrics about "twenty-three positions in a one-night stand."

James Garbarino of Cornell University argues that what physical toxins do to the body, social and cultural toxins do to the emotional lives of children. As he writes in *Parents Under Siege,* "A socially toxic environment contains widespread threats to the development of identity, competence, moral reasoning, trust, hope and other features . . . that make for success in school, family, work and the community."

Hanging out with teenagers reminds me of the extent of toxic lures that lurk in every urban and suburban neighborhood. One day I asked Phil the Philosopher to count how many kinds of drugs his classmates had used before coming to Swift River. He dashed off a list, starting with "alcohol and nicotine," then ticked off standbys such as pot, nitrous oxide, and mushrooms. Soon he started jotting down substances that my high school friends and I had never heard of, such as Ecstasy and snortable heroin. Then over-the-counter medicines, like cough syrup, whose potential hallucinogenic effects were unknown to us. I was struck by the number of prescription pills that we never knew about, painkillers like Percocet and OxyContin and antidepressants like Paxil. Within a few minutes, the list reached twenty-seven — more if you count Phil's helpful note at the end: "Plus other unknown sedatives, muscle relaxants, stimulants and various pharmaceuticals that kids didn't know the names of when they took it." There's plenty of money around for such recreation. Teenagers spend more than $24 billion on entertainment and another $23 billion on food and snacks a year. A third of teens have their own credit cards.

I have to shake my head when I read somber studies urging Americans to pay special attention to "at-risk" adolescents. What teenager in twenty-first-century Newark or Newport Beach, Raleigh or Des Moines isn't at risk? As I write this, I'm looking at my local newspaper, which has a story about teenagers in Amherst, Massachusetts. This is an affable, picturesque college town, a place so egalitarian it built tunnels under roads to ensure that salamanders won't get crushed while meandering during mating season. And yet a survey commissioned by Amherst's high school found that 23 percent of students reported feeling depressed for at least two continuous weeks; 12 percent had seriously considered suicide; and 7 percent had attempted it. (In an attempt to inject some positive news, the newspaper noted that these figures are lower than the state averages.)

Parents don't have to give in; they can try to counter many of the risks before trouble strikes. The old saws are worth repeating. We need to spend uninterrupted time with our kids. Sorry, no cell phones, no pagers, no checking e-mail on the Blackberry. We have to know the parents of our kids' friends, too. Although the students at Swift River pushed away adults in their lives, they admitted that they yearned for someone to reach out and ask what their classmates were like, where they went during recess, what happened at parties. The advice of singer Marilyn Manson is appropriate. In the movie *Bowling for Columbine,* Manson was asked what he would say if he could speak to students at Columbine. "I wouldn't say a single word to them," he replied. "I would listen to what they have to say and that's what no one did."

Listen and you'll learn about the secret world of teenagers. While volunteering as a writing teacher at Swift River, I jump-started class every few days by asking students to free-write about an array of topics. One day I gave a simple prompt: "Write about the friend back home you worry about the most." The descriptions were chilling — girls who purged three times a day or became pregnant at age fourteen, boys who drank whiskey while driving or hawked family heirlooms to buy Ritalin. A kid from a middle-class suburb told the story of his ex-girlfriend, who snorted cocaine daily. Her mother and father saw her as an unrepentant cokehead; her teachers saw her as irredeemably lazy. None of the adults realized that she had been raped. "Her parents and teachers look at her as a problem, not as someone who can be helped," the student wrote.

The parents of Swift River students say they wished they'd listened and watched more closely. They realize now that their kids displayed warning signs by eighth or ninth grade:

Low self-confidence. The kids didn't feel competent at anything. When describing themselves, they used negative images: "I'm fat . . . ugly . . . stupid . . . slutty . . . a weirdo." Peers or adults had labeled them so often that they had become the labels.

Poor social skills. They didn't know how to listen or absorb information; they couldn't take constructive criticism; they avoided looking someone in the eyes when talking.

Dwindling passion for sports and constructive pastimes. The kids had excelled at soccer, basketball, chess, or other activities but lost interest as they entered adolescence. Once they had dropped sports and extracurricular clubs, they didn't know how to fill their free time after school.

Few, if any, adults whom they could confide in. They didn't feel comfortable talking to their parents, and they lacked aunts, uncles, teachers, coaches, neighbors, or others whom they trusted.

A feeling of being an outsider in a family. The kids didn't have connections with their parents and, in many cases, their siblings. They felt like pariahs in their own houses.

Troubled friends. Many of the students had shed genuine, deep friendships of elementary school to fit in with kids who were floundering.

Constant lying. They gave dubious explanations for skipping classes, arriving home late, and not being at the house of the friend they were supposedly visiting.

Looking different. They tried to treat red eyes from pot smoking with Visine. They even smelled different, using perfume or cologne to mask the odor of cigarette smoke.

If children don't have high self-esteem, a strong sense of values, a passion for something constructive — if they don't have friends, relatives, and mentors to support them — they are like houses built on rickety foundations. They'll have difficulty withstanding the emotional hurricanes that hit during adolescence. Many kids can bear up under a single trauma, such as abuse or divorce. But it takes an exceptionally resilient teenager to deal with multiple traumas. By the age of seventeen, Bianca had had to cope with rape, miscarriage, the murder of a friend, the fatal car crash of another friend, her aunt's spinal-cord accident, her grandmother's breast cancer, and then her father's leukemia — all while she was trying to recover from the death of her mother.

In Queens, Tyrone Harriston's mother, Natalie, has developed quite a few sound theories about parenting. She always hugs Tyrone's neighborhood buddies whenever they stop by. If they flinch, she can tell they have something to hide. Also, a hug allows her to smell alcohol, pot, or cigarettes on their clothes.

Thousands of miles away, in a lush suburban enclave, Mary Alice's mother, Lillian Chambliss, has come up with her own theories. Lillian now believes she put too much pressure on her first-born daughter to succeed while offering too little compassion and support. She no longer chooses the friends and pastimes of her other three children. Instead, she encourages them to find their own passions, from riding horses to wrestling, as long as they are productive. She also sets clear rules about drug use and curfews. At night she lingers in the children's bedrooms to find out what's on their minds.

Sometimes her own kids don't want to open up. Lillian has found, though, that their friends are pining to talk to an adult. Several kids recently mentioned that a boy had done cocaine at a party in the Chamblisses' basement. Lillian called the boy's parents right away, as she often does when she hears something alarming about a kid. Assuring them that she doesn't want to spread gossip or be judgmental, Lillian relates what she's been through with Mary Alice. The mothers cry, the fathers stammer or go into denial — but inevitably they thank her for having the courage to call. "Parents need to have the information," she says. "What they do with it is up to them." She wishes that a concerned parent had phoned her several years ago to relay rumors about Mary Alice doing drugs.

In retrospect, Lillian understands that she was too eager to avoid conflict with her strong-willed daughter. She wishes she had established firm boundaries. "First," she says, "you have to be a parent, not a friend."

Although the Academy at Swift River is far from perfect, it offers some invaluable lessons for parents, schools, and community groups. The school gives kids plenty of time in the woods, away from video games, troublemaking peers, and other potentially harmful distractions. It insists that students clean dorms and classrooms and take responsibility for the campus. It pairs troubled boys and girls with successful kids who become tutors, mentors, and role models. It devises rituals — sweats, date nights, formal Sunday dinners — because adolescents love ritu-als. Counselors and teachers constantly remind students that actions have conse-quences: Good conduct and progress in school mean field trips to aquariums, museums, movies, restaurants; lying, taunting, and bullying mean extra chores. Just as important, kids who skip classes or scream at counselors or parents have to write about what's really troubling them and what they plan to do about it.

Above all, Swift River provides emotional education along with traditional academic classes. Emotional education involves teaching kids about the history of courtship and dating, helping them manage their anger, allowing them to express their feelings without being ridiculed. In seminars, they look at scientists' discover-ies about how the brain changes during adolescence, and why teenagers take risks. Many schools offer health education, sex ed, and drivers ed, but therapeutic schools encourage kids to learn about themselves — a subject they care deeply about and understand poorly.

As I wrapped up this book, I took a yearlong job teaching at Deerfield Acad-emy, a premier boarding school. Deerfield parents dream about their kids going to Yale, while Swift River's parents have nightmares about their kids going to jail. Yet there are similarities in the two schools. At Deerfield, students sing, tap dance, or recite poetry in frequent schoolwide meetings. At the end of classes each day, they must play competitive or recreational team sports or do community service. Not only are there appropriate consequences for kids who break rules, but there are chances to make amends and start anew. At Deerfield, as at Swift River, the admin-istration limits access to television, yet gyms, dance halls, ceramics studios, science labs, and libraries hum with activity at night and on weekends.

I am unnerved when I compare these two campuses to public high schools I've seen across the country. School boards prattle on about education reform, but most of the time they just mean standardized testing. Unions resist efforts to purge lousy teachers. Principals spend lavishly on wireless classrooms but won't hire enough competent guidance counselors to ensure that students have the hu-man contact they need. Administrations lock school buildings at 3:15 P.M. because they're so afraid of vandalism; they chain up playing fields so that no one will have an accident and sue the district. Although I've seen some innovations in my visits to public schools, I've seen a lot more retrenching. Communities are slashing bud-gets for music, art, and vocational education — the very pursuits that engage kids who have difficulty in traditional academic subjects.

The sad fact is that parents and teachers can do only so much. If we truly want to help adolescents, we need to change our priorities as a country. We can start by pushing insurance companies and social service agencies to make mental health services available to all teenagers and parents. We also need to rethink the way we plan communities, the way we build public spaces — even the way we de-sign houses.

I keep coming across places where adults treat teenagers like outcasts. Mall owners and downtown shopkeepers greet teens with a resounding No: No skate-boarding. No loitering. No groups of three or more teens allowed. For her book *A*

*Tribe Apart,* Patricia Hersch observed students in the prosperous suburb of Reston, Virginia. She showed how teenagers lived in the shadows, even in a planned town like Reston that prided itself on being "family friendly." "They are a tribe apart, remote, mysterious, vaguely threatening," she wrote. "America's own adolescents have become strangers."

We worship freedom of choice, but sometimes I wonder if we have too many options. Our unceasing search for choice in education has fragmented neighborhoods. On a typical block in a middle-class suburb, every morning you'll find children splintering off to private academies, parochial schools, Montessori schools, Waldorf schools, charter schools, magnet schools, language-immersion schools, and plain vanilla public schools. A child has different sets of friends from school, Little League, and the neighborhood. As parents of teenagers try to keep track of all those spheres, they have a tough time knowing whose mothers or fathers are around when the kids convene in someone's rec room. It's hard enough to recall the names and faces. Each year, more than 14 percent of Americans relocate — compared with 4 percent of Germans and 8 percent of Britons. Only a quarter of American teens expect to live in their hometowns as adults.

Forty years ago, the visionary architectural and social critic Lewis Mumford warned that suburban developments would bring about "an encapsulated life, spent more and more either in a motor car or within the cabin of darkness before a television set." Mumford, it turns out, understated the case. Today the isolation is not only between neighbors but within families. Inside the home, Americans are split into electronic fiefdoms, with dad checking news on line, mom sending e-mail, one sibling dueling with the PlayStation, and another IMing while watching ESPN. Recently the *Wall Street Journal* reported that open-floor house construction is giving way to compartmentalized designs that feature one-person "internet alcoves," locked-door "away rooms," and kids' bedrooms with 42-inch plasma televisions. There's even a separate room for the dog. These new designs are "good for the dysfunctional family," the research director of the National Association of Home Builders remarked. "We call this the ultimate home for families who don't want anything to do with one another."

Americans have gone too far. We must stop creating houses for dysfunctional families and start creating neighborhoods that help families function — tight-knit places with shops, restaurants, and parks at the center. We must stop slapping on labels that emphasize kids' shortcomings and start nurturing their passions for music, carpentry, or auto mechanics. We must stop turning schools into guarded, metal-detectored, closed-circuit-cameraed fortresses and start welcoming parents and community members into classrooms. We must revise zoning codes and use our imaginations to build high schools next to nursery schools, middle schools next to nursing homes — and then encourage the different generations to teach each other.

Most of all, we must change our attitude. Rather than viewing the twenty-nine million teenagers around us as problems, we must see them as the potential solutions to our problems. Then, finally, we can help adolescents — and ourselves.

# AUTHOR'S NOTE

This book grew out of an assignment that I tried my best to avoid. When an editor at *U.S. News & World Report* asked me to write about the rise of boarding schools that offered therapy, I worried that I'd have to deal with a bunch of rich, uppity brats. At the Academy at Swift River, though, I met humble, introspective kids, many of whom expressed remorse about their arguments with parents, their carousing, and other recklessness. I realized that they had a story to tell — a story about the complicated, troubling, dangerous lives of some teenagers. After the article ran in October 2000, the responses from readers reinforced my view that the subject deserved a broader canvas than four columns at the back of a newsmagazine.

Several authors had followed random teenagers, but I wanted to observe a therapeutic program, to see a group of kids learning about themselves and about one another. Initially, I planned to conduct my research at a nonprofit program so that questions about companies making a profit on adolescent mental health services wouldn't sidetrack the story. But no nonprofit started with a wilderness program and ended with a community service project, and I wanted to watch the kids responding to all sorts of challenges. Also, I came to see that any book about programs for teenagers should at least touch on the debate about the role of the corporations that are coming to dominate treatment.

In June 2001, I moved my family to Massachusetts and started observing as the admissions department selected the twenty-third group of students to go through the school. I asked parents to sign a release giving me permission to write about their children. I asked the kids to sign, although they were minors and didn't need to. I warned that participating in this project would be difficult, perhaps heart-wrenching. All sixteen sets of parents signed, including a couple of divorced parents who hadn't seen eye-to-eye on many other matters.

Although several of the students graciously offered to let me publish their real names, I decided to use pseudonyms for all the parents and children as well as their friends and acquaintances back home. I didn't want anyone to be identified years from now as "that kid in the book about messed-up teens." For the same reason, I suggested changing the hometown of one of the characters and slightly altering the profession of one parent (though a trial attorney, for example, did not become a tow-truck operator). I also changed the names of the schools that the students previously attended. The names of counselors and teachers have not been changed. These aren't composites but real people dealing with real life — rendered as realistically as possible.

After reading the manuscript, several colleagues speculated that I disliked Mary Alice and her parents. Far from it. Mary Alice quickly won me over by asking about journalism, then listening raptly (and by taking my son and daughter sledding on the Swift River campus). I loved talking to her mother and father; they were remarkably candid as they reexamined their parenting styles. I liked all the kids and parents, including Tyrone's dad, who spoke thoughtfully to me about fatherhood. Ashley, Andy, and Trevor were three of my favorites from base camp on. While writing, though, I had to set aside my affection for these folks. I'd feel like a nicer person if I airbrushed all the blemishes from the portraits, but this book wasn't about being nice. It was about letting readers learn from the mistakes that parents and kids make.

I cannot say enough about the courage and generosity of these parents and children. They opened their homes to me; they showed me letters and diaries; they reflected on their most painful memories. They shared their stories, their innermost secrets — their lives — in the hope that their painful experiences will help someone who reads this book.

Swift River's executive director, John Powers, allowed me to rove anywhere I wanted and to talk to any willing staff member or student. I insisted that anything would be fair game — if I learned that a counselor was abusing a student, no one could tell me it was "off the record." Swift River's privately held parent company, now called Aspen Education Group, took a gamble in allowing me complete access to every meeting, class, and activity on campus, in the wilderness camp, and in Costa Rica. Elliot Sainer, the CEO, understood that this would not be a hagiography of the staff or the institution. Still, he had enough confidence in the school to believe that the positive would outweigh the negative.

Aspen executives did not review the manuscript before publication, nor did they ask to. The company's risk-management division insisted on only two stipulations. First, I could not describe the four all-day workshops in enough detail to allow another program to steal intellectual property. That made sense to me as a writer because I wanted to focus on a few significant moments in three workshops rather than going into lengthy descriptions. The second stipulation proved to be prescient: I couldn't hold Aspen liable if I got injured. As it happened, I took a spill from a mountain bike in Costa Rica and ended up in the Osa Peninsula's only emergency room.

Swift River asked me to give something back by teaching writing. Realizing that accepting money from the school could cloud my objectivity, I decided to volunteer. Everyone on campus knew that I was primarily an author researching a book, not a teacher. I explained my role to new kids on campus; a newsletter informed parents.

In reporting this book, I hewed to the principles of the best authors of narrative nonfiction, including Michael Winerip, author of *9 Highland Road,* and Ron Suskind, author of *A Hope in the Unseen.* I used what Suskind calls "basic, block-and tackle standards of fact gathering." If someone is quoted, that means I heard the quote or I was told about it, then checked it with the speaker and others present. When I switch to a character's point of view, or summarize how he or she felt, that is because I've debriefed the person, usually for hours.

I observed many of the scenes in this book. When Tyrone went to dinner with his father, I sat a few booths away; at dawn two days later when D.J. and his dad climbed aboard a deep-sea fishing boat, so did I. When Bianca flew home after graduation, I shadowed her. Because I couldn't be at every late-night conversation between counselor and student, I relied on reconstructions by participants soon after the discussions took place. Sometimes, sensing that my presence would disrupt conversations, I stayed away. I decided against observing Bianca on "date night" in Northampton, for example, but I did ride in a van and tag along when another girl in the group went on a date night to see what it was like. Likewise, I base descriptions of childhood scenes on extensive interviews and, often, visits to the parks and schools, movie theaters and hospitals where the events happened.

When I started, psychologists urged me to focus on main characters struggling with learning disabilities or reeling from adoption, the death of a parent, or bitter divorce. I also wanted at least one kid who seemed to have it all — a loving family and plenty of money. In other words, I looked for archetypes that others could learn from. I was blessed to find sensitive, perceptive kids who had compelling stories yet who illustrated larger issues as well. Although I chose the four main characters after a few months of observation, many of the students at the school later told me they weren't sure which of the Group 23 kids I planned to highlight. I was lucky to be assigned to the group of a talented new counselor, Tanya Beecher. She worked with two tough-and-loving co-counselors, Jason Deni in the first half of the program, then Candice Porter in the second.

The counselors decided that, in most situations, I would distract the kids by wielding a notebook. A tape recorder was out of the question during group therapy. So I watched, then retreated to a favorite nook in the woods or the teacher's office to jot field notes about what I'd seen. After the group graduated, I spent months checking facts. I also taped interviews with several of the kids so I could get a sense of the cadence of their voices. Breaking my newspaperman's practice, I let kids and parents see portions of the text in advance. They weren't allowed to change my opinions, but they could, and did, help me correct errors.

Yes, the Heisenberg principle applies: The observer affects what is being observed. During my first days in base camp, the kids preened and strutted like peacocks. But time has a way of making even a balding six-foot-tall man invisible in a sea of teens. Many students have told me that I became just another one of the adults around them. Teenagers live in the present and have a hard enough time thinking about next week or next month; a book scheduled for publication three and a half years later was an abstraction.

Initially the staff regarded me as a novelty. Thanks to my constant presence, though, I became about as remarkable as a table lamp. I know this because often a counselor would start to describe a revelation in group therapy or a confrontation in a hallway a day earlier.

"I remember," I'd interject. "I was there."

"Really? I didn't see you."

At one point, a producer for a well-known TV newsmagazine heard about my project and inquired if she could send someone with a miniature video camera. The publicity could have been a publisher's dream. I thank Houghton Mifflin for saying that a camera, no matter how unobtrusive, would ruin the integrity of this project.

In many ways, I had to unlearn what I'd learned during my twenty-two-year career covering wars, coups, and quakes. A journalist wants to know the facts before everyone else. For once, I didn't care about scoops, so I asked students not to approach me with exclusive or confidential disclosures. If the kids' innermost horrors were going to come out, that needed to happen the way it normally does in a therapeutic program — during writing assignments or talks with counselors and peers. I made it clear that if anyone told me of a plan to run away or hurt him- or herself, we would go to a counselor immediately. While runaway plots and suicidal ideation did come to light during my time at Swift River, I was never the first to know about them.

I've managed to bury my emotions when writing on deadline about famine in Ethiopia, massacres in Colombia, and a plane crash in Detroit; journalism taught me to be dispassionate in order to get the job done. In the last four years, I unlearned that lesson, too. Listening to the Swift River students describe rapes, abuse, and attempted suicide brought me to tears. I had the pleasure of getting to know, and care about, subjects in a way I had found impossible in hit-and-run journalism.

On Sundays, I showed up on campus with my own rambunctious children — who were two and five at the start. I marveled when I watched my daughter drawing or my son playing checkers with the teenagers — teenagers who had committed credit card fraud or even slugged their parents. Involving my children gave me insights that I would have missed if I'd taken the typical journalist approach and kept my family at bay. The first time I brought Benjie and Tatiana, in the summer of 2001, a girl cooed, "They're so cute."

"Yeah," a boy grumbled, "we were cute once, too."

They were, and they are. Beneath that cool, hardened, "troubled teen" veneer, these boys and girls are empathetic and smart and creative, and enchanting. I hope that this book will remind parents, teachers, and others that adoring kids thrive somewhere beneath those inscrutable adolescent exteriors, just to be summoned.

# ACKNOWLEDGMENTS

IT TAKES A VILLAGE to write a book. It takes several villages to raise someone's children while the book's author is busting deadlines and fretting over "just one more revision." I've been an itinerant journalist for two decades, and I treasure the encouragement I've received from friends in my adopted homes of Providence; Palm Beach and Miami; Dallas and El Paso; Mexico City, Bogotá, and Rio de Janeiro; Silver Spring, Maryland; and Boston, Amherst, and Deerfield, Massachusetts. Researching this book convinced me that I didn't want to raise my son and daughter in suburbs where there's no *there* there. That meant leaving a wonderful job at *U.S. News & World Report* and setting out for small-town, great-for-kids-but-forget-about-a-job New England.

No place has ever made me feel at home as much as Northampton, a little city that still has locally owned coffee shops and bookstores; the 110-year-old Forbes Library provided a sanctuary. The Smith College Campus School community and the Almost Monthly Book Group cheered our family during this adventure. Sarah Berwieser, Missy Wick, and Norm Sims of the University of Massachusetts tore apart early drafts. David Wilensky offered legal advice; the team at the Restaurant plied us with sushi, and Bill Dwight at Pleasant Street Video wouldn't allow us to pay for rentals.

This book started with a story suggestion from Steve Smith, the editor of *U.S. Editors Brian Duffy and Peter Cary encouraged me to follow my passion. I knew what compelled me to drive twenty hours round-trip to a therapeutic while reporting the article in the summer of 2000, but I'm glad I stopped to and Gina Kanter on the way back. They listened to my cockamamie book how Patinkin of the *Providence Journal* was my sharpest critic, musing about away have mangled Dr. Seuss. Mimi McGloughlin held my hand from far John and to find the story amid my stacks of notes. The *Wall Street Journal's* 2002 Be and Dottie Gaiter, my mentors in life, toasted me over tastes of the loosen up s. My hero, Mike Winerip of the *New York Times*, encouraged me to Other ee the wit that's inevitable when teenagers gather.

honored me, or gallantly did their best to dissuade me, as I gave up my salary, health insurance plan, and remaining sanity to pursue this project. These souls include Angie Cannon and Susan Headden of *U.S. News*; David Shribman of the *Pittsburgh Post-Gazette*; Holden Lewis of Bankrate; Tim Padgett of *Time*; Steve Sternberg and Marco della Cava of *USA Today*; Chris Marquis, Peter Applebome, and Jacques Steinberg of the *New York Times*. Jim Collins and Kristen Laine invited me to lead a writing seminar, then gave me pointers instead. In recent years, I've learned from wonderful colleagues and bosses, including Doug Clifton of the *Miami Herald*; the ever-curious Bob Mong of the *Dallas Morning News*; the *Boston Globe*'s Phil Bennett and Peter Canellos, as well as the beloved Elizabeth Neuffer, who died in Iraq as I worked on this project.

My agent, Andrew Blauner, responded with unflagging enthusiasm whenever mine flagged. At Houghton Mifflin, the amazing Eamon Dolan burnished his reputation as the keenest editor around (don't scrawl "vague" on that sentence, Eamon). Christina Smith, Megan Wilson, Peg Anderson, Ed Cone, Lois Wasoff, and Anne Seiwerath stayed patient as the clock ran out.

A few fellowships kept us afloat. The Nieman Foundation and its legendary curator, Bill Kovach, showed me that uncovering the stories of America could be as thrilling and engrossing as covering a foreign country. A tip of the Master-Card to the helpful folks at the Casey Journalism Foundation at the University of Maryland, the Woodrow Wilson National Fellowship Foundation, the University of Redlands in California, and Alma College in Michigan. I finished polishing the manuscript while a Wallace Wilson Visiting Fellow at Deerfield Academy, a true sanctuary. In this era when schools everywhere are cutting budgets and saying no, Headmaster Eric Widmer and Dean of Faculty Rich Bonanno always found a way to say yes. The students taught me how to teach.

At Smith College, the provost's office and the Department of Education and Child Study gave me office space, library privileges, and the use of rowboats on the appropriately named Paradise Pond. The irrepressible professor Sam "What's the Theme?" Intrator took me on as a project. For fact checking and Web design, I relied on an army of interns: Bonnie Obremski and Peter Harkawik of Hampshire College, Lynn Greenhut of Smith College, Sophia Tsoupas of the University of Massachusetts. Thanks also to the teen research whizzes Ben Levy, Ben Feinberg-Gerner, Emily Chapman, and Elliott Smith, as well as my coach, Jonathan Goldin.

Several mental health experts read portions of this manuscript for accuracy: Andrew Malekoff, associate executive director of the North Shore Child and Family Guidance Center in Roslyn Heights, New York; Judith Souweine, Ed.D., of the Children's Clinic in Northampton; Roger Friedman, a family therapist in Silver Spring, Maryland; and Stuart Bicknell of Deerfield's counseling department. Dr. Barry Sarvet, chief of child psychiatry at Baystate Medical Center in Springfield, Massachusetts, explained eating disorders as we rode bikes through pine forest. I'm indebted to others, whom I've listed at www.DaveMarcus.com. While every I've mentioned chipped in with perceptive criticism, any errors are entir fault.

This book, in many ways, is about risks. The Aspen Education Group and its flagship school, the Academy at Swift River, took a risk in allowing me in. They want to assist families; I hope that this book will further their goal. At Swift River, I was fortunate to find dedicated counselors and teachers, including Tanya Beecher, Candice Porter, Jason Deni, Chris Soto, Gennarose Pope, and Chris Locke. My heartfelt gratitude goes to the kids and parents of Peer Group 23, who opened their homes and hearts to me. I can never repay their kindness. They are an inspiration for families struggling in these complicated times.

Writing this book took four enthralling and agonizing years. Oodles of thanks and hugs to Migdalia and my parents, Alice and Lloyd Marcus, as well as my in-laws, Jesus and Gladys Martinez. Jim and Ellen Marcus never lost faith in my storytelling ability. John and Lisa Marcus were calming influences. It's ironic that the very research that deprived me of time with my children reminded me of the importance of spending time with my children. Benjie and Tatiana, maybe someday you'll read this and say the stressful moves and long hours were worthwhile.

When I needed a respite, Brook Larmer and Hannah Beech sent a plane ticket to lure me to their wedding in Shanghai. I waited till the last minute to request a visa, so my mother ended up going to the Chinese consulate in New York to pick it up. This prompted more than a few wags to question whether I will ever emerge from adolescence. I wonder, too.

*After I wrote these pages, I was distressed to learn of the death of the boy I called Tanner, Peer Group 23's beloved rapper. It wasn't coincidence that his e-mail address started with "Sincere." All of us who spent time on Swift River's campus in 2001 and 2002 will remember the tender way he mentored so many kids. We will never forget the sight of his parents beaming while watching him rap in the great room. We reminisce about his swimming in Costa Rica despite his fear of sharks, and we treasure the memories of him in that electric-blue suit at graduation, sharing his gusto for life.*

*This book is dedicated to his memory.*

To Shane A. Reardon
AKA "Teddy Bear"
1984–2004

# Sources

I observed dozens of the scenes in this book, from the admissions interviews to graduation. Occasionally — during "date night," for example — I skipped an event because my presence would have been a distraction. When I didn't watch something, I reconstructed it by interviewing the participants extensively and reading letters, diaries, and, in one case, a police report. I visited the houses and high schools where most of the key events took place. In the section that follows, I explain how I put together the longer scenes and where I found the historical information and data. For more information about the books and experts cited here, see the Bibliography and the Author's Note.

### Prologue
This scene is typical of the way I researched parts of the book that I was unable to observe myself. Because I couldn't possibly have been in Mary Alice's condominium when her father found the diary — that occurred several weeks before she was sent to the Academy at Swift River — I pieced together what happened by talking to Mary Alice and then, separately, to her father and mother. About ten months after I'd gotten to know Mary Alice, she showed me the Garfield diary.

### Introduction
I don't mean to be an alarmist about teenagers; most are doing well and many are exemplary. But there are some disturbing trends in binge drinking, sex, and sexually transmitted diseases, according to studies by the Alan Guttmacher Institute and the Henry J. Kaiser Family Foundation. The statistics about adolescents' problems are from the Centers for Disease Control (www.CDC.org); Monitoring the Future (www.monitoringthefuture.org); and Hersch, *A Tribe Apart*. The clearest source I found for summaries of statistics about drug use and the effects of drugs is Ketcham and Pace, *Teens Under the Influence*, pp. 23–63. Positive trends are cited in Angie Cannon and Carolyn Kleiner, "Teens Get Real," *U.S. News & World Report*, Apr. 17, 2000.

My article about therapeutic boarding schools, "The Toughest Cases Find a

Home Away," ran in *U.S. News* on October 2, 2000. Professor Mike Nakkula of Harvard's Graduate School of Education convinced me that "parenting by proxy" can help some kids. Talks with several other experts helped crystallize my thoughts about alienation: Professor Sam Intrator of the Smith College Department of Education and Child Study; Dan Kindlon of Harvard Medical School; author Patricia Hersch; and Roger Friedman, a family therapist in Silver Spring, Maryland. Thought-provoking books include Putnam, *Bowling Alone;* Kunstler, *The Geography of Nowhere;* and Hersch, *A Tribe Apart.*

The industry of adolescent treatment programs is so vast that it isn't monitored. There are more than one hundred short-term wilderness programs in the United States alone, according to Keith Russell of the University of Idaho Wilderness Research Center. He estimates that more than a hundred programs in the United States "may generate $200 million per year in revenues"; his 2001 executive summary is available at www.obhic.com. During my years as an education reporter, I became familiar with IDEA, the federal plan to make special services available to students who need help. Marsha Stevens, Swift River's special education consultant, and academic dean Peter Stevens (not related to Marsha) explained how IDEA applies to emotional troubles.

### 1. "I Hate You, Dad"

The scene of Bianca being taken away is based on interviews with her, her father, and her educational consultant as well as on two written versions of her life story. She and I retraced the route from the airport to her house and walked around the airport. I observed D.J.'s admissions interview at the Academy at Swift River. From what I could find, the book D.J. mentions is Joseph G. Ansfield, *The Adopted Child* (Springfield, Ill.: Charles C. Thomas Publishers, 1971). I watched Tyrone start to walk out, then left him alone. Susan Trudeau, the intake coordinator who walked to the woods with Tyrone, helped flesh out anecdotes, as did the student volunteer. The student's descriptions of Special K jibe with those in Ketcham and Pace, *Teens Under the Influence.* Mary Alice and her parents described her last night at home, and she showed me around the house. I learned details about the way she pawned toys for drug money after she wrote her truth letter.

### 2. Psychological Scavenger Hunt

The summary of troubles in therapeutic boarding schools comes from interviews I conducted with disgruntled family members for my *U.S. News* article. The most harrowing story came from Paul Lewis, who called me at *U.S. News* one day to tell me about his fourteen-year-old, Ryan, a Boy Scout who committed suicide at a therapeutic program in West Virginia. His story is summarized in Charles Shumaker, "Son Dies in Wilderness Camp, Parents Sue," *Charleston* (West Virginia) *Gazette*, Dec. 20, 2002. Typical criticisms surface in articles about the DeSisto School: "Two Staffers Charged in Medication Overdose at Private School," Associated Press, Jan. 28, 1999; Jessica Bennett, "'Serious Risks' Cited at School for Teens," *Boston Globe*, Feb. 23, 2004; "Curbs Placed on School for Teens," ibid., Mar. 17, 2004;

and David Abel, "Rapped by State, Special-Needs School to Close," ibid., Apr. 13, 2004. Typical articles about overseas schools include Dana Tims, "Costa Rica School Called 'Horror Story,' " *Oregonian,* July 5, 2003; and "Costa Rica Seizes U.S.-Owned Center for Troubled Youth," *St. Petersburg Times,* May 23, 2003. A story about methods at the Elan School is Brian MacQuarrie and A. J. Higgins, "Moxley Case Puts School's Methods on Trial," *Boston Globe,* July 3, 2000. Other articles about controversial programs include Michael Janofsky, "Boot Camps Proponent Becomes Focus of Critics," *New York Times,* Aug. 9, 2001; Martha Tod Dudman, "Desperate Parents and Dangerous Choices," *New York Times,* July 7, 2001; and Tim Weiner, "Program to Help Youths Has Troubles of Its Own," *New York Times,* Sept. 6, 2003. Parents' comments come from educational consultant Lon Woodbury's Web site, StrugglingTeens.com. I found criticisms of therapeutic schools at TeenLiberty.org; to learn more about the purposes of the Web site I contacted the founder but never received a response.

During my first visit to Swift River, for the *U.S. News* article in June 2000, I learned about the qualifications for students from Brian Ray, the admissions director at the time. Swift River was so popular in 2000 and 2001 that it turned away dozens of applicants. I observed Rudy Bentz during the admissions process, and I was present during the admissions interviews in the summer of 2001 that I describe. Jonathan Edwards is cited in Ketcham and Pace, *Teens Under the Influence,* p. 81.

Descriptions of the problems during Swift River's first year are drawn from interviews with Swift River executive director John Powers, teacher Jeremy McGeorge, and former staff members Andy Coe and Chris Locke (the poet and waiter who became Swift River's first teacher). Allegations of improper techniques at Swift River are in Stephanie Kraft, "Hard Lessons," *Valley Advocate* (Springfield, Mass.), May 21, 1998; and "Frightened Parents, Big Business," ibid.; and several stories by David S. Reid in the *Union-News* (Springfield, Mass.): "Academy Probed by State," Jan. 16, 1998; "School Fights State over Abuse Claims," Mar. 22, 1998; and "Two State Officials Barred by School," Apr. 25, 1998. While I respect the publications for having the guts to pursue critical stories about a potential advertiser, ultimately I felt that Swift River's transgressions were minor.

Therapeutic boarding schools present a quandary to state regulators because they don't fit into convenient categories: they're neither traditional college prep schools nor residential treatment centers. Although I believe that the programs should be regulated to ensure safety, I think many regulators don't know how to distinguish between the bad programs and the good ones. An employee complained of sleep deprivation and shouting during workshops — but after all, these were teenagers who barely slept at home and did plenty of shouting before being sent away. During my time at Swift River, I saw several counselors lose their tempers briefly, but I didn't see any inappropriate behavior. Swift River administrators gave me free access to every part of campus, which straddles the border of Cummington and Plainfield.

I could not find a comprehensive history of therapeutic boarding schools, so

I constructed my own based on interviews with Lon Woodbury and former staff members of CEDU, including Rudy and Jill Bentz; Michael Allgood; and Linda Houghton, who developed CEDU's parent program. They all knew Mel Wasserman. CEDU's Web site, www.cedu.com, confirmed some of the basics.

Descriptions of mental disorders come from the *Diagnostic and Statistical Manual for Mental Disorders,* fourth edition (*DSM-IV*), as well as Empfield and Bakalar, *Understanding Teenage Depression;* Ketcham and Price, *Teens Under the Influence;* and conversations with Dr. Barry Sarvet.

The information about the Swift River student who later committed suicide comes from Rudy and Jill Bentz, who knew him well, as well as former teacher Chris Locke, who taught him English and drama. Historical information about the Swift River property comes from interviews with Bill Dwight, representative of the Northampton City Council, and others who have kept track as the property changed hands. Supplemental information came from the Northampton Historical Society and from Jacqueline Walsh, "Former Inn Bought for $2 Million," *Union-News* (Springfield, Mass.), June 7, 1997. "The McCallum Farm in Cummington," *Daily Hampshire Gazette,* Nov. 6, 1917, is a front-page story with photos of the dairy on the property. Descriptions of the layout of the campus are based on what visitors saw in the summer of 2001. Later the school reconfigured dorms and offices and added buildings.

### 3. BACK TO BASICS

I went into base camp for three-day shifts when teams of counselors rotated in. The kids allowed me to read the letters they exchanged with their parents. I started attending group therapy with the kids during base camp and continued on campus. Although I was not allowed to take notes during group, I wrote field notes in the evenings while confirming events with counselors. I arrived just as base camp underwent a change in leadership. Outgoing supervisors Michael Pease and Chris Soto (who later left to attend Harvard's Graduate School of Education) and the new leaders, Jim Markham and Paul Brennan, helped me decipher the rituals of base camp. I received an education during my discussions around the embers of the campfires with wilderness counselors Joe Keefe, Hannah Price, Mark Malinak, Amanda Pyle, and Joyce Muktarian. Several students from Groups 22 and 24 who overlapped in base camp with Group 23 were insightful; to ensure their privacy I have not included their names, but thanks especially to J.M., S.P., T.S., Z.E., A.K., and D.B.

Some readers have asked whether Swift River intentionally put together a model group that would impress a writer. The answer is an emphatic no. Because it took me time to relocate my family to Massachusetts and then draw up releases for families, I wasn't sure until the last minute whether I would observe Group 21, 22, 23, or 24. In any case, the admissions process is too chaotic to be manipulated. Families constantly change their plans until the last minute (and afterward). Some get cold feet about sending a child away; others abruptly decide they cannot afford a therapeutic boarding school. Still others sign up but then realize the child needs a more intensive residential treatment program. I can say with near certainty that no family backed out because of my presence. Parents and children were not obligated to sign releases. For this project to succeed, I figured I needed 70 percent of the families to cooperate. Within a few months, all sixteen families signed.

Anyone who has worked with teenagers knows that, in the age of e-mail and instant messaging, good spelling and grammar are passé. In the excerpts from letters and journals here, I cleaned up small errors and repetitions for clarity. In Tyrone's case, because the grammar and syntax showed how far he had to go in school, I left some of the original misspellings and syntax.

### 4. THE COUNSELOR AND THE TEACHER
Scenes of the job interviews are based on interviews with Rudy and Jill Bentz and academic dean Peter Stevens as well as Tanya Beecher and Gennarose Pope, who let me read their application letters. Beecher shared her favorite textbooks as well as her thesis for the master's program at Smith College's School of Social Work.

### 5. MARY ALICE: "EVERY PARENT'S WORST NIGHTMARE"
The life stories of the students are based on interviews with them and their parents, their writings at the time, and the accounts they wrote later. "Lone Star Youth Ministry" does not resemble the real name.

### 6. BIANCA: "I CAN'T DO ANYTHING RIGHT"
Besides the usual sources for life stories, I read the police report of Bianca's arrest at the movie theater. Like most students, Bianca revealed many key facts about her life months later, when she felt more comfortable telling the counselors or the group. Some details — such as the plan to run away with her boyfriend — she never mentioned to others. I changed the name of Bianca's high school but not other details.

### 7. STONERS, WIGGERS, AND WANNA-BES
It took months to decide who I would focus on in Group 23 (shortened from Swift River's term, Peer Group 23), which ultimately had sixteen students. I wanted to highlight kids with different troubles, and I wanted to show a variety of backgrounds and geographic regions. At first I paid close attention to nine students, then winnowed that down to six and finally to four. I let the kids choose their pseudonyms, but I changed some because they turned out to be middle names or names that would sound unbelievable (D.J. chose "Strife" as his last name, for example). To protect the privacy of some of the secondary characters who might be easily identifiable, I decided not to name their hometowns. I thought that was better than fudging the details of their actions or their families.

While watching staff meetings, I ended up with information that students didn't know. For example, they weren't aware that counselors had named them the Brady Bunch. Geoffrey Tiernan of Marlboro College helped with descriptions of cliques and clothes. Two years after the Swift River students described "Robo-tripping," I read about it on the front page of a national publication: Donna Leinwand, "Latest Trend in Drug Abuse: Youths Risk Death for Cough-Remedy High," *USA Today*, Dec. 29, 2003. For information about 4-20, I consulted articles in college newspapers, including "What Time Is It? It's 4:20!" *Oregon Daily Emerald* (University of Oregon), Apr. 18, 2003.

### 8. "Y'ALL HAD NO CLUE"
Because I did not want to alter the "solo" experience, I did not observe the kids during their time alone. I relied on their memories and counselors' descriptions of the solos as well as letters they wrote during the two-day stints.

### 9. TYRONE: "LONELY ONCE AGAIN"
Writing about Tyrone proved difficult. His mother and stepfather insist that his father used drugs and stole money. His mother has bank records and other paperwork to show that thousands of dollars disappeared during the last years of their marriage. But Tyrone maintains that his mother is far too critical of his father. And his father, whom I met once in New York, says his ex-wife constantly lies. Ultimately, the reader must decide whom to believe. Statistics about Tyrone's high school come from the New York City Board of Education Web site.

### 10. BACK TO PATTERN
I was present in the woods on 9/11 as D.J. and others finished in base camp. The front-page article mentioned is Sara Rimer, "Parents of Troubled Teens Are Seeking Help at Any Cost," *New York Times*, Sept. 10, 2001; and Rimer, "A Family's Story: The Long Road from Desperation to Graduation," ibid.

### 11. PH.D. IN MANIPULATION
On campus, as at base camp, I witnessed many of the scenes described in the book. I had help with details from the counselors named earlier, as well as James Murray, Kathy Blackburn, Coretia Fernandez, Peter Williams, and Bob Picariello, and supervisors Julie Haagenson, Vince Schmidt, and Tom Moore. Human resources manager Gerry Wilcox is the school's institutional memory. Former supervisors Andy Coe and John Klem confirmed several anecdotes.

Descriptions of eating disorders come from Ketcham and Pace, *Teens Under the Influence,* and Maine, *Father Hunger,* as well as from interviews with Dr. Barry Sarvet; Dina Zeckhausen, Ph.D., executive director of the Eating Disorders Information Network, based in Atlanta; and Wendy Harris, M.D., associate director of the Wilkins Center, a psychiatric clinic that specializes in eating disorders in Greenwich, Conn.

### 12. D.J.: "THE BAD THING THAT HAPPENED TO GOOD PEOPLE"
As wonderful as D.J. was, he was about as communicative as most fifteen-year-old boys. His story emerged slowly. During hikes in Costa Rica, he clarified some of the

incidents I describe here. His parents helped with details. Insights came from Anna Mulrine, "Are Boys the Weaker Sex?" *U.S. News,* July 30, 2001.

### 13. STORMING, NORMING, AND FORMING

My discussion of the emotional-growth theories of Swift River is based on interviews with Rudy and Jill Bentz and with executive director John Powers. I consulted frequently with Andrew Malekoff, a psychologist and the author of a book that several Swift River counselors used, *Group Work with Adolescents: Principles and Practice.* Tanya Beecher, the head counselor for Group 23, worked for the first half of the program with co-counselor Jason Deni and for the second half with Candice Porter. To avoid inundating readers with extraneous details, in some scenes they are not named. Both Jason and Candice helped me with anecdotes. I mention that twenty people were packed into the sweat lodge; I was one of them.

### 14. "I'M ANGRY AT MYSELF FOR BEING BORN"

I observed all four of the daylong workshops and chose to write about three of them. The students were so focused on their activities that I was able to sit on the side and take notes. Swift River requested that I avoid describing all the parts of the workshops; they didn't want other schools to imitate them. (While I understand the desire to safeguard intellectual property, the reality is that counselors frequently move from one school to another, and there are no trade secrets. In addition, Rudy Bentz says that many features of Swift River's workshops came from the therapeutic programs at which he previously worked, CEDU in California and Hidden Lakes Academy in Georgia.)

### 15. FALLING IN LOVE AGAIN

I observed the four parental visits to campus and took notes. I also observed a family therapy session at each visit (the families were split into several groups for therapy, so each time I chose one group). "Spanked Rather than Spocked" comes from a fascinating history of twentieth-century parenting theories, Hulbert, *Raising America,* p. 6. I read portions of *Raising America,* then relied on two perceptive reviews for a summary: Stacy Schiff, "Because I Said So," *New York Times,* Apr. 17, 2003; and Nick Gillespie, "Child Scare," *Washington Post,* May 4, 2003.

### 16. WINTER OF THE UNDERGROUND

Because I concentrated on the counseling side of Swift River, I relied on teachers for descriptions about the academics. Especially helpful interviews and conversations took place with teachers Gennarose Pope, Kate Simmons, Jeremy McGeorge, Abi Onafowokan, and Christa Parravani. The Swift River staff complained that administrators raised the projected enrollment several times after the school opened in 1997. The complaints jibe with interviews with former employees and news accounts such as Daniel Miller, "Plainfield School Helps Teens Cope: Swift River Planning to Enroll 85–88," *Union-News* (Springfield, Mass.), July 21, 1997. I condensed many incidents that happened in the winter of 2001–2. Swift River's counts of expulsions sometimes differed from the counselors' counts because families often pulled students out just before they were formally expelled. The figure I cite, of eleven expulsions, came from Rudy Bentz.

### 17. DISCLOSURES
I was present during the groups when Trevor made the disclosure about sexual abuse, when Mary Alice discussed the incident with the two seniors, and when Tanner received his old suicide notes. Tanner later shared the notes with me.

### 18. MAKING CONNECTIONS
Teacher Kate Simmons, who left Swift River, helped fill in the details about D.J. Science teachers Steve Anderson and Odianosen Iyamabo of Deerfield Academy double-checked my facts.

During the weekend that students spent time in hotels with their parents, I drove from town to town, observing Bianca and her family, then D.J. and his parents, and finally Mary Alice and her parents and siblings. The kids' journals of their visits were helpful in fleshing out details. Descriptions of bipolar disease come from Empfield and Bakalar, *Understanding Teenage Depression*, pp. 43–45.

### 19. DATING, DUMPING, AND DRY-HUMPING
Statistics about dating and sex are based on information gathered by the Swift River staff from published reports. I verified the figures with information from Anna Mulrine, "Risky Business: Teens Are Having More Sex — and Getting More Diseases," *U.S. News*, May 27, 2002, which cites three of the most reliable sources: the Alan Guttmacher Institute, the Henry J. Kaiser Family Foundation, and the U.S. Centers for Disease Control and Prevention. One example: nearly one in ten kids reported losing his or her virginity before the age of thirteen, a 15 percent increase from 1997.

### 20. A CASE OF THE "FUCK-ITS"
The account of D.J.'s brief escape from his dorm is based on interviews with D.J. and the friend who initiated the runaway, as well as Swift River incident reports. John Klem helped by describing his work with D.J. Adoption studies are cited in Verrier, *The Primal Wound*, pp. xv and 3.

Many newspapers ran articles about the Food and Drug Administration's warnings about increasing use of antidepressants for children and teenagers, especially after an FDA study was released on March 22, 2004. I relied especially on Gardiner Harris, "Regulators Want Antidepressants to List Warning," *New York Times*, Mar. 23, 2004; and Shankar Vedantam, "Antidepressants Called Unsafe for Children," *Washington Post*, Apr. 23, 2004. While CEDU originally prohibited psychiatric medicines, the school now allows them, according to Rudy Bentz, who worked there. Dr. Ralph Cohen, who oversees Swift River's consulting psychiatrists, says he and his colleagues prescribe meds judiciously and then regularly monitor the students' health. And to be precise, he said, when a medicine causes a kid to be constipated, the psychiatrists recommend "stool softeners" rather than laxatives. I decided to be less graphic in my description.

In an interview in June 2004, Cohen also informed me that Swift River had recently stopped using Neurontin, the antiseizure medication. The previous month the drug's American manufacturer, Warner-Lambert, pleaded guilty and paid a large fine when the FDA accused the company of illegally and fraudulently promoting use of Neurontin for the treatment of bipolar mental disorder, attention deficit disorder, and other disorders; the background appears in "Warner Lambert to Pay $430 Million," Department of Justice press release, May 13, 2004: www.usdoj.gov/opa/pr/2004/May/04_civ_322.htm.

## 21. REAL FRIENDS
The supervisors mentioned in the sources for Chapter 11 helped me piece together the anecdotes in this chapter. So did several Swift River students who volunteered to let me use their real names. I declined.

## 22. RETURN TO INNOCENCE
I was allowed to sit on the side of the room and take notes during the psychodramas. Later, counselors and supervisors provided their interpretations. I used the nickname for counselor James Murray — "GQ James" — that a couple of kids from another group had surreptitiously bandied about. Bianca, Mary Alice, Tyrone, and D.J. were kind enough to allow me to use their childhood photos.

## 23. "THIS IS NOT A TEST, THIS IS YOUR LIFE"
For the first home visit, I decided to focus on two students who lived within an hour of each other. I rode to New York with Tyrone and his mother and watched as he adjusted to being home that evening. The next night, I observed the reunion with his father; I sat at a table with his mother at the Chinese restaurant. I then accompanied D.J. and his father on their fishing trip. Bianca and Mary Alice and their families recounted their visits. The headlines and opening sentences of articles about the deaths of Bianca's friends are from articles in the *Palm Beach Post;* I left out names of the friends in order to protect Bianca's identity.

## 24. MORE THAN LABELS
Watching the Swift River students as they played music at the Art Barn coffeehouse in Shelburne Falls on a Friday night, I was struck by how "normal" they appeared. It would take an entire book, at least, to write about the growing use of psychiatric medicines among children and adolescents. I tried to give a sense of it. Laura Jones, a nurse at Swift River, helped with descriptions of the medicines. John Powers provided the estimate of the percentage of students on meds. I also learned about labels in discussions with T. R. Rosenberg, who was later promoted to director of counseling. Helpful resources include Diamond, *Instant Psychopharmacology;*

Howard Chua-Eoan, "Escaping the Darkness," *Time*, May 31, 1999; Gardiner Harris, "Antidepressants Seen as Effective for Adolescents," *New York Times*, June 2, 2004; Harris, "New York State Official Sues Drug Maker Over Test Data," ibid., June 3, 2004; and Barry Meier, "Two Studies, Two Results, and a Debate Over a Drug," ibid.

### 25. "I Love That Kid"

I observed the consultants' visit, but because of a schedule conflict I missed the speech by Elliot Sainer, CEO of the Aspen Education Group, which owns Swift River. An admissions officer taped the speech for me. At this consultants' gathering and a later one, I gave a speech to the visitors but declined the usual honorarium that Swift River offers to speakers. Several of the consultants said they thought the "extravaganza" sent the wrong message to students. But when I called them for fact-checking, most of these consultants didn't want to be quoted because they do a lot of business with Swift River and other Aspen programs.

I observed the student services meeting about D.J. (I didn't include myself when I mentioned the thirteen people in the room). By a voice vote, the participants allowed me to tape the meeting, but because of poor acoustics, some of the tape was garbled. I supplemented this account with my notes and with follow-up interviews with John Powers, Candice Porter, Marsha Stevens, Gennarose Pope, Julie Haagenson, and John Klem. Although I thought the observations about Huck Finn were original, I later came across the same idea in Smith and Nylund, *Treating Huckleberry Finn.*

### 26. "Laugh Now, Cry Later"

I accompanied the group during the boulder hike and the final workshop. Supervisor Tom Moore allowed me to record the boulder hike and the discussions that followed in part because it was almost impossible to take notes outdoors at night. This was the only workshop at which I was allowed to tape discussions.

### 27. Life's a Permanent Party

Tanner's mother provided the lyrics to his rap. Berkshire Hills Productions taped the personal challenge. Tanya provided Leonard Beecher's poem.

When Tyrone's mother revealed the information about her own history to Ashley, I was not present; I was observing a different session of family therapy. I probably never would have known about it if Ashley hadn't mentioned it to me a few weeks later. I reconstructed the conversations after extensive interviews with Ashley, Tyrone, Tyrone's mother, and Tanya Beecher. Their accounts were so similar that I felt I didn't need to interview others who were in that group.

### 28. Pura Vida

I accompanied the fifteen kids to Costa Rica for the five-week visit, participating in the farm stay, the kayak trip, and other activities. I paid my own way. I swam, hiked, and rode horseback with the kids. To give them some space, I left them alone every few days. The history of the Costa Rica program is based on interviews with Eric Russman and Helaine Wemple, who, like many original staff members, have moved on to other jobs. Statistics about the Osa Peninsula come from *Frommer's Guide to Costa Rica* and *Costa Rica Insight Guide*. I translated interviews from Spanish to English. The key Costa Ricans in the program, Luis Quintero and his cousin Esteban Lopez, helped with a couple of anecdotes about Group 23 and past Swift River groups, as did Marco Loaiciga, the guide known as Taboga. Because it has become a major transshipment country for drugs passing from South America to the United States, Costa Rica is plagued by cocaine and other narcotics. I didn't dwell on this in the text because most of the Swift River kids didn't know enough Spanish to learn about this twist.

### 29. "I CAN'T GO THROUGH THIS AGAIN"
The kids allowed me to read portions of their Costa Rica journals. Anita Deeg, coordinator of the Costa Rica program, helped with fact-checking, as did counselors John Nicholson, Dan Lefco, Sylvia Lang, and Tom Hutten. Anecdotes about Bianca and Ashley were confirmed by Candice Porter and Spanish teacher Kate Comeau, both of whom joined the group during the first half of the Costa Rica trip.

### 30. "YOUR CHILD IS NOT FIXED"
I observed Mary Alice as she started the home stay and throughout the five days. I watched when her parents came to see the house where she had stayed. The anecdotes were confirmed by her host family, especially Virginia Guerrero (Doña Virginia), the matriarch. I was present at the late-night meeting when Ashley and Andy told the group about their dalliance and rule-breaking.

### 31. CONQUERING HEROES
Nurse Sandy Gallerani confirmed Trevor's scam. The accounts of Ashley's runaway attempt come from interviews with counselors Tanya Beecher, Erica Thiessen, Mike Charnley, and Candice Porter as well as students in Group 23. Predictions about Group 23 members arose in my conversations with counselors and, in some cases, when the counselors talked among themselves. Administrators at Swift River and other therapeutic programs might disagree with me about the unreliability of success claims. Nonetheless, the National Association of Therapeutic Schools and Programs has not been able to cite a therapeutic school that uses a thorough, scientific way of defining and assessing success rates. Lynn Luckenbach, president of the Independent Educational Consultants Association (IECA), says there is no such study; Phyllis Steinbrecher, an IECA founder, says admissions offices fear that precise numbers would contradict claims of overwhelming success.

Keith Russell has found a high success rate for wilderness intervention programs for adolescents, as I mention later in this chapter. But I feel I cannot rely on his data because the studies are sponsored by some of the wilderness programs that have a stake in the outcome. Details of the findings and the funding of the University of Idaho study of outdoor programs are from "UI Wilderness Therapy Study Reveals Benefits to Adolescents," Dec. 13, 2001 (www.obhic.com).

## 32. "You Have Your Little Girl Back"

I observed the graduation; Ben Levy transcribed the speeches from a video by Berkshire Hills Productions. Rudy Bentz gave a fairly similar pep talk to every group, so I selected excerpts from several of those speeches. A day later, I followed Bianca and her family when they flew home to Florida, and I observed her during her first afternoon back home. The statistics on the enrollment growth at her high school come from her father. Because I was an education reporter for the *Miami Herald*, I found such statistics very familiar.

## Epilogue: "So Many Fake People in the Real World"

The information about Rudy and Jill Bentz is from a Swift River press release, "Organizational Changes at Academy at Swift River," Sept. 18, 2003. Descriptions of the main characters after graduation are based on interviews with them and their parents. Bianca and another girl from the group told me about the funeral of the gentle young man I call Tanner. His mother gave me permission to use Tanner's real name in the hopes that his story will educate others. His family has set up a fund to help families with struggling teenagers. Donations can be sent to the Shane Reardon Memorial Foundation, 7100-39 Fairway Drive, PMB 400, Palm Beach Gardens, FL 33418.

## Memo to Parents

My thinking in this section, as in the Introduction, was shaped by the trenchant observations about adolescence and community in Hersch, *A Tribe Apart*. I found useful information in the articles on adolescence in the May/June 2002 issue of *Knowledge Quest*, a journal for school librarians. Statistics about Amherst Regional High School are cited in Michal Lumsden, "ARHS Students Tested for Risky Behaviors," *Daily Hampshire Gazette*, May 8–9, 2004.

My remarks about what kids lack — and what parents should provide — were shaped by talks with a New York child psychiatrist, Dr. Herman Roiphe, and with the experts mentioned above in the notes to the Introduction. The "cultural anxiety" quote is cited in Hulbert, *Raising America*, p. 4. The Lewis Mumford quote comes from Kunstler, *The Geography of Nowhere*, p. 8. Statistics about Americans' mobility are cited in David Brooks, "Our Sprawling, Supersized Utopia," *New York Times Magazine*, April 4, 2004. The Manson quote comes from the 2003 film *Bowling for Columbine*, directed by Michael Moore. Although I'm critical of public high schools, I should mention that I became a writer because of Vic Leviatin and Jill Gluckson, who coordinated an innovative program at my public school. Now in its third decade and renamed the Wise Individualized Senior Experience, the program is battling senior slump at more than seventy high schools. In 1982 I wrote my college thesis on Americans' search for community; Professor Howard Chudacoff of Brown University inspired me on a lifelong intellectual journey.

# BIBLIOGRAPHY

American Psychiatric Association. *Diagnostic and Statistical Manual for Mental Disorders,* 4th ed. (*DSM-IV*). Washington, D.C.: American Psychiatric Press, 1994.

Aries, Elizabeth. *Adolescent Behavior: Readings and Interpretations.* New York: McGraw-Hill/Dushkin, 2001.

Armstrong, Thomas. *ADD/ADHD Alternatives in the Classroom.* Alexandria, Va.: Association for Curriculum Development, 1999.

Blais, Madeleine. *In These Girls, Hope Is a Muscle.* New York: Warner Books, 1996.

Brooks, Robert, and Sam Goldstein. *Raising Resilient Children: Fostering Strength, Hope and Optimism in Your Child.* New York: McGraw-Hill, 2001.

Diamond, Ronald J. *Instant Psychopharmacology,* New York: W. W. Norton, 2002.

Dudman, Martha Tod. *Augusta Gone: A True Story.* New York: Simon & Schuster, 2001.

Empfield, Maureen, and Nicholas Bakalar. *Understanding Teenage Depression.* New York, Henry Holt, 2001.

Ferguson, Gary. *Shouting at the Sky: Troubled Teens and the Promise of the Wild.* New York: St. Martin's Press/Thomas Dunne Books, 1999.

Garbarino, James, and Claire Bedard. *Parents Under Siege.* New York: Free Press, 2002.

Hersch, Patricia. *A Tribe Apart: A Journey into the Heart of Adolescence.* New York: Fawcett Columbine Books, 1998.

Hine, Thomas. *The Rise and Fall of the American Teenager.* New York: William Morrow, 1999.

Hulbert, Ann. *Raising America: Experts, Parents and a Century of Advice about Children.* New York: Knopf, 2003. (My digest of her thesis is drawn largely from Stacy Schiff's perceptive review in the *New York Times,* April 17, 2003.)

Ketcham, Katherine, and Nicholas A. Pace. *Teens Under the Influence: The Truth about Kids, Alcohol, and Other Drugs.* New York: Ballantine Books, 2003.

Kindlon, Dan, and Michael Thompson. *Raising Cain: Protecting the Emotional Life of Boys.* New York: Ballantine Books, 1999.

Kunstler, James Howard. *The Geography of Nowhere: The Rise and Decline of America's Man-Made Landscape.* New York: Simon & Schuster, 1993.

Lara, Adair. *Hold Me Close, Let Me Go: A Mother, A Daughter, and an Adolescence Survived.* New York: Broadway Books, 2001.

Maine, Margo. *Father Hunger: Fathers, Daughters and Food.* Carlsbad, Calif.: Gurze Books, 1991.

Malekoff, Andrew. *Group Work with Adolescents: Principles and Practice.* New York: Guilford Press, 1997.

Marshall, Peter. *Now I Know Why Tigers Eat Their Young: Surviving a New Generation of Teenagers.* Vancouver: Whitecap Books, 1999.

Pertman, Adam. *Adoption Nation: How the Adoption Revolution Is Transforming America.* New York: Basic Books, 2000.

Pipher, Mary Bray. *Reviving Ophelia: Saving the Selves of Adolescent Girls.* New York: Putnam, 1994.

Putnam, Robert. *Bowling Alone: The Collapse and Revival of the American Community.* New York: Touchstone Books, 2001.

Smith, Craig, and David Nylund, eds. *Treating Huckleberry Finn: A New Narrative Approach to Working with Kids Diagnosed ADD/ADHD.* New York: Jossey-Bass, 2000.

Sternberg, Robert J., and Elena L. Grigorenko. *Our Labeled Children: What Every Parent and Teacher Needs to Know about Learning Disabilities.* Boston: Perseus Books, 1999.

Verrier, Nancy Newton. *The Primal Wound: Understanding the Adopted Child.* Baltimore: Gateway Press, 1993.

Zere, Kathryn. *The Body Betrayed: A Deeper Understanding of Women, Eating Disorders and Treatment.* Carlsbad, Calif.: Gurze Books, 1995.